SYSTEMATIC
TREATMENT
SELECTION

Toward Targeted
Therapeutic Interventions

BRUNNER/MAZEL INTEGRATIVE PSYCHOTHERAPY SERIES, NO. 3

SYSTEMATIC TREATMENT SELECTION

Toward Targeted Therapeutic Interventions

by LARRY E. BEUTLER, Ph.D.
and JOHN F. CLARKIN, Ph.D.

BRUNNER/MAZEL *Publishers* • New York

Library of Congress Cataloging-in-Publication Data
Beutler, Larry E.
    Systematic treatment selection: toward targeted therapeutic
interventions/by Larry E. Beutler and John F. Clarkin.
        p. cm.—(Brunner/Mazel integrative psychotherapy series:
    3)
    Includes bibliographical references.
    ISBN 0-87630-576-1
    1. Psychiatry—Differential therapeutics.   I. Clarkin, John F.
II. Title.   III. Series.
    [DNLM: 1. Decision Making.   2. Mental Disorders—therapy.
3. Psychotherapy. W1 BR917I v. 3/ WM 400 B569s]
RC480.52.B48   1990
616.89'14—dc20
DNLM/DLC
for Library of Congress   89-71203
                                                               CIP

Published by
BRUNNER/MAZEL, INC.
19 Union Square West
New York, NY 10003

Manufactured in the United States of America

10 9 8 7 6 5 4 3 2 1

To our wives Elena and Audrey,
and to our children
Jana, Kelly, Ian, Gail, Kevin, and Brian.
We love you.

Contents

Preface...xi
A Note on Case Examples xv

PART I. BACKGROUND AND INTRODUCTION

1. INTRODUCTION 3
   A History of Eclectic Psychotherapy..6
   Contemporary Eclectic Theories 10
   Summary and Comment...12
   Suggested Readings..13

2. A MODEL OF DIFFERENTIAL TREATMENT SELECTION 14
   Contributing Viewpoints 14
   An Integrative Model 20
   Summary and Comment...27
   Suggested Readings..27

PART II. PATIENT PREDISPOSING VARIABLES

3. DIAGNOSTIC CONSIDERATIONS 31
   Critique of Diagnostic Concepts...32
   A Practical Critique 36
   Seeking a Role for Diagnosis in Treatment Planning 40
   Summary and Comment...55
   Suggested Readings..55

4. PATIENT PERSONAL CHARACTERISTICS............................57
   Patient Expectations 58
   Coping Ability..63
   Patient Personality...66
   Summary and Comment...80
   Suggested Readings..82

5. ENVIRONMENTS AND CIRCUMSTANCES............................83
   Environmental Stressors 84
   Environmental Resources...86

Summary and Comment...96
Suggested Readings...97

PART III. THE TREATMENT CONTEXT

6. THE TREATMENT SETTING 101

Least Restrictive Treatment Settings.......................................102
The Psychiatric Hospital 104
Restrictive Settings for the Acute Patient................................105
Restrictive Settings for the Chronic Patient............................107
Alternatives to Hospitalization 108
Treatment Settings vs. Treatment Programs............................109
Summary and Comment...111
Suggested Readings........:...112

7. TREATMENT MODE AND FORMAT................................113

Psychosocial Modes and Formats 114
The Treatment Mode of Medical Management.........................133
Summary and Comment...139
Suggested Readings..140

8. TREATMENT FREQUENCY AND DURATION...................141

Treatment Duration 141
Interrelationships of Frequency and Duration.........................152
The Decision Not To Treat..155
Summary and Comment...161
Suggested Readings..162

PART IV. RELATIONSHIP VARIABLES

9. THERAPIST-PATIENT PERSONAL COMPATIBILITY 169

Persuasion and the Therapeutic Alliance.................................171
Dimensions of Compatibility..174
Summary and Comment...184
Suggested Readings..185

10. ENHANCING AND MAINTAINING THE THERAPEUTIC ALLIANCE 186

Role Induction 187
In-Therapy Environmental Management 196
Summary and Comment 205
Suggested Readings 206

PART V. TAILORING STRATEGIES AND TECHNIQUES

11. SELECTING FOCAL TARGETS OF CHANGE......................211

Differences Among Psychotherapy Methods............................212
A Model for Matching Therapy to Patient...............................222
Formulating Focal Treatment Goals.......................................224
Summary and Comment...234
Suggested Readings..237

12. SELECTING THE LEVEL OF INTERVENTION AND
THE MEDIATING GOALS OF PSYCHOTHERAPY.............238

Types of Psychotherapy Experiences.......................................239
Mediating Goals and Phases of Psychotherapy.........................253
Summary and Comment...263
Suggested Readings..264

13. CONDUCTING THERAPEUTIC WORK 265

The Dimensions of Specific Procedures..................................266
Treatment Manuals and the Four Steps...................................279
Summary and Comment...283
Suggested Readings..284

PART VI. TRAINING DIRECTIONS

14. TRAINING IN DIFFERENTIAL TREATMENT
SELECTION...289
with John C. Norcross, Ph.D.

Critique of Conventional Training 290
Ideal Training Models..293
Recurrent Obstacles in Integrative Training 297
Clinical Supervision 300
Conclusions and Recommendations 304
Suggested Readings 307

References 308
Index..352

Preface

This book is designed to facilitate the integration and systematic prescription of mental health interventions. It represents an effort to apply what we know about "when, what works for whom" and to enhance the application of technical procedures to specific kinds of patient and problem presentations. It should be said, however, that this is not a manual on how to become a clinician or psychotherapist, nor is it a manual on how to conduct psychotherapy. Rather it is a manual on how to select appropriate interventions. There are many manuals on how to implement various procedures, both somatic and psychosocial; this volume may be complemented by reference to these manuals. Accordingly, we have provided suggested readings at the end of each chapter to assist in this process.

We intend the system of clinical decision making and treatment selection presented in this book to do more than simply provide a basis for the application of technology, however. We also hope that this book will facilitate the development of a certain thought process, one that is sufficiently flexible to accommodate an expanding array of therapeutic styles.

Just as treatment specification defies precise definition by a finite set of rules that are invoked at any one point in time, so too do available and potential treatments defy description by reference to brand-name labels. Therefore, rather than concentrate upon how and when to prescribe classes of medication or global psychotherapies (e.g., psychoanalytic, cognitive, behavioral therapies), the array of which will certainly change by the time this book is published, we will direct our comments both at more general and at more specific levels than can be indicated by reference to these titles. We will present decisional criteria for designing individualized psychosocial treatment programs that are responsive to the multiple objectives and contextual interactions which comprise both treatments and patients.

To accomplish our objectives, this volume is divided into six sections. Part I provides the background for the development of a prescriptive decision model for assigning mental health treatment. Chapter 1 introduces the history of eclectic thinking in mental health treatment with special emphasis upon psychotherapy and psychotherapy research. Without such a historical perspective, it is too easy to lose sight of the similarities which bridge different viewpoints and to compare these viewpoints merely in terms of their differences.

In concert with the foregoing perspective, Chapter 2 provides the historical foundations of our particular approach to the problem of differential treatment selection. These foundations are firmly implanted in a history of empirical research and integrative thought. We outline in Chapter 2, the skeleton of a model for treatment assignment (Figure 2.1). To this skeleton, we attempt to add the muscle, bone, nervous system and soul in the subsequent five sections of this volume. This is a complex process. Indeed, our fear is that it is too complex to hold the reader's interest. We have wrestled with the dilemma of balancing the simplicity of technology with the complexity of the clinician's art, and finally have concluded that the problems with which we are dealing are sufficiently important to not be oversimplified.

To help the reader as we develop our logic and rationale, the introductions to Parts II through V include a figural elaboration of the basic outline presented in Chapter 2. These figures serve as a pictorial overview of the chapters within each section. Collectively, these figures provide a relatively detailed outline of this book.

Part II outlines the predisposing characteristics of patients that will subsequently be invoked in structuring a prescriptive approach to treatment selection. In Part III, we develop the initial relationships between these patient predisposing qualities and the context in which treatment is offered. Within the broad framework of mental health treatment, it is our intent to blend clinical and empirical wisdom in order to go beyond the bounds of specific modes and formats of treatment, as if they were frozen in time, to encompass a larger view of the helping process.

While the decisional processes described in this book encompass the array of mental health treatments, our focus ultimately centers on psychotherapy. This focus will become obvious in Part IV. Our decision to concentrate on psychotherapy is based upon our belief that psychotherapy epitomizes the complexity of influence forces, objectives and sources of resistance with which patient and practitioner must contend in any health treatment. Psychotherapy is, by its very nature, the medium through which all mental health interventions are applied, as well as a set of treatment procedures in its own right. Based upon our belief in the critical importance of the human relationship to the healing process, Part IV concentrates on the nature of developing and enhancing the relationship that comprises the helping alliance or collaborative therapeutic relationship.

Part V culminates our movement from the general to the specific in differential treatment assignment. The chapters of this section detail the decisional criteria for making moment-to-moment decisions about the psychotherapy process. It is here that therapist flexibility in applying the guidelines is most important and it is also here that our formulations require the broadest interpretation. The best psychotherapeutic decisions are based upon an accumulation of knowledge about the patient's unique history, the demand characteristics of the treatment context, and the nature of the existent treatment relationship. Only if taken within this broad perspective can effective psychotherapeutic decisions be made. Hence, Part V outlines the dimensions of psychotherapy technology, and these in turn represent both a capstone to the treatment decisions previously made and a potentiator for the construction of subsequent treatment decisions.

Part VI departs from the intensity and specificity of the previous sections in order to explore the implications of our presentation for training. Here we provide suggestions by which training programs might facilitate evolution of the inquiring and flexible attitudes among their students that are so important for an "eclectic" viewpoint.

Preparing this book has been a challenging task. At least for L. E. B., the process was eased by the support provided by a grant from the National Institute of Mental Health (MH 39859) to study the differential effects of psychotherapy. In addition, many people have contributed to the production of this volume. Our secretaries, Mary Anne Bescript, Lillian Conklin, and Linda Fowler have been especially important to this process. We also owe a great debt to J.I., M.V., S.B., J.C., A.D., C.A., H.D., G.B., M.D., M.S., P.O., N.K., and all the other pseudonamed patients whose stories are partially and incompletely shared throughout these pages. We owe special thanks to our colleagues and friends in the Society for Psychotherapy Research (SPR), since it was through these (too numerous to mention) associations that we came to know and appreciate each other, and it was before these colleagues that we were challenged to defend and refine our ideas. And, of course, none of this would have been possible without the support of our many colleagues outside of SPR who also provided feedback and critique, those authors (see reference list) whose ideas influenced our own, and our families who gave us (almost) unending patience as well as confronting us with experiences that challenged our capacities to be "eclectic."

L.E. Beutler
J.F. Clarkin

A Note on Case Examples

Throughout this volume, we follow several patients, to whom we refer with fictitious initials. These patients are used to exemplify some of the principles of prescriptive treatment assignment. To facilitate the task of remembering the continuing case examples as they unfold, we are providing a quick description of the identified patient and a reference to the chapter and page on which a more detailed description of the patient initially is provided.

J.I.   (Chapter 1, Page 3). This 34-year-old woman initially presented with Post Traumatic Stress Disorder secondary to an automobile accident. Her history also included an early assault and attempted murder from which she had emerged paraplegic, suspicious of men, and with considerable difficulties in establishing intimacy. Her case is followed closely throughout the book.

J.C.   (Chapter 3, Page 43). This 24-year-old male college student presented with auditory hallucinations and the delusional belief that he was Jesus Christ. He reported being controlled by radio waves broadcast by the CIA and indicated some significant suicidal ideation should his "mission" not be completed by the time he turned 33.

A.D.   (Chapter 3, Page 45). This patient was a 57-year-old physician who initially was referred by his estranged wife. The patient presented with compulsive rituals, hoarding, checking, and preoccupation with poverty. The patient was the only member of his family who had survived the holocaust.

C.A.   (Chapter 3, Page 48). This 36-year-old woman presented suicidal ideation and recurrent Major Depression. The patient had been disowned by her family, had lost her inherited wealth, had been raped, and had observed the violent murder of her fiancé.

H.D.   (Chapter 3, Page 50). This 44-year-old unemployed but highly educated man presented with a long history of alcohol abuse. His prominent family had assisted him through a doctoral level education in spite of his problem, but the patient remained unemployed because of his inability to refrain from alcohol. He represents an example of an individual with conflicted dependencies upon his family.

M.D. (Chapter 3, Page 53). This 27-year-old woman presented with a Borderline Personality Disorder. She had a history of being over protected and sexually molested as a child. Her adult life was characterized by a recurrent pattern of unstable and intense relationships with married men.

M.S. (Chapter 4, Page 77). This 25-year-old graduate student in anatomy presented with obsessions and ritualistic behaviors. Rituals revolved around cleanliness and were associated with a germ phobia. The extremeness of her symptoms resulted ultimately in her leaving graduate school and threatened to disrupt her marriage.

PART I

Background and Introduction

1

Introduction

J.I. was a 34-year-old woman who presented with symptoms of Post Traumatic Stress Disorder (PTSD). She had nightmares, panic attacks, flashbacks, and suicidal thoughts. She came to the therapist's office in a wheelchair, having been paraplegic since age 13, secondary to being stabbed in the back and left for dead by an unknown assailant who also raped and killed the patient's girlfriend during a family outing. For four hours, the patient had lain motionless, unable to move and afraid to call for help.

J.I.'s family provided tentative initial support to the patient, but had taken the position that these events were a potential embarrassment and best ignored. They refused to discuss the incident and criticized the patient for her residual "helplessness." Through years of struggle, J.I. had overcome her major fears of social contacts and gained at least marginal control of her recurrent suicidal ideation. She had achieved an education and a good job and had gotten married a few months before presenting herself to psychotherapy.

She had been in psychodynamically oriented psychotherapy for the two years immediately before the present occasion, largely motivated by free-floating anxiety and depression, and had achieved moderately good results. Now her symptoms of anxiety had been reactivated within the past month after a drunk driver had run a stop light and hit her car, destroying her only "place of safety and control." To complicate things, J.I.'s marriage was struggling, as it had been since its inception. Her inability to give up a degree of interpersonal control and her longstanding failure to develop a feeling of intimacy toward men had provoked many arguments and

3

power struggles, all of which now threatened the survival of the relationship.

When presented with such case material, the clinician must decide what form of initial intervention would be most productive. Most clinicians would probably agree that the exacerbated and trauma-induced anxiety symptoms deserve first attention if for no other reason than that they may impede changes that are considered to be more important. However, the method of intervening with these symptoms would probably vary widely. Some would offer reassurance and support, others desensitization, and still others anxiolytics or antidepressants. Moreover, once the anxiety symptoms have abated, as they almost surely would do with any of these treatments, should the patient be continued in treatment and if so for how long, with what goals and by what means? Would symptoms alleviate any faster or for a longer period with one treatment rather than with another? On what basis could one justify opening the door to explore old wounds in one who seeks only relief from immediate stress and who has learned to live a productive life by putting aside the memories of her early trauma?

These are some of the questions facing the mental health practitioner and these are some of the questions that we seek to answer in this volume. We do not believe that simple answers to these questions are possible. Nor do we believe that information derived from symptom presentations alone or at any one point in time provides great assistance in deriving these answers. To provide consistent and predictable interventions, the practitioner must engage in an ongoing process of assessing patient problems, existent supports and contexts, and available treatments. This process begins with understanding the patient and the patient's environment and proceeds to understanding the nature of the available treatment resources, the characteristics of the patient-clinician relationship upon which treatment is being built, and the efficacy of the procedures that are being utilized to achieve treatment goals and subgoals.

As the foregoing suggests, the processes of assessment and treatment are inseparable. As information and knowledge unfold, new decisions are made by both clinician and patient. At each decisional step, the clinician must be open to the prospect of incorporating into those decisions a very wide array of possible treatment responses, preferably unfettered by parochial adherences to narrow theories. In order to prevent treatment from becoming an interminable, random trial-and-error selection of interventions, the clinician must have a guiding theory that governs treatment decisions. Within the framework of this theory, he or she must be willing and able to balance pragmatism with abstract theoretical concepts in order to translate the resulting plan into time-efficient interventions.

The usual term referring to the type of integration of treatment procedures to be described here is "eclecticism." However, the term "eclectic," at least as it has been applied to mental health treatment, is much maligned. Yet we know of no better term by which to describe the various efforts to bring the numerous viewpoints that characterize mental health treatment into some common and practical framework.

There are really several different types of eclecticism. The particular type to which this volume is addressed has been referred to as "technical eclecticism" (Lazarus, 1981; Norcross, 1986c). Technical eclecticism maintains that integration among various treatment approaches should take place at the level of specific procedures, rather than at the level of theory. That is, a technically eclectic clinician endeavors to select the best and most useful procedures for a given patient from the hundreds of procedures available, irrespective of the theories from which these procedures derive. "Theoretical Integrationism" is a second major type of eclecticism and practitioners of this philosophy are distinguishable from the practitioners of "technical eclecticism" by their desire either to combine concepts from different theories or to translate the terms used by one theory to those employed by other theories (see Norcross & Prochaska, 1988; Wolfe & Goldfried, 1988, for a discussion of these terms).

Some technical eclectic approaches have developed specific guidelines to help the clinician determine the procedures to be selected. These approaches are collectively referenced by attaching the adjective "systematic" to the term "eclectic" (Norcross, 1986a; Beutler, 1983). The approach to treatment selection to be presented here represents a form of systematic, technical eclecticism. Moreover, the methods we propose are also "prescriptive" and "differential" in that they are designed to allow the selective assignment of patients to treatments, settings and therapists on the basis of anticipated responses to those assignments. These latter terms, however, also carry unwanted meanings because of their association to medical treatments and traditional diagnoses. "Differential assignments" and "prescriptive" applications of psychotherapy are not the same as "differential diagnosis" and "prescriptive" applications of antihistamines. In psychotherapy, the treatment prescribed is as often a particular relationship between the treatment environment, the treater, and the treated as it is a specific type of medication or brand of psychotherapy.

In this initial chapter, we will explore the history and basic concepts of contemporary eclecticism. Several of the major contributors to this movement will be presented briefly. A more detailed analysis of the contributions of those who are most relevant to the current volume will be saved for presentation in Chapter 2.

A HISTORY OF ECLECTIC PSYCHOTHERAPY

This volume, we believe, is the first of the second generation of descriptive treatises on "technical eclecticism." The first systematic effort to define a technical eclecticism for mental health treatment was made by Arnold Lazarus (1967, 1971, 1976, 1981). In breaking from the tradition of behavior theory to which he had become prominently identified, he dared to say out loud what many of us silently believed—that theoretical procedures were not intrinsically bound to their spawning theories. It was Lazarus who subsequently defined the parameters that have since guided the technical eclectic movement.

Though the term "eclectic" itself has remained controversial, the movement it describes reached a level of clear respectability with the publication of *Psychotherapy: An Eclectic Approach* by Garfield (1980). Following in this wake, numerous others published and presented eclectic models of treatment in the ensuing decade (see Norcross, 1986a, 1986b for a review of many of these approaches). These early efforts to develop eclectic views of psychotherapy either extracted the most effective procedures from extant theories of psychotherapy or sought ingredients which were shared among them to account for the similarity of therapeutic effects. From these analyses, the more technically oriented theorists and writers attempted to derive second-order systems for integrating the numerous specific procedures so that they could be applied in their diversity without the need to commit their loyalties to the theories which spawned the procedures.

Unlike the first generation of technical eclectic systems (to which we both have contributed), in this volume we are seeking integration among the various eclectic models of treatment selection themselves, rather than from among the primary theories of psychotherapy and psychopathology that provided the basis of discussion for previous eclectic efforts. Thus, the model presented in this volume represents an effort to integrate certain of the prior models of psychotherapy integration.

Eclecticism in Theories of Psychotherapy

Every theory is, in reality, an amalgamation of previous viewpoints. When we speak of one theory or another as "a different perspective," we forget that it derived developmentally from others. When a "new theory" is developed and compared with an old one, the comparison dims one's awareness of the fact that the new theory has incorporated some of the common knowledge to which the earlier theory contributed. Reichenbach (1964) refers to this creative integration as the "context of discovery" and distinguishes it from the later scientific enterprise of "confirmation." To the degree that we accept that no new knowledge arises in a vacuum, but is an amalgamation of prior knowledge, all scientific discovery is "eclectic."

Because of the process of theory amalgamation and borrowing, the history of eclectic psychotherapy begins before the formalization of psychotherapy. Across time, each evolving viewpoint in psychotherapy incorporated salient ingredients of prior philosophies, often extending beyond the realm of the healing arts. Even Freud was "eclectic" within this limited meaning of the word, incorporating principles of Newtonian physics and the mechanics of energy transfer into his view of neurology and psychopathology. The physics of energy conservation and transfer of Freud's day was transported to psychopathology through a hydraulic metaphor when he presented instinctual urges as accumulating impulses that could be either discharged or diverted, but not eliminated.

As the practice of psychotherapy evolved, it did so by extending the realms of experience and knowledge which theorists attempted to incorporate within the still developing psychoanalytic theory. When Freud's students broke with his teachings, they did so as often because of an adherence to different values, teachers and religious doctrines as they did because of advances in scientific knowledge. They placed a different value upon quasi-religious concepts of motivation (e.g., Adler), symbols (e.g., Jung) and goals (e.g., Horney) than did Freud. Neo-Freudians integrated, selected, and refined psychoanalytic principles with the western world's emerging interest in social behavior. From these efforts arose the social psychiatry movement as well as existential and object relations theories.

The first major departure from the progressive evolution of psycho-analytic theory through the assimilation of new social viewpoints came with the advent of Client Centered Therapy (Rogers, 1951). Unlike earlier theorists, Rogers attempted to develop a new foundation for psychotherapy, rather than simply to append or modify the old one. While he was quite successful in divorcing himself from psychoanalysis, Rogers was an eclectic, nonetheless. Coming from a forgiving, American Protestant tradition, he incorporated concepts of "free will" and Christian acceptance into a view of personal change. With these quasi-religious concepts in place, Client Centered theory proposed relationships which established Rogers as an independent theorist.

The pervasive tendency among theory builders to incorporate the new into the newer (a frequently unrecognized form of "eclecticism") is nowhere better illustrated than in the fact that Rogers' proposals have become incorporated into the literature of most psychotherapies. Even recent applications of psychoanalytic theory have assimilated into their workings the relationship and collaboration values inherent in Client Centered Therapy (e.g., Strupp & Binder, 1984; Luborsky, 1984).

Behaviorism has been no more successful at escaping the pull of eclecticism than other theories. While Behavior Therapy arose ostensibly from atheoretical laboratory observations as a "pure" set of empirical principles that disparaged mentalistic causal elements, its application was far from being either value-free, cognition-free, or atheoretical. Eclectically assimilated theoretical notions extracted from neurology (Pavlov) and social perception (Tolman) were used to explain the effects of behavioral interventions. The relationship between values, cognitions, and behavioral principles became clear in Skinner's (1971) *Beyond Freedom and Dignity*. Acknowledging the impossibility of selecting targets of change atheoretically, some authors, such as Mowrer (1953), even explicitly incorporated religious concepts such as "sin" and "repentance" into the rationale for applying behavioral interventions. Other authors tried to remain value-free by eclectically refiltering the new behaviorism until it emerged in psychoanalytic terms (e.g., Dollard & Miller, 1950; Stampfl & Levis, 1967). Efforts to integrate the apparently contradictory theoretical perspectives of behavior therapy and psychoanalytic theory have persisted in more recent efforts to find rapprochement by contemporary behavioral and psychoanalytic theorists (e.g., Arkowitz & Messer, 1984; Goldfried, 1982; Wachtel, 1977).

Out of the same type of effort to accommodate new knowledge arose the group of interventions collectively considered to be Cognitive Change Therapies. From their inception, these cognitive therapies were eclectic. In part, they were developed because of the persistent concern, expressed by relationship and insight therapists, that behaviorism failed adequately to account for the role of thinking, early experience, and unconscious processes in altering behavior.

Other developments that pushed behaviorism to become both cognitive and eclectic were more empirical than those instigated by dissatisfied psychotherapists. Behavioral theorists themselves became aware that thoughts exerted an interactive influence on the environment in which a behavior occurred (Bandura, 1977): thought processes actively changed and were changed by the environment to which a person responded. More than simply adding a cognitive dimension to established principles of behavior therapy, however, the more elaborate forms of cognitive therapy (e.g., Beck et al., 1979) incorporated a view that unconscious processes founded in early experience continued to exert a guiding influence in one's life and were legitimate spectra on which to implement change efforts. These unconscious products of early experience were incorporated into cognitive therapy theories under the scientifically respectable label of "schema" (Beck & Weishaar, in press; Edwards, in press). These schema, it was proposed, were formed early in one's experience and, once incorporated as organizing rules of behavior, were forgotten.

While the historical roots of cognitive therapy were rather obvious, early writings said little about the similarity of cognitive and insight therapies. More recently, it has again become respectable to discuss these similarities. Both Beutler and Guest (in press) and Beidel and Turner (1986), for example, have recently pointed to the focus upon cognitive awareness as deriving from psychoanalytic principles of insight. Edwards (in press) states the case even more directly, observing that understanding the etiology of primitive cognitive systems may be necessary to support long-term changes in serious and chronic problems.

Eclecticism in Psychotherapy Research

Research does not advance knowledge simply by passively following the lead of great thinkers; it sets directions in its own right. For example, both behavior and cognitive therapies were the direct product of research applications of treatment models. Yet, research itself borrows from other fields of knowledge in order to develop these new directions, and in this process becomes eclectic in its applications.

This creative borrowing of methodologies in empirical research was seen in the early influence that hypnosis research had on Freud. From the research and observations of Charcot and Janet directly arose Breuer and Freud's (1955/1895) theories of hysteria. Similarly, research on behavior therapy paved the way for the theoretical development of cognitive change therapies (cf. Anderson, 1980). In each case, research highlighted apparent deficits in existent theories and thus made it necessary that the theories themselves be modified to account for observed discrepancies.

The inconsistency between therapists' theoretical viewpoints and their in-therapy behavior became apparent through psychotherapy research and resulted in what has become a major revolution in psychotherapy training. The foundation for this movement was in the joint observations that (1) therapists of equivalent experience but different theoretical positions behaved quite similarly to one another (Fiedler, 1950; Sloane, Staples, Cristol, Yorkston & Whipple, 1975), and paradoxically, (2) there was great diversity in therapeutic behaviors and outcomes among therapists who were of the same theoretical orientation (e.g., Lieberman, Yalom & Miles, 1973; Luborsky et al., 1975).

If the methods espoused by different theories were practiced so differently by different practitioners and if experience washed out many of the differences among treatments, how could one hope to evaluate the increasing number of theoretical models constantly becoming available? Obviously, the problem was one of methodological control in comparative studies of different psychotherapies, but the very awareness of this problem also raised critical questions about how to assure competence in the course of clinical training and subsequent practice.

Collectively, the methodological and clinical concerns resulted in an effort to operationally define and standardize treatments (Luborsky & DeRubeis, 1984). "How to do it" manuals soon appeared for Cognitive Therapy (Beck, Rush, Shaw & Emery, 1979), Interpersonal Psychotherapy (Klerman, Weissman, Rounsaville & Chevron, 1984), Psychoanalytic Psychotherapy (Luborsky, 1984; Strupp & Binder, 1984), Gestalt Therapy (Daldrup, Beutler, Greenberg & Engle, 1988), and various forms of group and family therapies (Jacobson & Margolin, 1979; Freeman, 1983; Sank & Shaffer, 1984).

The first noteworthy test of manual-driven therapies was the NIMH Collaborative study of depression (Elkin et al., 1985). Numerous studies followed the lead of this large-scale, multisite project and their methodologies extended the application of manualized treatments to the study of specific subgroups of subjects, such as those with concomitant depression and psychogenic pain (e.g., Beutler, Daldrup, Engle, Guest & Corbishley, 1988), anxiety disorders (e.g., Borkovec et al., 1987) and the depressed elderly (e.g., Thompson, Gallagher & Breckenridge, 1987). As these initiatives have caught on, manuals are becoming more clinically oriented and less often geared only to specific research applications. This has resulted in a plethora of manuals for the application of various models of therapy to particular populations (e.g., Blanchard & Andrasik, 1985; Calhoun & Atkinson, 1986; Clark & Bemis, 1982; Daldrup et al., 1988; Dangler & Polster, 1985; Fuchs & Rehm, 1977; Gallagher & Thompson, 1981; Marks, 1985; Yost, Beutler, Corbishley & Allender, 1986).

CONTEMPORARY ECLECTIC THEORIES

As we have illustrated, all theories of mental health intervention, by their nature, are eclectic. Nonetheless, only recently has "eclectic" become a term with which one would comfortably identify one's treatment position to colleagues. Given the role of borrowing and assimilation occurring in the natural course of theory development, the exponential increase in the number of discrete theories of psychotherapy, and the necessity of defining both the similarities and differences among applied theories in order to conduct empirical research, the eventual and formal acceptance of eclecticism may have been inevitable. In any case, by the mid 1970s, eclecticism was the approach to treatment most preferred by most psychologists (Garfield & Kurtz, 1976a), if not other practitioners. But this was a largely undefined or "haphazard" eclecticism, being based upon individual preferences, inclinations and momentary impressions.

The early forms of eclecticism were aimed primarily at defining the common principles which accounted for the effects of all mental health treatments. Frank's (1973) observations that successful healing consisted of overcoming demoralization, instilling hope, and providing a corrective emotional experience through benevolent persuasion carried a clear eclectic message. This "common factors" eclecticism, while one of the earliest developments, is far from being outmoded (e.g., Garfield, 1980; Orlinsky & Howard, 1987). Current research has not moved us far from Frank's basic conclusions (e.g., Lambert, Shapiro & Bergin, 1986; Parloff, 1986), although it has begun exploring the interactive relationship between specific and common ingredients (Jones, Cumming & Horowitz, 1988).

The challenge to formal models of mental health treatment has always been to increase the benefit above and beyond that attributable to the common characteristics of the successful treatment setting and relationship. Contemporary eclectic approaches consist of several relatively independent movements, each identified with a group of adherents, each reflecting different objectives, and each expanding upon a somewhat different aspect of the history of eclecticism.

"Technical Eclecticism" is a relatively new entrant to the eclectic scene, coming somewhat later than but existing concomitantly with contemporary theoretical, eclectic efforts. The Multimodal Psychotherapy of Lazarus (1976) and the prescriptive treatments of Goldstein and Stein (1976) were the first innovative efforts to accomplish this task by applying systematic and planned logic to assign patients to treatment. These innovations marked the beginning of a movement from an idiosyncratic and often undefined amalgamation of guiding philosophies and interventions toward a systematic decision-making process for selecting interventions.

With the early efforts of Lazarus (1976, 1981) and the more recent efforts both by our own research groups (Beutler, 1983; Frances, Clarkin & Perry, 1984) and by others (cf. Norcross, 1986b), the principles of "common factors" and "technical" eclecticism have themselves become integrated and quite well accepted. These integrative efforts have continued to progress through the development of increasingly specific decision rules and guiding principles.

The movement from haphazard eclecticism to theoretical integrationism and then to pragmatic and technical eclecticism has been one of increasing openness to the value of empirical work and to the decreasing value of theory-based discipleship. Accordingly, contemporary eclecticism frequently has close ties to empirical research, and relies on research findings to define the effectiveness of its postulates and to validate the means of its application.

As a witness to the timeliness of the concept of eclectic integration, the past decade has seen the development of a major journal (*Journal of Integrative and Eclectic Psychotherapy*) devoted to the eclectic movement and the organization of at least two professional societies which hold as their principal purpose the furthering of eclectic thought. The International Fellowship of Eclectic Psychotherapists (IFEP) evolved from these forward-looking ideas and continues as an international body whose function is to recognize, through invited fellowship in the organization, individuals whose ideas advance the cause of eclecticism.

Concomitantly, the Society for the Exploration of Psychotherapy Integration (SEPI) was organized by a group of researchers for whom the idea had evolved from workshops on issues of integrating theories and procedures at consecutive annual meetings of the Society for Psychotherapy Research (SPR).

SUMMARY AND COMMENT

In this chapter, we have described the historical roots of "eclecticism." Aside from simply clarifying the historical bases for the current volume, there are several points to emphasize from this review.

First, mental health treatment generally and psychotherapy research and practice specifically have been inherently eclectic fields. Treatment application has progressed, both as a scientific and as a professional activity, by merging contemporary knowledge with established clinical principles. While disagreements as to what constitutes either "knowledge" or an "established clinical principle" have been pervasive (some might say, "perversive"), the field has maintained a lively rate of growth. Formalizing the principles of eclecticism has been a recent development in this growth process. Its recognition acknowledges and legitimizes the differences which exist among psychotherapies, therapists, and patients. Indeed, the emergence of eclecticism as a legitimate field of inquiry directly marks the end of adherence to the myths of patient and treatment uniformity (Kiesler, 1966).

Second, some of the observations that have been elucidated by our consideration of the historical roots of eclectic efforts have become the foundation stones for distinctions among contemporary efforts to increase treatment efficacy. We have noted evidence of (1) considerable variability among the treatments and outcomes of therapists from a given school of treatment, and (2) an unexpected degree of similarity among equally competent therapists from different schools. Some theorists have attempted to resolve this discrepancy by identifying the common qualities that exist among effective practitioners regardless of their theoretical allegiances (i.e., common factors eclectics), others have responded by clarifying the similarities that exist among theories (i.e., theoretical eclectics), and still others have attempted to achieve resolution by establishing clear and nontheory-bound bases for applications of procedures (i.e., technical eclectics).

It is likely that even the "purists" among clinicians practice some form of eclecticism. They may justify these approaches at a pragmatic level (i.e., it works), they may develop a new concept to justify their practice, or they may borrow some theoretical concept from elsewhere. In any case, the very need to extend one's practice beyond the limits of convention emphasizes the limited relationship that theory has to treatment procedure for most therapists.

The significance of the foregoing observations to the current applications of eclectic theory will become clear in the following chapters. Suffice it to say, at this point, that we have acquired from the history of psychotherapy: (1) the belief that an effective system of treatment prescription must account for the common ingredients of change (e.g., common factors theories), (2) a respect for the diversity of theories and values that characterize clinicians, and (3) a faith that there are benefits to be derived from tailoring specific treatments to the needs of specific patients. In the following pages, we present the dimensions which we consider to be most relevant to retaining a respect for these three principles.

SUGGESTED READINGS

Garfield, S. L. (1980). *Psychotherapy: An eclectic approach.* New York: John Wiley.
Lazarus, A. A. (1981). *The practice of multimodal therapy.* New York: McGraw-Hill.
Norcross, J. C. (1986c). Eclectic psychotherapy: An introduction and overview. In J. C. Norcross (Ed.), *Handbook of eclectic psychotherapy* (pp. 3–24). New York: Brunner/Mazel.

2

A Model of Differential
Treatment Selection

Portions of this chapter were presented as a presidential address to the Society for Psychotherapy Research, June, 1987, Ulm, West Germany, and are published in *Psychotherapy* (Beutler, in press). Reprinted with permission.

Clinical wisdom has always held that patient and problem variables dictate the use of specific treatment approaches. Moreover, such lore maintains that therapist variables interact with the selection of treatment procedures in a way untapped by most controlled research. From the clinician's viewpoint, the failure of research evidence to reveal the presence of differential indicators for introducing specific interventions is a function both of a coarse-grained diagnostic system and a tendency for research to rely on criteria that are different than those actually used by clinicians in treatment. In order to evaluate clearly the proposal that there are predisposing patient, therapist, and technique contributors which optimize treatment outcomes, a fine-grained and interactive analysis of patient, therapist, and treatment procedures is necessary.

This chapter presents the background and an overview of a sequentially stepped, eclectic model upon which the remaining chapters of this book will expand. This model extracts and combines relevant principles from prior models which have been developed to facilitate the assigning and tailoring of treatments. The model proposes that treatments should be assigned with consideration given to predisposing patient characteristics, the contexts in which treatments are provided, patient-therapist personal compatibilities, and the matching of patients and technological interventions.

CONTRIBUTING VIEWPOINTS

In the past decade, a number of efforts have been devoted to constructing theoretical and empirical models for improving the effectiveness of assigning treatments. These efforts are usually associated with the contemporary *Technical Eclectic* movement which was described in Chapter 1. The integrative model proposed here derives from the progressive movement toward prescriptive assignment of psychotherapies. Our model combines the clinical wisdom and empirical underpinnings of four theories—two historically significant perspectives of eclectic treatment (Common Factors and Prescriptive Psychotherapy) and two specific, contemporary theories of technical eclecticism (Differential Therapeutics and Systematic Eclectic Psychotherapy)—along with input from several additional, contemporary developments. Each of these theories lends unique wisdom to the effort to define the parameters for effectively assigning treatments to patients. We believe that the formulations presented here both represent a common ground among several contemporary theoretical models and combine the unique strengths of each.

General Roots

While the model to be proposed in the current volume derives directly from two contemporary theories of technical eclectic psychotherapy, both its historical and contemporary roots actually are more broad-reaching. The historical roots of our model extend to and encompass the common factors theories of therapeutic integration (Chapter 1) and spawn from at least one earlier effort at systematic integration (i.e., the prescriptive psychotherapy of Goldstein and Stein, 1976) which was too far ahead of its time to receive the recognition it deserves.

Common Factors Eclecticism. The common factors theories of eclectic intervention (cf. Frank, 1973; Garfield, 1980; Kazdin, 1983; Parloff, 1986; Wilkins, 1979, 1984) highlight the role of "nonspecific variables" in facilitating treatment outcomes. While it is clear that many variables are common to diverse psychotherapies and account for a preponderance of the changes associated with each, the degree to which they are characteristic of the therapists who most frequently use these approaches and the degree to which they can or should be made an integral part of various therapies have been points of considerable debate. It is our contention that common treatment ingredients are created by specific and controllable communication patterns inherent to caring therapists, by the technologies which such therapists employ, and by the sensitive ways with which those procedures are applied. This view of common factors, in other words, holds that the empathic, credible, supportive, and caring aspects of the therapeutic relationship represent underlying but created experiences in effective treatment; therapists have a reasonable amount of control over the development of these experiences and can be trained to use that control effectively.

Prescriptive Psychotherapy.   Prescriptive psychotherapy was a concept introduced by Goldstein and Stein (1976), who initiated a systematic effort
to specify the relationship between symptom presentation and specific
treatments. The authors undertook the novel task of providing a set of
treatment principles and procedures for each of several symptomatic conditions. Their prescriptions were adapted for neurotic disorders (e.g., phobic disorders, depression, obsessive-compulsive disorder), psychophysiological disorders (e.g., asthma, colitis, hypertension), sexual disorders, a
variety of habit disorders (e.g., smoking, obesity, insomnia) and psychosis.
While these prescriptions were largely derived from principles of behavior
therapy, this was because these approaches more closely coincided with
the authors' desire to rely on empirical data where possible than did the
nonbehavioral approaches of the time.

Behavior therapy had (and largely still has) the strongest empirical basis
from which specific patient-treatment characteristics could be identified
at the time. Behavior therapy has always had a relatively strong investment
in identifying the characteristic patterns and behaviors which respond to
discrete interventions. Research on relationship therapies, reflecting the
perceptual system of these psychotherapists more generally, have traditionally been relatively inadequate in defining the discrete problems that might
serve as the objectives for intervention.

The kinship between the prescriptive psychotherapy of Goldstein and
Stein and more recent technical eclectic approaches is notable in several
respects. Prescriptive psychotherapy was the first noteworthy effort to define specific relationships between discrete interventions and selective targets of change, using empirical knowledge. It also acknowledged the
persuasive role of therapist variables in enhancing treatment response, and
it specifically encouraged research on clinical decisional processes as a
means of improving treatment assignment. Given today's enthusiasm for
developing decisional models for applying theories or procedures, one
cannot help but admire the wisdom and foresight which guided the development of these early ideas.

Specific Roots

Differential Therapeutics.   Differential Therapeutics is a term which was
first used in the context of psychotherapy assignment and applied in a
consistent way to treatment issues by Frances, Clarkin, and Perry (1984;
see also Perry, Frances & Clarkin, 1985). The ideas presented in this
formulation were also used as a model for treatment decisions by the
American Psychiatric Association's (1982) commission on treatment
effectiveness.

Differential Therapeutics combines the clinical wisdom of experienced practitioners and an ample array of clinical examples to define the enabling factors and indicators for a wide range of treatments. These indicators include diagnostic, characterological, and environmental variables. From these indicators, we can define contraindicators and enabling factors for predicting the probable response to be derived from different treatments. The treatments considered extend far beyond psychotherapy, thus partially accounting for the appeal of this approach to practicing clinicians, and include an array of treatment settings (e.g., partial and residential hospitalization), the selection of medications, and the assignment of treatment mode, frequency, duration, and format. These variables are rarely considered in other existing integrative models.

Aside from the advantage represented by the breadth of treatment procedures addressed by this model of technical eclecticism, it also presents a point of view which is intuitively familiar to mental health practitioners and is presented in a way that is both clear and straightforward. As applied to the particular (and often peculiar) methods of the psychotherapies, however, Differential Therapeutics is less specific than some other technical eclectic efforts and relies predominantly upon a common factors approach to describing the effectiveness of psychotherapy. If, as we propose here, even the common qualities that exist among the psychotherapies can and should be selectively applied by the therapist, then a more finely tuned assessment of the relationship between specific treatment activities and outcomes is warranted.

Systematic Eclectic Psychotherapy. Systematic Eclectic Psychotherapy, as presented by Beutler (1983) has its foundations in the general rationales of technical eclecticism, as outlined by Lazarus (1981), and social persuasion theory (e.g., S. S. Brehm, 1976, 1986; Brehm & Brehm, 1981; Goldstein, 1966; Strong, 1978). Systematic Eclectic Psychotherapy represents an effort to develop decisional criteria for the assignment of discrete treatment procedures, independently of the theories which gave rise to them. The specificity of this approach to the discrete operations of psychotherapy adds to the concepts of Differential Therapeutics and thus refines psychotherapy decisions beyond the specification of the format, setting, strategies, duration and frequency, and the use of medication.

Systematic Eclectic Psychotherapy proposes three patient or problem dimensions which are matched with three complementary aspects of psychotherapy technique. These patient/problem dimensions include: (a) symptom complexity or severity, (b) defensive style, and (c) interpersonal reactance level. The first of these dimensions is used to determine if treatment should be symptom or conflict focused. The second dimension determines whether cognitively, behaviorally, or affectively oriented procedures will be selected. The third dimension determines the degree of therapist directiveness to be used. Treatment menus are derived based upon patient status on these dimensions and are adjusted across time as patient/problem status changes.

Systematic Eclectic Psychotherapy is closely tied to empirical literature and has developed some empirical support for at least some of the dimensions (Beutler & Mitchell, 1981; Calvert, Beutler & Crago, 1988). The weakness of the model is its failure explicitly to provide for selecting treatment setting, format, duration, and frequency, as Differential Therapeutics does. Together, these two models provide a rough signs and symptoms approach to the assignment of treatments ranging from the general (whether or not to treat) to the specific (what psychotherapy intervention to make at a given point).

Ancillary Roots.   There have been a number of important theoretical and clinical advances in the area of treatment integration since *Differential Therapeutics* (Frances, Clarkin & Perry, 1984) and *Systematic Eclectic Psychotherapy* (Beutler, 1983) were published. To keep the current model abreast of these developments, several additional theories and formulations are also incorporated into the model presented here. While these do not have the salience and visibility in our proposal as the foregoing ones, their limited roles are important and bear some mention at this point.

Stages of Change.   A number of authors whose work has centered upon developing greater treatment specificity have taken the view that differential treatment applications must be at least partially dependent upon the stage or phase of treatment (Beitman, 1987; Fuhriman, Paul & Burlingame, 1986; Prochaska, 1984). These authors have attempted to identify the characteristic stages through which treatment proceeds and then to link these stages to corollary characteristics of different psychotherapies. While we will be drawing on the wisdom of several of these efforts from time to time, our model most heavily relies on the stages of normal problem resolution (a patient characteristic) defined by Prochaska (1984; Prochaska & DiClemente, 1982) and the stages of psychotherapy (a unique aspect of psychotherapy process) described by Beitman (1987).

Four sequential problem-solving processes characterize the *phases* through which people go when solving personal problems, according to the Transtheoretical model of Prochaska: *precontemplation, contemplation, action,* and *maintenance.* Research support for these phases has been quite consistent, enough so that Prochaska and his colleagues have determined that an orderly sequencing of these stages characterizes most individuals' behavioral change, whether or not this change takes place within the context of formal treatment.

Beitman (1987) has suggested that all individual psychotherapies inherently involve certain means-to-ends objectives. These objectives are sequential and constitute process (i.e., mediating) goals that are thought to lead efficiently to desired treatment outcomes. As such, they constitute the *phases* of treatment: (1) engagement or relationship building, (2) a search for patterns in the patient's responses, (3) the instigation of personal and/or interpersonal change, and (4) preparing for termination. We believe these simple definitions of the treatment process are sufficiently universal across treatment modes (i.e., somatic as well as psychological) and formats (i.e., group and family approaches as well as individual treatment) as to provide a framework on which the practitioner can prioritize even more specific mediating treatment goals within each phase. In turn, the nature of these *mediating goals* determines the treatment orientation taken and directs the therapist in selecting ways to keep the treatment moving forward.

Core Conflictual Focus. Quite a separate series of developments have recently been addressed to the problem of directing and focusing therapeutic procedures. Therapists typically orient their treatment objectives around formulations of the problem based upon their own particular theoretical models. However, these formulations often become clouded and uncertain as interesting material surfaces and accumulates. By applying a standard procedure to determining them, the treatment focus may remain clear over time and the power of our procedures may be intensified as a result. In seeking ways to preserve the constancy of treatment, we find much of value in recent writings devoted to clarifying the thematic patterns that underlie much of disturbing and distressed behavior.

Unlike the concept of treatment phases, the concept of *conflictual focus* does not derive from a treatment model that proposes to be eclectic in nature; neither is it represented in the work of a single author. Thematic conflicts are most clearly described in the writings of psychodynamic (especially psychoanalytic) psychotherapists, and their methods of operationalization derive directly from the work of Malan (1976). Today, the most systematic and empirically based methods for assessing conflictual themes derive from *Time Limited Dynamic Psychotherapy* (TDLP) outlined by Strupp and Binder (1984) and *Expressive Psychoanalytic Psychotherapy* as presented by Luborsky (1984). These authors have developed methods for identifying the recurrent themes that function as a guiding thread in treatment during relationship and insight oriented psychotherapy. The theme around which conflict oriented treatments focus can be expressed as four dimensions: (1) acts of the patient him or herself, (2) expectations about others' reactions, (3) actual acts of others toward the patient, and (4) consequential conclusions that the patient draws about these patterns (Strupp & Binder, 1984, pp. 76–77).

AN INTEGRATIVE MODEL

The model of treatment selection and therapeutic intervention presented in this volume emphasizes that effective treatment is a consequence of a sequence of increasingly fine-grained decisions. No effective treatment can be developed from information that is available at one point in time nor from decisions made on the basis of a static set of patient characteristics. There are at least four temporally related classes of variables which must be considered and which serve as enabling or activating characteristics that guide the selection of treatment dimensions. The relationships among these variable classes are presented in Figure 2.1.

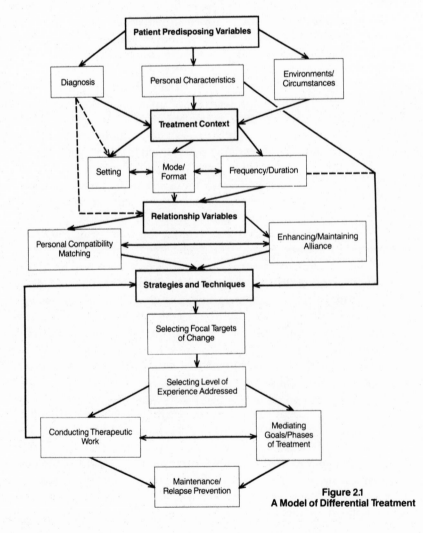

Figure 2.1
A Model of Differential Treatment

Previous models of assigning treatment have treated one or another of these sequential classes of variables as being of signal importance while minimizing those representing the other classes. Common Factors eclecticism focuses upon the role of relationship variables, Systematic Eclectic Psychotherapy emphasizes specific therapeutic interventions, while Differential Therapeutics attends most closely to predetermining variables and treatment contexts.

Each of the four classes of variables presented in Figure 2.1 includes dimensions that effectively will direct treatment decisions at subsequent points in the treatment selection process. Conversely, decisions that are made at any single point in time will be most useful if they incorporate the knowledge gained and decisions made at earlier points in the assessment and treatment process. As Figure 2.1 suggests, maximal treatment gain accrues when variables of each temporal or sequential class are considered as only links in a chain of decisions and when all previous classes of variables are considered to contribute synergistically to effective change.

While clinicians have long been aware of the complexity of these temporally sequenced influences, psychotherapy research has unfortunately restricted itself to a consideration of one or another of these temporal categories, and has seldom explored them in sequence as they interact and compound their influences. It is our intention to cast the speculations presented in ways that will facilitate their empirical exploration.

To facilitate the reader's understanding of the following chapters, we will briefly describe each of the major classes of variables that must be addressed at each decision point. These variables concepts will be explored in greater depth in the following chapters, in a format that coincides with the general outline provided here.

Patient Predisposing Variables

Patient Predisposing variables are defined as those characteristics that characterize the patient and his or her environment at the time they enter into treatment. Predisposing patient variables can be grouped into three general classes, specific aspects of which we will consider for assigning treatment at the three subsequent levels of our model. These three classes include diagnostic dimensions, dimensions of personality and conflictual style, and dimensions of the patient's environment.

(1) Diagnostic Dimensions (Chapter 3). Even though we question the value of diagnoses in assignment of psychotherapy and specific psychotherapy strategies, diagnostic labels have proven themselves useful in the selection of chemical interventions and hospitalization. Hence, their value as predictors of treatment setting and mode may be seen most clearly. Indeed, when applied to medical diseases, symptom-syndrome-based diagnostic

systems have been used both as treatment indicators and as benchmarks for assessing progress. In mental health, however, the distinctions among what are truly disturbances of metabolism, electrochemical transmission and neurological integrity, on the one hand, and those which reflect only exaggerations of normal behavior in the face of low social tolerance, on the other hand, are not easily made.

When applied to psychotherapy, symptom-based labels may occlude important patient distinctions and patient-therapist interaction variables that are relevant to assigning the most specific treatment procedures. With the wide array of possible treatments available to the psychotherapist, we believe that it is imperative to attend both to symptomatic presentations and to more subtle dimensions of patient presentation and therapist characteristics when developing a treatment response.

(2) Personal Characteristics (Chapter 4). While numerous authors have reviewed the patient characteristics which are related to successful mental health treatment, few of these variables have consistently been found independently to predict the clinical efficacy of any given treatment (e.g., Garfield, 1986; Orlinsky & Howard, 1986; Beutler & Crago, 1987). Patient variables operate in concert with variables associated with treatment selection, therapists and types of outcome. However, certain aspects of patient styles seem to have some limited importance in facilitating effective treatment assignment. These variables may contribute both to selecting the context (i.e., setting, format, modality, duration, and frequency) of treatment and to the selection of specific psychotherapy interventions.

Treatment-relevant personality characteristics include such nondiagnostic variables as problem severity and defensive style, capacity to form a relationship, and the specificity of the conflict or symptom presented. These dimensions are seldom incorporated into Axis I diagnoses and are only indirectly represented in some Axis II diagnoses.

As a general rule, patient demographic qualities (i.e., gender, age, SES, ethnicity), expectations, capacity to relate to others, and selective attitudes assist in selecting desirable treatment formats, settings, relationships, and durations more than they do in the selection of specific treatment strategies. Similarly, patient personality and coping styles comparatively may be invoked more strongly when selecting characteristics of the psychotherapeutic interventions and objectives than they are in the selection of treatment context.

(3) Environments and Circumstances (Chapter 5). The third class of patient predisposing variables is composed of those that determine patient perceptions and abilities to sustain treatment gain. These variables include personal support systems, work/school environments, family patterns, the

setting or relationship in which dominant conflicts occur, and the social forces which apply pressure and support. Certain of these environments will be conducive to the conduct of psychotherapy and others will not. In some situations, the contribution of a failing support system may influence the choice of family therapy as a treatment format. Likewise, the availability of supportive systems will determine the duration of treatment, the maintenance of effects, and the intensity of the treatment applied. A history of common environments and social systems may also be relevant to predicting the likely compatibility of patient and therapist.

Treatment Contexts

Characteristics of the Treatment Context are assigned from a knowledge of treatment-relevant predetermining patient qualities. You will recognize the concepts of *Differential Therapeutics* (Frances, Clarkin & Perry, 1984) in selecting treatment assignment at this level of decision process. We will consider treatment contexts under three general headings: (1) treatment settings, (2) treatment modes and formats, and (3) treatment duration and frequency.

(1) Treatment Setting (Chapter 6). Treatment settings range from inpatient to outpatient facilities and from closely monitored to unstructured situations. The setting selected may partially determine the nature of the treatment itself, the procedures used, and the nature of the outcome. Yet, for most purposes, treatment settings also allow a range of additional decisions which become apparent as the setting is selected and as patient predisposing characteristics are kept in view. These decisions apply to the other aspects of treatment context as well as to later decisions about specific interventions.

(2) Treatment Mode and Format (Chapter 7). Like the selection of setting, decisions about mode and format are based on predisposing patient characteristics, and also must be responsive to the nature of the setting in which treatment is provided. These decisions usually occur in two stages: selection of broad treatment modes, represented as somatic or psychological interventions, followed by the selection of the more specific format.

The selection of treatment mode reflects the desirability of implementing psychotherapy, pharmacotherapy, or some combination of these treatments. Selection of treatment format, on the other hand, is predicated upon the assignment of a psychological treatment mode in addition to patient predisposing variables and treatment setting. The formats available include combination treatments, group interventions, individual treatments, and interventions which involve the family or its subgroups.

Clinical wisdom suggests that the indicators and contraindicators for group, individual, psychopharmacological, and combination treatments are different (e.g., Frances, Clarkin & Perry, 1984). Treatments often cut across disorders so that predisposing variables like motivation, psychological mindedness, and relationship skill may significantly affect the selection of the treatment format more than does the patient diagnosis or symptom complex.

(3) Frequency and Duration (Chapter 8). Like mode and format, frequency and duration of treatment are interrelated concepts. Together they comprise a nonexclusive index of treatment intensity. Treatment duration ranges from single, crisis-oriented sessions to long-term intervention. While decisions about the frequency of sessions are not completely nested with the duration of treatment, normally both crisis-oriented and very long-term treatments are applied at higher frequencies than treatments of medium frequencies.

Recent years have seen increased interest in planned short-term treatments. Yet, the notion of short-term treatment is not new. Most mental health treatment is short-term, either by design or circumstance (Koss & Butcher, 1986). Indeed, the modal number of mental health treatments is one (1) and the mean varies from five to eight sessions depending upon setting (Koss & Butcher, 1986; Koss, 1979; Orlinsky & Howard, 1986). Nonetheless, most therapists prefer and intend to practice long-term treatments and, in fact, are most influenced by those patients who do seek long-term interventions. While only 16 percent of the patients who seek mental health treatment account for over half of the costs and services provided (Horgan, 1985; Taube, Kessler & Feuerberg, 1984), it is these 16 percent who set most practitioners' expectations. Indeed, a decision frequently omitted from considerations of treatment length is whether or not to provide any treatment at all. The therapist must be aware that there are instances in which a decision not to treat at all is the optimal decision for the patient's well being.

The selection of treatment frequency and duration is a complex function of predisposing characteristics of the patient, the setting of the intervention, and the format offered and accepted by the patient. The overall task is to select that frequency and duration which will exert the greatest effect on the most relevant and comprehensive problem and at the least prohibitive cost.

Relationship Variables

A compatible and productive treatment relationship evolves from the combined influences of patient characteristics, the selected treatment, and the qualities of the therapist. Managing the therapeutic relationship requires attention both to incoming compatibilities between patient and therapist and those interventions that can be used to activate the relationship potential.

(1) Therapist-Patient Compatibility (Chapter 9).   It is generally agreed that of all the things a therapist can provide, a caring, respectful, and understanding relationship is the most important. However, such a relationship, along with the therapeutic alliance it is designed to facilitate, is not the prerogative of the therapist alone. It is a simple but seldom discussed fact that not all patients and therapists "fit." There are, in fact, certain mixes of patient and therapist characteristics that are more conducive to developing an understanding and caring relationship than others. Therapist-Patient matching is possible through attention to those characteristics of both that contribute to compatible interactions. Treatment effectiveness can probably be enhanced by matching patient and therapist for compatible backgrounds and relationship styles. The process proposed in this volume incorporates both background, belief, and treatment format variables in proposing compatible matches.

(2) Enhancing the Therapeutic Alliance (Chapter 10).   In addition to selecting patients who are capable of establishing facilitative relationships and assigning them to therapists who are able to bring these qualities to fruition, therapists have the power to augment relationship qualities by both preparing the patient for what will transpire and altering the treatment environment to accommodate patient expectations. Role-induction procedures are designed to prepare patients for treatment, and session-enhancement procedures build upon and reinforce preexisting expectations and hopes. Collectively, these considerations facilitate the therapeutic alliance, from which effective treatment procedures can be employed.

Tailoring Strategies and Techniques

While various types or modes of psychotherapy are associated with distinctive therapeutic processes, only a few dimensions are necessary to describe most variations among psychotherapy orientational strategies (Sundland, 1977). Strategies and techniques are assigned from a fine-grained analysis of how these dimensions affect psychotherapy transactions. The assignment progresses through four levels of specificity.

(1) Selecting Focal Targets of Change (Chapter 11).   Defining and formulating the nature of the patient's problem in a way that allows a consistent focus over time is central to efficient treatment. From whatever theoretical posture a therapist comes, at least general consistency in the definition of the goals of treatment over time is important in order ultimately to assess how successful intervention has been.

While variation in the selection of specific outcome goals is necessary to attend to patient differences, treatment strategies can be divided roughly into two groups depending upon the breadth of their targeted influence. Some strategies emphasize and may be most effective for initiating symptomatic changes, while others emphasize the value of and are appropriately addressed to changing underlying conflicts.

Patients, in turn, present problems that vary in complexity and, therefore, may be more or less appropriate for treatment within the context of symptom change and conflict change strategies. Effective treatment assignment will match the nature and complexity of the patient's problems with the nature of the targeted aims and the strengths of the selected procedures.

(2 and 3) The Level and Mediating Goals of Treatment (Chapter 12). The level of experience valued and accessible through different treatment procedures represents the second level of treatment specificity. By matching the patient's style of coping with threatening experience to the level of experience affected by different procedures, menus of relatively specific treatments can be constructed.

The third level of treatment specificity defines the mediating tasks around which the procedures used in different phases of treatment will be organized. At this level of specificity, interventions are assigned by virtue of their ability to fit the sequential subgoals of treatment to the patient's progress through the problem-solving stages.

Just as a treatment plan must accommodate variations in the ultimate goals of intervention, it must also recognize that these different goals will be met most efficaciously by following different paths. Conflictual goals entail a different set of intermediate steps and require a different level of intervention than symptomatic goals. The therapist's formulation of the problem must be consistent with the type of problem to be addressed. Effective treatment also will be adjusted to the set of mediating goals that are likely to most directly lead to the desired treatment objectives.

The demands of specific procedures require that we alter the procedures selected as patients and circumstances change. The stages of psychotherapy outlined by Beitman (1987) offer some suggestions about how the subgoals of treatment might be prioritized and distinguished. Likewise, the phases of behavioral change (precontemplation, contemplation, action, and maintenance) proposed by Prochaska's (1984) Transtheoretical Psychotherapy illustrate the orderliness of people's struggle with conflicts and decisions. We suggest that the various ways that patients progress through these stages may be indicative of their compatibility with various formats and durations of interventions.

(4) Conducting Therapeutic Work (Chapter 13). The most specific level of

matching the therapeutic procedure to the patient occurs within the changing environment of the treatment session itself as one conducts therapeutic work. While the therapist can develop a general treatment plan and can select general goals that will remain quite constant throughout treatment, there are many decisions that must be made within the moment-to-moment interactions of the psychotherapy process. These decisions are designed to direct the patient's focus and to maintain movement toward productive ends. Here, the therapist makes decisions about the directiveness of the intervention, the degree to which he or she should increase or reduce the patient's arousal level, and when to address topics outside and inside of the therapy session. Specific decisions rest upon observing the patient's level of reactance (i.e., resistance), the amount of impairment produced by the symptoms, and the point reached in the patient's efforts to change behavior. These patient, treatment, and environmental patterns periodically are reevaluated to modify the treatment as effects are noted and as one plans procedures to prevent relapse.

SUMMARY AND COMMENT

This chapter has provided a brief overview of the treatment selection and application model which is to be developed in this volume. This model derives from the lack of consistency currently present in clinical settings and the inadequacy of diagnostic- and symptom-based systems alone to lend themselves to defining and refining the interventions that effectively can be applied to patients seeking mental health services. The model presented in this volume considers dimensions of patients, environments, treatment settings, therapists, therapies, and outcomes to be sequentially built. Each set of temporal variables, therefore, can be used to select the next level of treatment intervention. In turn, each treatment decision is based upon the maximal information available from each and all preceding temporal sets. This is not a novel idea; it parallels what is done in clinical practice at all levels.

Rather than presenting new information, we hope to lend systematization to the process of treatment selection. It is our intent to make explicit the processes that effective clinicians probably use intuitively. In this process, we hope both to provide the guidelines by which clinicians might learn to use this process systematically and to make explicit a method and rationale for systematic treatment planning which spans settings, theories, and disciplines.

SUGGESTED READINGS

Beutler, L. E. (1983). *Eclectic psychotherapy: A systematic approach.* New York: Pergamon.

Frances, A., Clarkin, J. & Perry, S. (1984). *Differential therapeutics in psychiatry.* New York: Brunner/Mazel.

Norcross, J. C. (Ed.). (1986b). *Handbook of eclectic psychotherapy.* New York: Brunner/Mazel.

Parloff, M. B. (1986). Frank's "common elements" in psychotherapy: Nonspecific factors and placebos. *American Journal of Orthopsychiatry, 56,* 521–530.

PART II

Patient Predisposing Variables

In Part I we presented a basic model of treatment selection. In the remaining pages, it is our task to expand upon this rough structure in order to address the problems of making meaningful treatment assignments. Part II provides the initial background in the form of a critical exploration of the patient variables that form the basis for treatment selection. The reader will quickly see that the three chapters in this section are not intended to provide guidelines for treatment selection. The delay may initially seem unnecessary to the impatient reader. However, these chapters are necessary since they specify patient and environmental dimensions on which the treatment decisions to be described in Parts III, IV, and V rely.

Figure II.1 provides an outline of the concepts to be discussed in Chapters 3, 4, and 5. It also displays the primary (solid arrows) and secondary (dashed arrows) relationships among these patient predisposing characteristics and subsequent treatment decisions that will be discussed in later sections of this volume.

One will note from the figure that predisposing patient characteristics are listed under three general categories (Diagnosis, Personal Characteristics, and Environments) corresponding to the titles of Chapters 3, 4, and 5. The directional arrows suggest that patient diagnoses and environments have a rather direct bearing upon decisions about treatment context (setting, duration, and format) while personal qualities (personality, coping styles, problem severity, etc.) bear upon selection of treatment relationships and the selection of specific strategies and techniques. The way that patient characteristics are utilized in selecting treatment contexts and treatment strategies will be illustrated in depth in the later sections that are devoted to these aspects of treatment.

Figure II.1

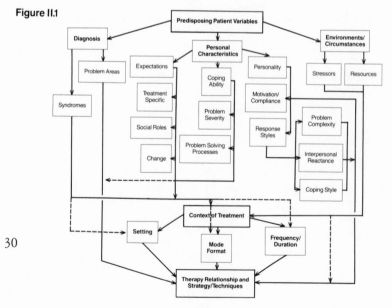

3

Diagnostic Considerations

"What treatment, by whom, is most effective for this individual with that specific problem, under which set of circumstances, and how does it come about?"

—Gordon Paul (1969)

Our level of knowledge has increased tremendously since Gordon Paul framed the question that has since become the litany of psychotherapy research and eclectic practice. Yet, we can still only begin to answer this pithy question in a factual way. The closest we can come to a consensual conclusion from available research is that the characteristics that the patient brings to the treatment experience are the single most powerful sources of influence on the benefit to be achieved by treatment. Even the therapy relationship, as potent as this variable is in determining treatment effectiveness, occupies a lower rung than preexisting patient qualities in the hierarchical arrangement of contributors to outcome (e.g., Lambert & DeJulio, 1978; Garfield, 1986).

To set the stage for applying differential treatment selection, we must emphasize our belief that the nature, breadth, and severity of a patient's problem should planfully determine the nature of the treatment assigned. If this does not happen, then the practitioner's favorite treatment will be applied indiscriminately to every problem that is presented. The traditional road to accomplish these ends in medicine has been to arrive at a "diagnosis" that, in turn, provides a target for intervention. Developments in psychopharmacology have reinforced the ideology that this same approach can be applied to mental health.

The search for biological contributors to emotional disorders supported and motivated the introduction of the criterion-based DSM-III in 1980. It

Portions of this chapter were presented as a presidential address to the Society for Psychotherapy Research, June, 1987, Ulm, West Germany, and are published in *Psychotherapy* (Beutler, in press). Reprinted with permission.

31

was reasoned that little progress in developing condition-specific treatments could be expected without ensuring that diagnoses could be reliably made across settings. The psychiatrists who spearheaded the movement for DSM-III were, by and large, clinical researchers who were interested in efficacy studies of psychopharmacological interventions. The diagnostic system itself reflected these interests, being largely based upon symptoms and clusters of symptoms that responded to somatic interventions.

While an accurate diagnosis allows the medical practitioner to account for relevant aspects of the patient's problem when developing a treatment program, diagnosis provides less useful information for the mental health practitioner. Consider, for example, J.I., the 34-year-old woman described in Chapter 1. The diagnosis of PTSD provides little to reflect the fact that this patient's anxiety following a car accident represented a recurrence of a similar reaction that followed the failed rape and murder attempt that had left her paraplegic 20 years earlier. Would a patient with this history warrant the same treatment as a 45-year-old male transient whose diagnosis of PTSD derived from the trauma of the war in Viet Nam? While the pharmacotherapist might recommend very similar somatic treatments for these two patients (usually antidepressants and sedatives), any given clinician would probably suggest very different psychosocial interventions for them.

Diagnostic systems are based on the assumed treatment specificity of certain symptoms and signs. While somatic treatments have benefited from this level of analysis, psychosocial treatments have expanded and developed without the assumption that they are diagnosis-specific; in fact practitioners of these treatments usually assume that their methods cut across most diagnostic conditions. For example, we find it interesting that recent surveys of psychotherapists' treatment preferences (e.g., Garfield & Kurtz, 1976; Norcross & Prochaska, 1988; Norcross & Wogan, 1983) give no attention to the therapist's considerations of how varieties among patient diagnoses might affect the selection and use of these strategies, techniques, and theories. This lack of attention to the match between treatment strategies and patient problems might be due in part to the dissatisfaction, both politically and academically, with diagnostic systems.

To place the issue of diagnosis and treatment planning in perspective, it will be helpful to review both the history of the diagnostic and statistical manuals as created by the American Psychiatric Association in this country and the sociopolitical implications of the debate over the medical model in clinical psychology and psychiatry.

CRITIQUE OF DIAGNOSTIC CONCEPTS

DSM-III (APA, 1980) defines a mental disorder as "a clinically significant behavioral or psychological syndrome or pattern of behavior that occurs in an individual and is typically associated with either a painful symptom (distress) or impairment in one or more important areas of functioning (disability)" (p. 6). The authors of DSM-III note an important implication of this definition: There is present a behavioral, psychological, or biological dysfunction which cannot be reduced to a simple relationship between the individual and the society. However, it is noted that the etiology of this "dysfunction" is not known for most disorders. Indeed, the authors of DSM-III specifically strove to avoid speculating about the etiology of disorders.

Given the state of our knowledge of etiology, the turf issues in mental health, and the lack of research on behavioral typologies, the authors of DSM-III are to be applauded for their effort to achieve reliable classifications of problems by seeking and applying clinical descriptors at the lowest level of inference. Nonetheless, we agree with Morey and McNamara (1987) in our belief that the assumptions underlying psychiatric classification must be carefully inspected if the mental health field is to move beyond simple description to the level of treatment planning.

The Politics of Nosology

There have always been disagreements about what constitutes emotional disorders, and diagnostic labels have changed both as social values have changed and as our sensitivities and tolerances for different behaviors have evolved. Contemporary sexual preferences have been particularly influential in altering our concepts of mental disorder. For example, homosexuality, which was considered to be a "mental disease" prior to the early 1970s, was "cured" by vote of the American Psychiatric Association when this latter body was petitioned by vocal groups who resisted being identified as "ill." Though not for its sexual implications directly, even "neurosis" was redefined in DSM-III and excluded from recognized diagnostic consideration by committee vote. Less sanguine writers than we might express regret that neither diagnostic committees nor special interest groups have yet applied their curative vote to cancer and heart disease.

With tongue in cheek, Ellenbogen (1986) illustrated the tendency to classify as a "disease" anything that is at variance with our own values when he suggested adding "Vegetarian Personality" to DSM-IV in recognition of the pathology of those who persistently avoid eating "sinewy flesh." The salience of this point was further emphasized when Smoller (1986) observed that "childhood" also represented an insidious and progressive mental disease characterized by congenital onset, dwarfism, emotional immaturity, knowledge deficits, and "Legume anorexia" (i.e., children almost never eat their vegetables) (p. 5).

Applying a less humorous note to the issue, a number of authors (e.g., Langer & Abelson, 1974; Herbert, Nelson & Herbert, 1988) have documented the tendency for diagnostic labels to distort the clinician's view of "normal behavior." Eysenck, Wakefield, and Friedman (1983) succinctly have summarized a number of other scientific difficulties with DSM-III.

> DSM-III includes many behaviors which have little or no medical relevance and belong properly in the province of the psychologist, e.g., gambling, malingering, antisocial behavior, academic and occupational problems, parent-child problems, marital problems, and the curious "substance use disorders," which apparently would bring almost any kind of behavior within the compass of psychiatry—drinking coffee, having sex, eating wiener schnitzel (p. 189).

These authors go on to emphasize that, given the group process that went into the generation of the document and the need for compromise during its development, DSM-III should be considered a *professional*, and only secondarily a scientific manual. They point out that the decision to create a document that does not deal with etiology and that contains no treatment recommendations was made explicitly to avoid offending the proponents of the various schools of treatment.

We believe that the lack of a conceptual link between diagnosis and treatment outcome introduces unneeded instability into our diagnostic manuals. At the same time, we recognize that at least two additional factors contribute to the lack of correspondence between diagnoses and treatment response. The first of these is the almost haphazard increase in the number of treatment systems espoused as effective. Over the past two decades, we have witnessed a huge growth in the number and variety of psychotherapies, behavior therapies, antidepressants, anxiolytics, and neuroleptics. We also have seen a significant growth in the number and variety of diagnoses, starting with 66 categories in DSM-I and increasing progressively to 111 in DSM-II, 206 (including appendices) in DSM-III, and currently to 261 in DSM-III-R. Moreover, DSM-III-R contains an appendix of "Proposed Diagnostic Categories Needing Further Study" which sets the stage for a further expansion of diagnoses in DSM-IV.

A second factor that may have contributed even more directly to the lack of correspondence between the specific effects of psychotherapy and diagnosis is the tendency of governmental agencies (at least in the United States) to fund only studies which define samples in terms of current diagnostic groupings. This latter bias virtually has forced psychotherapy research to look for differential treatment effects in the same dimensions that form the basis for diagnosis rather than in dimensions that are more consistent with the cross-cutting principles of psychotherapeutic treatment. The expansion of brief and creatively integrative psychosocial intervention strategies, stimulated by the reduction of the value of the health care dollar, is increasingly hard to research because of the diagnostic bias among funding agencies. As a result, new models of psychotherapy, especially brief psychotherapies, far outstrip our knowledge of their effects.

Effective treatment planning must link symptom descriptions with treatment interventions. The focus of various DSMs on specific, definable, and measurable symptoms is a necessary first but not sufficient step in the explication of relevant problem areas around which to plan treatment. More specifically, DSM symptom-based clusters are relevant for assessing treatment *efficacy* among symptom-focused treatments (i.e., they have criterion relevance), but they are not sufficient to serve as dimensions for prescriptive *assignment* of either symptom- or conflict-focused treatments.

We are not alone in suggesting the inadequacy of diagnoses to serve as prescriptive dimensions of treatment assignment. Behaviorally oriented clinicians (e.g., Barlow & Waddell, 1985) call for a functional analysis of symptoms that goes beyond the information contained in a diagnosis. This analysis specifies the cognitions, feelings, and/or behaviors that accompany target symptoms themselves in order to arrive at a statement of the antecedent and consequent behaviors that are related to problematic symptoms. By the same token, those in the interpersonal and dynamic traditions look for the interpersonal and intrapsychic meanings attributed to the problem behaviors. From whichever of these viewpoints one addresses human problems, information beyond DSM diagnosis is required.

Problems vs. Syndromes—The Level of Abstraction

Treatment is generally focused on either a symptom complex or a conflict pattern. DSM-III-R is almost exclusively oriented to symptom descriptions and groupings. In fact, concepts that implied the presence and importance to the presence of inferred conflicts and coping styles were explicitly excluded from DSM-III and III-R (e.g., Neurosis) even though those practitioners who preferred psychotherapeutic to somatic treatments objected to this exclusion.

By excluding inferred concepts such as "neurosis" and "conflict," DSM-III-R perforce became more relevant to the assignment of pharmacological than to psychosocial treatments. Given the nature of the DSMs, it is no surprise that among the psychosocial treatments, diagnoses are more helpful to those that are symptom-focused rather than conflict-focused. Even when psychosocial treatments are symptom-focused, diagnosis is inadequate to guide treatment; there must be a model of the condition that provides a rational assessment of precipitating and consequent conditions in order to structure interventions.

Barlow's (1988) symptom-focused treatment of panic and agoraphobia is a good illustration of the need for a model of both the symptom complex and the treatment approach even when dealing with symptoms alone. This model of the etiology of panic disorder includes biological vulnerability, stress, false alarms, and learned alarms leading to psychological vulnerability and agoraphobic avoidance. From these factors evolve a specific treatment plan of self-directed exposure to feared situations, and the use of self-monitoring techniques to anticipate the experience of panic. The symptoms described by the DSM diagnostic systems are neither specific enough to describe the function of antecedents and consequences to be of much value to the behavioral clinician nor sufficiently concerned with motivation and defense to be of value to the psychodynamic psychotherapist.

The gap between DSM-III-R and treatment planning is even larger when psychotherapy is conflict-focused. Since the very notion of conflict involves hypothetical constructs beyond actual observation, these are excluded from DSM-III-R. The closest DSM-III-R comes to any description of conflict is in scattered items suggesting repetitive patterns that occur in the patient's relationships with others, and these are all contained in Axis II, rather than in Axis I definitions.

The multiaxial approach to diagnosis of DSM-III-R is helpful in distinguishing different aspects of the person and focusing the clinician's attention on them: clinical symptoms (Axis I), personality disorders (Axis II), covarying medical conditions of significance (Axis III), psychosocial stressors (Axis IV), and prior level of functioning (Axis V). This approach to diagnosis helps the clinician keep in mind the complexity of factors that potentially contribute to the patient's presenting symptoms.

It should be recognized that the authors of DSM-III and its derivatives noted the limitations of the diagnostic criteria for treatment planning, observing that DSM-III diagnosis is only an initial step in a comprehensive treatment planning process. They acknowledge that each clinician, guided by his or her own theoretical preferences, will need to gather additional information in order to plan and select relevant treatment.

A PRACTICAL CRITIQUE

The foregoing paragraphs have suggested a number of weaknesses in the diagnostic systems. These points collectively suggest that the content and structure of diagnoses do not lend themselves readily to prescriptive treatment selection. The primary points can be elaborated as follows:

(1) Axis I diagnoses do not adequately reflect variations in problem complexity. Patients' problems vary in complexity, some being quite symptom-specific while others reflect a complex array of underlying conflicts and struggles. In parallel fashion, treatments vary in *breadth* of impact. Some treatments are very symptom-specific while others attempt broad-ranging changes. Hence, prescription of different treatments requires that the clinician assess the complexity of patient problems, rather than simply relying on the degree to which the symptoms fit a defined syndrome.

The diagnostic nomenclature is much more consistent with the tradition of symptom change than with the tradition of specifying underlying conflicts and meanings. This symptomatic specificity is both an asset and a liability. Symptoms can be reliably rated and this aids in interclinician communication. Doing so also enables the development of drug trials for the treatment of specific symptoms. The liability of this cross-sectional view of symptom clusters is that it gives one little information about the multiple causative paths to these symptom states, and is of decreasing value as one's preferred treatment becomes relatively more oriented to recurrently manifest conflicts and relatively less interested in overt manifestations of these hidden processes (cf. Schulberg & McClelland, 1987).

For most disorders, DSM-III, III-R and IV may be more useful at the level of specific diagnostic criterion (i.e., at the criterion level) than at the level of treatment planning. At the criterion level, many of the behaviors constituting a diagnostic category could be useful in defining some treatment objectives.

(2) *Diagnoses primarily address areas of weakness and deficit to the exclusion of areas of strength.* Central to treatment planning is defining the strengths of the individual that can be called upon in order to cope with the problem areas. In recognition of the importance of these areas, Frances, Clarkin, and Perry (1984) introduced the concept of "Enabling Factors" to the process of prescriptive treatment assignment. Not to be confused with a similarly labeled concept that has been applied to the behaviors of dependents and codependents in addictive disorders, enabling factors as described by Frances et al. are those characteristic strengths and resources that patients bring to the situation which allow them to take advantage of the treatment available.

For example, contributions to family systems and stable work contributions are given little consideration in diagnoses. Yet, these activities not only index strengths, they construct important contextual environments that provide important sources of support that can enhance the patient's prognosis and support recovery.

(3) *The interpersonal context of the patient's environment is largely ignored by the current diagnostic system.* With an overriding emphasis on the symptoms of the individual, the diagnostic system provides little information about the patient's salient environment, or hypotheses about how the environment interacts with other variables to influence the treatment plan. There is some recognition of the environment in the ratings of stress on Axis IV, and some "v" codes indicate the presence of such environmental events as marital conflict.

The immediate family of the patient can provide an important variable in understanding etiology, maintaining pathology, and developing the treatment plan. An example of important family involvement is the rela-

tionship between marital conflict and symptom (e.g., depression) formation among family members. The family is most crucial for symptomatic
children and adolescents, and for older adults who reside with those family
members who provide care for them.

The relationship between diagnosable symptoms and types of family
contextual stressors needs careful clinical assessment in the process of
planning treatments. For example, even when the family members are not,
themselves, manifesting or directly contributing to a diagnosable condition
in other family members, the non-symptomatic members may be an integral part of the treatment plan, especially as one plans for long-term maintenance of gains.

Even diagnostically similar patients require distinctly different treatments, depending in part upon the nature of the family support system
and the multicausality of psychological difficulties (e.g., Schulberg &
McClelland, 1987). A functional analysis of similar symptoms will often
reveal quite different causal patterns and every patient's unique strengths
and family environment will serve as enabling or restraining conditions
upon which to predict differential treatment responses.

(4) *Diagnostic systems exclude many problems for which people seek help.* In
spite of its increasing extension (some would say, "intrusion") into the
domain of problems presented by the "worried well," DSM-III diagnoses
still do not capture many of the problems presented by most of those
seeking assistance (Howard, 1988). This lack of coverage means that there
are many more clinical situations that present to clinicians than those that
are tabulated in the diagnostic code.

It is unlikely that disease labels should be placed either on normal
behaviors that occur in abnormal environments or on all the transient
distresses for which people seek counsel and advice. The extent to which
DSM-III adequately describes the range of known human difficulties is an
important criterion, often forgotten, upon which to judge the adequacy of
a prescriptive, treatment-based diagnosis, however. The traditional DSM
diagnostic system is more narrow than the myriad of difficulties that are
typically presented to clinicians, especially in the area of interpersonal
difficulties (McLemore & Benjamin, 1979; Horowitz & Vitkus, 1986).
Unfortunately, as long as clinical practice and research are geared exclusively to considering symptoms as "diseases of individuals" rather than as
the behaviors of systems, the relevant structure of the environment will be
neither examined carefully nor used systematically when treatment decisions are made.

(5) *DSM-III diagnoses lack construct- and criterion-related validity.* It's surprising that in spite of their common database and methods DSM-III does
not correspond closely with the several systems that it is designed either
to replace or to supplant. For example, Klein (1982) reports inconsistency

of diagnoses among 46 cases of schizophrenia, consecutively admitted to an inpatient unit, each of whom was diagnosed by seven different sets of diagnostic criteria: the Research Diagnostic Criteria (RDC) (Spitzer, Endicott & Robins, 1978); the DSM-III; the Flexible System from the World Health Organization International Pilot Study of Schizophrenia (Carpenter, Strauss & Bartko, 1973); the Feighner criteria (Feighner et al., 1972) as modified by Tsuang and Dempsey (1979); the criteria of Taylor, Greenspan, and Abrams (1979); and Schneider's first-rank symptoms (FRS) as defined by Carpenter and Strauss (1973). The intercorrelations among the seven systems ranged from –.21 to .89. The DSM-III diagnosed 28 percent of the sample as schizophrenic, while the other sets ranged from a low of 24 percent for the Feighner criteria to a high of 63 percent for the WHO system. There were only nine patients who were diagnosed as schizophrenic or non-schizophrenic uniformly by all seven systems.

Clarkin and colleagues (1983) noted that given the method of diagnosing borderline personality disorder in DSM-III there are 93 possible ways to arrive at the diagnosis (five or more of eight criteria). In a sample in a large outpatient clinic, it was found that empirically there are five typical symptom patterns that yield a borderline diagnosis, several of which would call for different treatment plans. Furthermore, there was a significant number of patients who just missed the borderline diagnosis (met four of eight criteria), but these criteria must be addressed in the treatment plan, nonetheless.

Such studies as the foregoing lend credence to observations (e.g., Gillis, Lipkin & Moran, 1981; Gillis & Moran, 1981) that treatment setting, country, and therapists' previous treatment recommendations are more predictive of treatment assignment than patient diagnosis.

(6) DSM diagnostic systems do not serve as equivalent indicators of somatic and psychosocial treatments. Even without criterion validity, the presence of internal reliability may be sufficient, if clear and consistent relationships were present, to indicate that diagnoses either predicted treatment response or indicated the probability of a treatment's success. Garfield (1986a) argues that if a diagnostic system is not linked in important respects to prognosis and treatment it has little utility.

While other research on more representative patient samples suggests stronger relationships between DSM-III diagnoses and treatment response than those reported by Klein on schizophrenics, diagnostic criteria are not equally predictive for somatic and psychosocial interventions. For example, utilizing a problem-oriented record, Longabaugh and colleagues (Longabaugh, Stout, Kriebel, McCullough & Bishop, 1986) coded treatment problems, DSM-III diagnoses, and treatment interventions among psychiatric inpatients. In a stepwise multiple regression analysis, both diagnoses and problem descriptions were found to be robust and significantly related to outcome when the patient was treated with medication, but were not strongly related to the prediction of benefits received from psychotherapy. Moreover, specific problem types were better indicators of the value of psychosocial treatments than were diagnoses, indicating that psychological treatments do not exert their strongest effects at the level of abstraction captured by DSM-III.

Most psychotherapists would agree that knowledge of the patient's unique history and coping pattern is a better indicator of what treatment to apply than either diagnosis or a listing of presenting problems. Consider again the case of J.I., our 34-year-old paraplegic patient whose presentation of post traumatic stress symptoms presents a rather colorless view of the nature of her condition. Can or should one treat this patient without at least a knowledge of her early history of traumatization? Most would answer "No," but neither problem descriptions nor diagnoses capture this important history.

SEEKING A ROLE FOR DIAGNOSIS IN TREATMENT PLANNING

Although we have criticized the limitations of DSM-III in planning treatment, we do not wish to conclude that it is valueless. For example, conventional diagnostic labels quite effectively (1) provide targets for the pharmacological treatments, (2) identify some targets of change for symptom-oriented psychosocial treatments, (3) identify symptom clusters that are differentially responsive to specific classes of medication, and (4) indicate that a treatment-worthy condition is present. These are important functions, and emphasize the need for obtaining a reliable diagnosis on all patients seeking treatment.

Beyond this, clinicians generally acknowledge the limitations of DSM-III and its derivatives for planning specific treatments, and have become sensitive to the types of information that are needed to supplement diagnostic information. For example, Hadley and Autry (1984) surveyed practicing clinicians to determine their beliefs about the usefulness of DSM-III. They concluded that diagnosis and severity of symptoms can determine short-term treatment goals, while information about prior functioning, degree of stress, psychological mindedness, and the developmental stage of the patient are needed to establish long-term treatment plans and to define the processes by which to reach the treatment goals.

Eysenck, Wakefield, and Friedman (1983) concluded their critique of DSM-III by suggesting that treatment decisions would be facilitated if: (1) the categorical diagnoses were replaced or supplemented with quantitative estimates of emotional qualities, since these better reflect the nature of psychological processes; (2) assessment of these qualities were considered in relationship to the requirements of available treatments; and (3) assessment were to reflect reliably observed behavior rather than idiosyncratic personal preferences of given clinicians.

Diagnoses, for all their problems, can contribute to selective treatment assignment as long as one does not expect more than is warranted. For example, when a patient carries a diagnosis of schizophrenia, major affective disorder, bipolar disorder, current substance abuse, or antisocial personality disorder, most clinicians would initially prioritize a set of options and considerations for the setting and modality of treatment. Knowledge of the diagnoses alone would result in most clinicians selecting general medication priorities from among the neuroleptics, anxiolytics, and antidepressants. Questions about hospitalization also would come to mind for schizophrenia, bipolar disorder, and major affective disorder, although this option would probably be assigned different weights for these three conditions. On the other hand, a rehabilitation setting would assume a higher priority for most clinicians confronting a patient with a substance abuse disorder or antisocial personality than one with Generalized Anxiety Disorder.

Given their use in selecting the treatment setting and the nature of somatic intervention, it may be unnecessary for diagnostic labels to carry a significant responsibility in defining the focus of treatment or treatment goals when applied to behavior therapy or psychotherapy. Nonetheless, the symptoms that comprise diagnoses, whether or not they are sufficiently specific to serve as the focus of the presenting complaints of the client, are of sufficient general and clinical significance that they must be incorporated into any treatment plan. One way of doing this is to translate these symptoms into more specific descriptions of problems and patterns.

Once one has a list of symptoms, recognizing that these symptoms often covary with one another, one can then use these to begin a functional analysis of the evoking situations and consequential behaviors. Ultimately, diagnostic labels will have value for psychosocial treatment planning only if and when they indicate several parameters: (1) a phenomenological description of the essential symptoms that will enable the diagnosis of the condition, and (2) a *model* of the disorder that specifies the variables and their relative weight and salience in the etiology and course of the disorder.

At this point, it is advantageous to introduce a distinction between the *final* and *mediating goals* of treatment, as these are crucial concepts in any treatment planning scheme. The final goals of most treatments are relatively similar and correspond to the alleviation of the symptoms and conflicts that initially brought the patient for help. On the other hand, it is the mediating goals of treatment, those goals hypothesized to be necessary steps en route to the final goals, that are differently posited by the various schools of psychotherapy, and that are crucial in planning psychotherapy variations.

An illustration of the foregoing point is in order. The final goal of the treatment of a patient with depression is the alleviation of the depression; this goal will be common across different therapeutic intervention strategies. However, the mediating goals to achieve the alleviation of the depression will vary, depending upon the individual characteristics (biological and psychological) of the patient, the characteristics of the patient's social environment and support system, the patient's progress in resolving the problems presented, and the theoretical stance of the therapist. All of these variables will contribute to a definition of the mediating goals of the treatment, those changes that are necessary steps in the alleviation of the depressive mood.

Common classes of mediating goals can be defined to the extent that there exists some uniformity among the stages through which successful treatment proceeds. Uniform stages of treatment are most easily observed in psychosocial treatments. Hence, we will return to this issue at greater length in Chapter 11 when we offer suggestions about the focus selected to guide psychotherapy toward desired outcomes, and again in Chapter 12 when we address the problem of selecting the levels of intervention and the tasks of treatment. It is sufficient here to emphasize that the mediating goals of treatment are not precisely dictated by the outcome goals; in prescriptive treatment selection, both the therapist's theoretical viewpoint and patient characteristics will combine with outcome objectives to determine these mediating goals and tasks.

Representative Diagnoses and Treatment Planning

As the field generates more empirical information about patients in each of the diagnostic categories (including etiology, contributing variables, course, response to treatment), we can construct models of the conditions/symptom clusters/syndromes that will help direct treatment interventions. In fact, one of the major difficulties in treatment planning at the present time is the paucity of information that would inform practitioners of the conditions being treated.

Models of major diagnostic groups such as schizophrenia (Nuechterlein & Dawson, 1984) and depression (Billings & Moos, 1982) have been generated. The typical model proposes the presence of interactions among personal cognitive, psychological, interpersonal, and biological attributes, as well as interactions of each of these with the environmental supports, resources, and stressors that lead to the disorder in question.

It is likely that the different disorders are influenced to different degrees by different etiological factors. For example, biological predisposing factors probably weigh more heavily in such disorders as schizophrenia and bipolar disorder than in unipolar depression, but interpersonal and cognitive variables probably play a more important role in the latter condition.

Likewise, it is unlikely that biological variables are of major consequence to most of the interpersonal conflicts (e.g., marital conflict, repetitive interpersonal conflicts) which most individuals bring to treatment (Howard, 1988).

There are a few cases in which DSM-III diagnostic categories contain information that facilitates making treatment decisions. For example, the response-relevant subtypes of alcoholics described by Morey and Skinner (1986) and the treatment-relevant schizophrenia subtypes described by Carpenter and Heinrichs (1981) allow for the development of general guidelines for intervention. While even in these conditions the diagnosis alone is not sufficient for treatment planning, it provides some general direction to the application of biological interventions, and to a lesser extent helps define the mediating goals of the treatment. A given diagnosis can be supplemented with relevant deficit and excess behaviors in order to refine diagnostic groupings and to construct treatment-relevant subtypes.

To illustrate the types of decisions that can be made on the basis of patient diagnoses, we will describe case examples and review some of the information currently available on a number of specific disorders. The case examples will be used in later chapters to illustrate treatment decisions.

Schizophrenia. J.C. was a 24-year-old male college student. He came to the attention of the mental health community after he approached a psychology professor at the university, asking where they kept the machines that sent him messages. On clinical interview, he reported that his name was "Jesus Christ" and that he had been sent by his grandmother, the Virgin Mary, to prepare the world for the coming of God. Moreover, he indicated that his grandmother (deceased) kept in contact with him through the CIA who maintained communication equipment in the basement of the psychology building. Finally, he indicated that if he was not successful in convincing the world that he was Jesus Christ by the time he reached the age of 33, he was commanded to kill himself.

The patient lived off campus with his widowed mother who reported that he had developed his peculiar beliefs during adolescence. He had received no previous treatment and had completed high school and four years of college. The patient was a graduate student in the Department of Physics. Students perceived him as "strange" and socially isolated, but they did not know of his special calling. Professors reported that his written examinations often contained phrases from the Beatles' albums, as well as drawings of disproportionate or disembodied people. Yet, the content of his answers was taken to suggest unusual creativity.

The concept of Schizophrenia in DSM-III-R is narrower than utilized earlier in this century, with a specified duration of symptoms required for the diagnosis (six months), excluding conditions without overt psychotic features, and excluding those patients with extended affective symptoms. Characteristic symptoms involve disturbance in content of thought (delusions); disturbance in form of thought (e.g., loosening of associations, poverty of speech content); disturbance in perception (hallucinations); flat or inappropriate affect; disturbed sense of self; paucity of self-initiated and goal-directed behavior; social withdrawal and emotional detachment.

DSM-III-R subdivides Schizophrenia into catatonic, disorganized, paranoid, undifferentiated, and residual (DSM-III-R) subtypes. Catatonia is rarely seen today, and most patients meet criteria for the paranoid and disorganized subtypes (Pfohl & Andreasen, 1986). Onset is usually in late adolescence and early adult years, somewhat earlier in males, with almost equal prevalence in both sexes. The course of schizophrenia is quite diverse, and suggests that the category in DSM-III-R probably covers a multitude of conditions.

In one of the best large-scale studies using criteria comparable to those of DSM-III (Tsuang et al., 1979), schizophrenics were assessed 30 years after initial diagnosis. Twenty percent of the patients were symptom-free, 25 percent had moderate symptoms, and 55 percent had severe symptoms. Other studies suggest that up to 40 percent of those with the diagnosis may be asymptomatic five or more years after onset (see Kendell et al., 1979; Bland et al., 1978; Harding & Strauss, 1984).

A diagnosis of schizophrenia is helpful in alerting the clinician to certain key treatment planning issues:

(1) Both patient and family will need information concerning the symptoms, causes, and possible course of schizophrenia.

(2) There will very probably be a need for the patient and family to cooperate in complying with medication.

Schizophrenia is a broad-band designation that needs further elaboration in order to be useful for treatment planning:

(1) Coping adequacy/problem complexity, coping style (including defenses), interpersonal reactivity, problem-solving cycle (as explicated in Chapter 4).

(2) The presence and severity of positive and negative symptoms (Pfohl & Andreasen, 1986).

(3) The nature and extent of the patient's social skills.

(4) The "co-morbidity" or presence of other diagnoses and problems that the individual with schizophrenia has, including drug and alcohol abuse.

Carpenter and Heinrichs (1981) argue that for early treatment planning the following subgroups are relevant: (1) good prognosis, nonparanoid patients; (2) paranoid and poor prognosis patients; (3) poor responders to antipsychotic medications; and (4) schizophrenics with depressive episodes. For long-term treatment planning, information about episodic patterns of illness, the presence of neurological risks, social and environmental supports, the duration of prior drug therapy, and history of treatment noncompliance is relevant.

McGlashan (1986) has observed that since schizophrenia is a very heterogeneous condition, a range of therapeutic strategies must be applied. These may differentially be assigned depending upon the phase (i.e., prodromal, active, residual) of the disorder, environmental factors, individual assets and weaknesses, and other nondiagnostic factors. The core of the treatment is a clinical relationship between the professional and the patient. The treatment should be open-ended and perhaps lifelong (*duration*). Brief hospitalization should be used when necessary, and structured aftercare programs with social skills training, structured activities, and vocational rehabilitation (*settings*) have demonstrated effectiveness (Harding & Strauss, 1985; Paul & Lentz, 1977). Family management has been found to be very effective in reducing relapses and helping the family cope with the condition. If used, individual therapy should be reality-oriented, pragmatic, adaptive (*format*).

Anxiety Disorders.   A. D. was a 57-year-old physician who sought consultation at the request of his estranged wife. The initial complaint was of compulsive rituals, primarily in the form of checking and hoarding. The patient's first marriage had also ended because of his inability to give up these rituals. A.D.'s early memories were of poverty and deprivation. He, his brother and his uncle were the only surviving members of his family and they had immigrated from Germany at the end of the Second World War. His family were Russian Jews and had been captured and interned in a concentration camp during the German invasion of Russia. They had been held for two years before being rescued at the end of the war.

From the time of his release, the patient had been given to performing hoarding rituals and these had become more severe with time. His wife reported episodes of secreting food, garbage, and other disposables in his closets and drawers. While the patient tended to minimize the significance of his hoarding, attributing this behavior to his desire to be prepared for any future needs, he acknowledged a ritual of checking doors, windows, and locks as many as 30 times each night before going to bed. Moreover, failure to perform any of these rituals resulted in considerable anxiety. Efforts on the part of his wife to control his behavior by removing his stores or reorganizing his possessions resulted in explosions of anger, and on one occassion he had been physically abusive. These episodes of rage were followed by profuse apologies and depression.

Axis I anxiety disorders, as described in DSM-III-R, are differentiated into five broad classes: panic disorder, phobic disorder, obsessive-compulsive disorder, post-traumatic stress disorder, and generalized anxiety disorder. Subtypes of these disorders are also identified. For example, phobic disorder includes subtypes, partially determined by the presence or absence of panic attacks (e.g., two of the four types of phobic disorders are agoraphobia with panic attacks and agoraphobia without panic attacks). Agoraphobia (with or without panic) involves marked fear of being alone or in public places and increasing constriction of normal activities until the fears and avoidance behaviors dominate the individual's life, without these features being caused by other syndromes such as depression, obsessive-compulsive behavior, paranoid personality disorder, or schizophrenia.

It is educational to explore the usefulness of the distinctions among anxiety disorders made by DSM-III-R. A critical question revolves around the question of whether there are distinctions among panic disorder, social and simple phobias, obsessive-compulsive disorder, post-traumatic stress disorder, and generalized anxiety disorder that make a difference in terms of treatment planning.

While DSM-III-R provides a descriptive listing of typical symptoms of anxiety, there is reason to question whether the categorical distinctions have treatment-relevant meaning. For example, panic attacks do not uniquely distinguish Panic Disorder; panic occurs frequently in all of the anxiety subtypes, varying from 83 percent to 100 percent (Barlow, 1988, p. 98). Likewise, generalized anxiety is extremely difficult to justify as a separate disorder. Generalized anxiety is a characteristic not only of all of the Anxiety Disorders, but of the depressive disorders as well. Finally, many of the symptoms of anxiety are present to some degree and intensity among normal populations, suggesting that anxiety may best be understood as a series of continuous dimensions rather than as categorical distinctions.

Barlow (1988) argues for the importance of identifying clusters of anxiety-related symptoms in treatment planning. He notes, as examples, that distinctive cognitive mediating processes distinguish performance and social phobias from other phobias. Likewise, blood and injury phobias are characterized by a physiological response that distinguishes these phobias from other simple phobias. Barlow also points out that treatment plans may differ depending on the presence or absence of depression among those individuals having obsessive-compulsive disorder.

Agoraphobia. Agoraphobia (fearful avoidance of certain places and situations) usually occurs in women, with onset in late adolescence or early adulthood, and has a prevalence rate of between six and 260 per 1000 depending upon which study one accepts. The temporal development of agoraphobia is characterized by one or more initial and seemingly spontaneous panic attacks, followed by the increasing development of phobic avoidance (Thyer & Himle, 1985).

Barlow (1988) has argued cogently that agoraphobic behavior is a complication of less specific forms of anxiety, involving an initial panic attack and subsequent, anticipatory fear of the recurrence of panic. The nature of panic/agoraphobia suggests that both a biological vulnerability and the occurrence of stress provoke the initial panic attack. This panic attack may be associated with environmental cues and becomes related to learned alarm signals that exaggerate psychological vulnerability. In turn, this vulnerability is manifest in apprehension and sensitization to signals from the environment. This hypervigilence and vulnerability are accompanied by autonomic and cognitive symptoms of anxiety which could precipitate instances of agoraphobic avoidance.

Barlow also observes that the development of agoraphobic avoidance may reflect culturally-induced sex role behaviors. While equal numbers of men and women experience panic attacks, approximately 75 percent of agoraphobics are women. Barlow suggests that men and women learn to cope differently with the experience of panic, with men being prone to develop alcoholism and women to engage in agoraphobic avoidance. The cultural etiology of the relationship between sex and agoraphobic avoidance is emphasized by the observation that, independent of one's actual gender, individuals who score relatively low on masculine scales of sex role identification tend to be likely to exhibit agoraphobic behavior (Chambless & Mason, 1986).

Agoraphobia has been successfully treated with behavioral approaches, most notably prolonged exposure *in vivo* (Emmelkamp, 1986). Based upon the model of agoraphobia as explicated above, the typical mediating goals to which the treatment of agoraphobia may attend include:

(1) Education about the prevalence, symptoms, and treatability of the disorder,

(2) Assessment of possible confounding conditions, including depression, panic attacks, depersonalization,

(3) Encouragement of and preparation for exposure *in vivo,*

(4) Exposure *in vivo,*

(5) Elimination of anxious thoughts and use of coping self-statements, and

(6) Support of spouse/family.

A number of differential treatment planning issues arise with agoraphobia. In terms of treatment format, group exposure is about as effective as individual treatment, and provides cost-effective benefits. One of the most interesting issues is the role of marital treatment among those whose agoraphobia is coincidental with marital conflict. Barlow, O'Brien, and Last (1984) have advocated the use of the spouses of agoraphobic women as co-therapists, perhaps with some particular benefit to this subgroup of maritally distressed women.

Generalized Anxiety Disorder.   The essential feature of DSM-III-R Generalized Anxiety Disorder (GAD) is the presence of excessive and unrealistic anxiety, worry, and apprehension about life's circumstances. This apprehension and worry are often accompanied by motor tension (e.g., trembling, muscle tension, restlessness), autonomic hyperactivity (e.g., shortness of breath, palpitations, sweating, dry mouth), vigilance, and scanning of the environment.

Barlow and colleagues (1984) have attempted to develop a diagnosis-specific treatment for GAD that comprehensively involves biofeedback and relaxation, stress inoculation, and cognitive therapy for anxiety. The 18-session treatment has proven successful in reducing psychological and physiological indices of anxiety. Confirming our position that few treatments are diagnosis-specific, it is notable that Barlow and colleagues have found that patients with Generalized Anxiety Disorder and those with Panic Disorder appear to respond in a similar way to the treatment. The specificity of the treatment beyond these two groups of patients is as yet unassessed.

Mood Disorders.   C.A. was a 36-year-old woman who reported suicidal preoccupation and recurrent depression. The patient had been reared in a wealthy family as the oldest of five children. The patient's first depressive episode occurred shortly following her father's death. This death necessitated that the patient leave a lucrative business that she had built herself and return to the family home to take care of her mother and to manage the family finances.

In the two years following her father's death, the patient encountered a number of additional environmental stressors, each of which evoked a depressive episode. These included two surgeries for injuries incurred in an automobile accident and an episode of rape by an unknown assailant. The surgeries left her with a permanent limp and the rape left her feeling defeated and rejected, a feeling that was exacerbated by a decision not to disclose the incident in order to protect the family name.

Following the rape, C.A. left home. Within a few weeks she met a man whom she came to love. Her decision to convert to his religion resulted in her family disowning her. The depression from this event was magnified when her fiancé was shot to death during a holdup of his store. It was at this point that she sought treatment.

DSM-III-R subclassifies the mood disorders into Bipolar Disorders (including Bipolar mixed, manic, and depressed; Cyclothymia), and Depressive Disorders (including Major Depression and Dysthymia). Bipolar Disorders are characterized by symptoms and behavior of mania and hypomania. The bonding feature among these various conditions is the presence of depressed mood and diminished daily functioning.

Unlike the case of Anxiety Disorders, certain distinctions among the Mood Disorders are relevant for the selection of treatments. The presence of vegetative signs, severe motor retardation, and manic states is relevant in planning drug intervention with these conditions. Beyond some general decisional guidelines, however, the application of psychosocial interventions is not specific to any of the DSM-III criteria. For these interventions, a clinical evaluation and functional analysis of the generation of symptoms is required. Indeed, for discriminating treatment to occur even among those with vegetative signs, careful distinctions must be made between those with unipolar, single episode depressions; unipolar, recurrent depressions; bipolar depressions; those with coexisting affective or organic illnesses; depressions mimicking a medical disorder; depressions indicative of a true medical disorder; and depressions that are reactive to a medical disorder (Schulberg & McClelland, 1987).

Nonpsychotic Depressions. The 1980's have been an era of much attention and successful clinical research on the psychotherapeutic treatment of mild to moderate, nonpsychotic depressions in ambulatory patients. The manualized treatments of depression postulate different models of mood disturbance, and consequently focus their interventions on different mediating goals. While all accept the alleviating of depression as an end goal, they differ in the relative weight given to psychodynamic, behavioral, and interpersonal goals. Thus, the DSM-III-R diagnosis selects a group of patients, homogeneous for certain depressive symptoms but heterogeneous for stressful life events, marital conflict, interpersonal problems, social skill deficits, and depressive cognitive thought patterns. In turn, all of these dimensions of heterogeneity are the primary targets of one or more of the intervention packages.

Mild to moderate levels of nonpsychotic depression in outpatients have been successfully treated with individual brief behavioral (McLean & Hakstian, 1979; Bellack, Hersen & Himmelhoch, 1983), cognitive (Kovacs, Rush, Beck & Hollon, 1981), and interpersonal (Klerman, Weissman, Rounsaville & Chevron, 1984) therapies. The often disparate mediating interventions in these treatments of depression include:

(1) Education about the symptoms, prevalence, and treatment of depression,

(2) Decrease of specific environmental stressors,

(3) Increase of positive environmental reinforcers,

(4) Decrease of marital/family conflict, and other salient interpersonal conflicts,

(5) Resolution of grief,

(6) Identification of depressogenic thoughts and replacement with coping self-statements, and

(7) Self-control procedures.

At this point in our knowledge, there is no clearly "superior" manual for the treatment of depression. While it is quite likely that some models are more relevant to some individuals than others, it is also clear that diagnostic distinctions do not assist in predicting this differential effect.

Alcohol Abuse. H.D. was a 44-year-old, unemployed man. He had been raised in a prominent family. His father was the president of a small Lutheran college and disdained alcohol use. The patient himself had received a divinity degree from a prestigious eastern university, as well as a Ph.D. in English literature.

H.D. began drinking when he was 14 years old. His parents discovered his transgression when he was 17 years old, but by this time the patient was drinking daily and becoming drunk at least four times per week. After completing high school, with significant intervention by his father with school officials, the patient went to college. He was discharged from seven different colleges before graduating from his father's alma mater.

H.D. was unable to control his drinking during his graduate work. He frequently missed class and nearly failed several courses. En route to his oral defense for the Ph.D. degree, he was picked up for drunken driving. After the intervention of his father, however, his committee elected to let him complete his defense and granted him a degree. He had since been employed and fired from several jobs and for the 15 years prior to entering treatment, he had been unemployed. His parents provided financial support for him and had paid for his treatment in several different settings.

DSM-III-R describes Psychoactive Substance Use Disorders as conditions of impaired control of alcohol use and abuse. "Impaired control" is defined as repeated substance intake and use despite adverse consequences. The consequences of alcohol abuse, in turn, include cognitive, behavioral, and physiological symptoms, as well as increases in interpersonal conflict. As with other diagnoses, a major problem with the categorical distinction among Alcohol Abuse Disorders is that such categories do not adequately reflect the continuity, generality, and lack of empirical support for the importance of many of the associated symptoms. For example, the distinction between "dependence" and "abuse" proposed by DSM-III-R has not been empirically found to be relevant or reliable (Schuckit et al., 1985).

On the other hand, there is some support for the presence of interdependence among behaviors that compose a Dependency Syndrome. This syndrome consists of a progressive increase in alcohol-seeking behavior, increased tolerance for alcohol, repeated withdrawal symptoms, seeking alleviation of withdrawal symptoms by further drinking, a compulsion to drink, and a tendency to relapse following abstinence (Edwards, 1986; Hodgson & Stockwell, 1985).

A number of descriptive models to account for the development of addictive behavior and alcohol abuse have been developed. These models typically propose that biological and genetic processes increase the risk of developing a dependency when they are accompanied by certain environmental factors (Connors & Tarbox, 1985). They also specify roles for classical and operant conditioning and both social learning and cognitive processes in setting the nature of patient patterns of drug usage (Brickman et al., 1982; Marlatt et al., 1988).

A number of diagnostic procedures and dimensions have been developed that parallel the multiple, complex processes that contribute to alcohol abuse. For example, Morey and Skinner (1986) have proposed a classification scheme which combines dimensional and categorical methods in order to make diagnosis more relevant to treatment decisions. A multilevel, sequential validation method was used to compare classifications generated by over 20 different strategies of cluster analysis. These classifications were then validated with personality, psychotherapy, intellectual, neuropsychological, socioeconomic status, and other variables relating to alcohol abuse. This model describes three types of alcohol abuse:

(1) *Early-stage problem drinkers* are those whose drinking pattern is characterized by beginning relatively late in life; they have relatively low average daily alcohol intake, and usually fail to perceive alcohol as a problem. Compared to other alcohol abusers, this group has relatively higher incomes and employment rates; most are married and living with spouse and children; they appear quite normal on most personality questionnaires and they have both self direction and high needs for mastery and accomplishment. They tend to progress to more severe stages of addiction.

(2) *Affiliative alcoholics* have drinking patterns characterized by brief periods of alcohol abstinence. Compared to early-stage drinkers, those in this group have more symptoms of depression, anxiety, thought disorder, and interpersonal problems. They are also characterized as affiliative, aggressive, impulsive, and possessing little desire for self understanding and little self-perceived control.

(3) *Schizoid alcoholics* have chronic and severe problems with alcohol, accompanied by a great sense of guilt, fear, and worry. They usually experience physiological and psychological effects when alcohol is withdrawn and tend to recognize drinking as a problem. They tend to drink in a solitary fashion, and among the three groups they have the lowest socioeconomic standing and self esteem, along with the greatest social instability and the highest incidence rates of depression, anxiety, and thought disorder. This group tend to have relatively antisocial attitudes and perceive themselves as being controlled by fate and others. They are prone to engage in risky and reckless action, even becoming extremely aggressive at times and very withdrawn at others.

Early-stage problem drinkers are thought to be responsive to a controlled drinking treatment strategy, while the affiliative and schizoid types are considered poor risks for such a tactic. In contrast, Alcoholics Anonymous (AA) with its strong group and sharing approach is considered to be suited to the affiliative type's style, while the schizoid type is hypothesized to be best treated through individual treatment formats.

Alcoholics who are impulsive and aggressive (i.e., externalized coping) drinkers have also been found to engage in very different and more dysfunctional marital relationships than those who are more introverted, introspective and steady (i.e., internalized coping) drinkers (Jacob & Leonard, 1988). This finding has implications for the observation that systems-oriented marital therapy has value for at least some alcohol abusers after the application of symptom-oriented treatments designed to reduce or eliminate alcohol intake (O'Farrell & Birchler, 1987).

More specifically, the potential value of planful sequencing of specific treatments for enhancing and maintaining symptom control suggests that the mediating interventions in the treatment of substance abuse may include:

(1) Detoxification
(2) Role induction into a structured treatment regimen including substance abstinence
(3) Aversion therapies (Cannon et al., 1986) and behavioral self-control training (Miller, 1987) for initial change in drinking behavior
(4) Social skills training (Hay & Nathan, 1982) and marital/family therapy (McCrady et al., 1986) for support of continued sobriety

The empirical investigation of the match between patient characteristics and the goals of treatment has focused on controlled drinking versus abstinence outcomes (Sanchez-Craig & Lei, 1986). Another area of patient treatment match is that between severity of drug usage and the specific focus or intensity of treatment. McLellan et al. (1983) have found that those patients with high levels of severity did poorly irrespective of the treatment parameters. In contrast, those with low levels of severity did well irrespective of treatment intensity. Matched cases showed significantly better outcome than mismatched cases in a nonrandom prospective design.

Personality Disorders. M.D. was a 27-year-old woman who presented with mixed anxiety and depression. She had been raised as the youngest of four sisters, and had always been treated as the baby of the family. She was nurtured and protected from anything that might have been harmful to her. Her father was a minister and regularly lectured his daughters on the evils of premarital sex. He favored his younger daughter openly and when she was 11 years old he began caressing and kissing her breasts and genitals. Ultimately, he asked her to stroke his sexual organ, and on some occasions this resulted in ejaculation. These sexual gestures and acts were followed by special favors and gifts, evoking the jealousy of M.D.'s sisters.

As an adult, M.D. described a long history of unstable and intense romantic relationships with married men, each ending when she became involved with another man. Following each incident, she had made a suicidal gesture. At the time of entering treatment, she had again become involved with a married man and was afraid that her current lover would find out. On evaluation, she met diagnostic criteria for Borderline Personality Disorder.

The multiaxial approach of DSM-III is conceptually helpful in guiding the clinician's diagnostic eye to distinguish between the symptom picture that may be temporary but which spurs the patient to seek help (Axis I disorders), and the more enduring personal and interpersonal traits of the individual (Axis II disorders). To some degree, the failure of Axis II to provide a solid basis for developing treatment, especially psychotherapeutic interventions, reflects flaws both in the construction of Axis II concepts and in the way that the diagnostic criteria are grouped.

On a conceptual and scientific basis, the organization of Axis II is a messy short story in need of a good editor. A review of individual criteria reveals that the items do not represent the same level of abstraction, they are not intercategorically consistent, and there is much interdiagnostic item overlap. The degree of item overlap among the Axis II diagnostic categories is at least one reason why many patients in empirical studies have been found to have multiple Axis II diagnoses. In addition, multiple qualifying diagnoses are simply an empirical demonstration that the 11 "diagnoses" presented in DSM-III Axis II are no more than conventional descriptions that mask the presence of an unknown and undetermined number of actual entities.

Marshall and Barbaree (1984) have redefined the descriptive features of DSM-III Axis II disorders into dimensions which promise to be more relevant to psychotherapeutic tasks and goals than the original groupings. By casting Axis II diagnoses into an interpersonal framework, these authors have addressed a concern expressed by many psychologists and object relations theorists—psychosocial treatment should be focused on the predominant interpersonal behaviors of the patient.

For example, McLemore and Benjamin (1979) and Horowitz and Vitkus (1986) have advocated the value of interpersonal diagnosis, and have begun to pilot self-report instruments to garner data that will be useful in treatment planning for the individual case.

Widiger, Trull, Hurt, Clarkin, and Frances (1987) also attempted to derive a *dimensional* model of personality disorders from the DSM-III categorical descriptions, utilizing the defining criteria. The presence of each of the DSM-III Axis II criteria for all the personality disorders was systematically assessed in 84 patients. The number of symptoms possessed by each patient, representing each of the personality disorders, was correlated across patients and subjected to a multidimensional scaling procedure. A three-dimensional solution was generated. The first dimension represented social involvement, with the schizoid and paranoid personality disorders at one pole and the dependent, avoidant, borderline, and histrionic categories at the other pole. The second dimension to emerge represented assertiveness along a dominance/power continuum with the narcissistic and histrionic personality disorders at one end of the continuum and the schizoid, passive/aggressive, avoidant, and dependent personality types at the other. The third dimension represented a continuum ranging from internal, anxious, and ruminative orientation defined by the schizotypal, compulsive, paranoid, and avoidant personality disorders at one pole, to externalizing and acting-out at the other pole, as defined by antisocial, passive-aggressive, schizoid, and borderline personalities.

Dimensions similar to those discovered by Widiger et al. (1987) have appeared throughout the history of the classification of personality and they provide a means by which to evaluate normal and abnormal traits along the same continua. As compared to the overlapping and conceptually inconsistent personality disorder categories of DSM-III, these dimensions of personality functioning may be more useful in assessment and treatment planning. These three dimensions may be foci or targets of change, or alternatively, they may help shape treatment planning since they closely resemble some of the nondiagnostic patient characteristics that will be discussed in the next chapter and that we believe are crucial for selecting among treatments.

Other Problem Areas.   There are multiple problem areas with which individuals present for assistance to mental health professionals that are included only in passing or subsumed under "other diagnostic categories." These problem areas deserve and require attention in treatment planning on an equal par with "diagnosis." We will mention only a few here: suicidal ideation and behavior, marital conflict, nonmarital interpersonal conflicts, coping with medical conditions such as insomnia, pain and cardiovascular disorders, work and study problems, anger and violent behavior. These conditions often present with symptoms of depression and anxiety, but not with enough severity to meet an Axis I diagnosis.

SUMMARY AND COMMENT

Effective treatment planning must involve the reliable and valid description of the problem areas that are the focus of intervention. The traditional way to describe problem areas is by an organized and agreed upon diagnostic system, the current diagnostic system being that of DSM-III-R as constructed by the APA (1987). DSM-III-R is helpful in its atheoretical and relatively objective description of symptom complexes that individuals who seek assistance report. However, whether the treatment is focused on symptom complexes or on more complicated conflict syndromes, one must have a model of the thoughts, feelings, and behaviors that are the focus of intervention in order to plan an organized, hierarchical intervention. DSM-III-R does not provide such a model.

Clinical research in the various areas of pathology are beginning to arrive at models that are useful in directing manualized treatments for these conditions. Because DSM-III and III-R were designed to achieve some compromise among various political influences, they do not reflect consistently any one theoretical model of psychopathology. Yet, this very compromise limits their usefulness in planning treatment, which is almost always based upon some theory of psychopathology. To organize treatment planning solely around a descriptive diagnosis is to assume that the diagnosis is the organizing kernel of the clinical thinking process. In contrast, we assume that there are multiple organizing kernels which must be in the forefront of the clinician's mind in planning treatment: patient variables (diagnostic and nondiagnostic), relationship variables, and therapy interventions (see Figure 2.1).

SUGGESTED READINGS

Beutler, L. E. & Crago, M. (1987). Strategies and techniques of prescriptive psychotherapeutic intervention. In R. E. Hales & A. J. Frances (Eds.), *American Psychiatric Association: Annual Review* (Vol. 6) (pp. 378–397), Washington, D. C.: American Psychiatric Association.

Eysenck, H. J., Wakefield, J. A. & Friedman, A. F. (1983). Diagnosis and clinical assessment: The DSM-III. *Annual Review of Psychology, 34,* 167–193.

Garfield, S. L. (1986a). Problems in diagnostic classification. In T. Millon & G. L. Klerman (Eds.), *Contemporary directions in psychopathology: Toward the DSM-IV* (pp. 99–114). New York: Guilford Press.

Widiger, T. A., Trull, T. J., Hurt, S. W., Clarkin, J. F. & Frances, A. (1987). A multidimensional scaling of the DSM-III personality disorders. *Archives of General Psychiatry, 44,* 557–563.

4

Patient Personal Characteristics

In the previous chapter we argued that diagnoses, in and of themselves, have limited relevance to the selection of specific procedures of psychotherapy. This chapter seeks to identify some of the nondiagnostic variables that can be used both to complement diagnostic information and for determining a range of conducive treatment contexts (i.e., setting, format, duration) and specific psychotherapeutic applications.

Patient characteristics which predispose how one will respond to treatment include sociodemographic background variables, dispositions to respond to environmental forces when they arise, and enduring patterns of personality. Age, gender, family structure, and learning history all work to establish certain expectations about treatment, self, and others that are significant to predicting and selecting treatment response. One's intellectual resources, prior successes, current distress levels, progress in solving current dilemmas, and general coping strategies (i.e., defensive and interpersonal styles) all reflect on what types of treatment environment and procedures will induce a positive effect (Garfield, 1978, 1986b).

For example, the diagnosis of PTSD applied to our patient J.I., whose traumatic history began this volume, sensitizes us to the presence of certain symptom clusters by which to evaluate progress and orients us to look for precipitating crises. More than her diagnosis, however, historical, personal functioning, and observational data will direct the format, nature, and patterning of treatment across time. Knowing that the patient is paraplegic subsequent to a rape and murder attempt many years earlier may direct us to consider the role of aborted grief and rage in her current symptoms; knowing that she has suicidal impulses may orient us toward the potential need for hospitalization; knowing that she has realistic expectations and prior positive experiences in treatment may assist us in establishing a prognosis; knowing how she copes with stressing events may tell us where to direct our interventions; and knowing that she is highly reactant to external control may sensitize us to the need to be nonconfrontive in our interventions.

For purposes of clarity, we have grouped the various nondiagnostic patient qualities that may contribute to treatment selection into three broad, somewhat arbitrary, and certainly interacting classes: (1) expectations, (2) coping ability, and (3) personality.

Patient *expectations* reflect the accumulation of wisdom gained through observed or experienced cause and effect relationships. Expectations may be situation-specific (states) or general (traits), but in either case, at least indirectly, bear a relationship to one's age, gender, social position, and personal background.

Coping ability reflects the *state* of the patient's efforts—proactively and reactively—to ward off stress. Coping abilities are captured in the severity of the problems and symptoms and the levels of problem resolution that have been achieved. While these response states, by their nature, are situationally specific, there also are enduring expectations and coping patterns that characterize patient responses in a variety of threatening situations. These latter response dispositions come to be identified as aspects of *personality*.

PATIENT EXPECTATIONS

Patient expectations accumulate from each person's unique personal history. They represent the translation of life views to current situations. These views in turn reflect the patient's accumulated observations within the sociodemographic environment to which they have been exposed. Expectations have been shown to play a role in determining both treatment outcomes and commitment to treatment (Garfield, 1986b), reinforcing the view that mental health treatment is a process of expectation and impression management (Corrigan, 1978; Corrigan, Dell, Lewis & Schmidt, 1980).

On the one hand, expectations may be specific to the therapy process and relationship, consisting of preexisting ideas of what is meant by "therapist," "treatment," and the nature of outcomes. On the other hand, however, there are social role expectations that extend beyond the treatment relationship. These latter expectations also affect how one will respond to interventions and influence what interventions will have a desirable impact.

Collectively, preexisting expectations are the building blocks both of coping ability and the enduring response patterns that we define as "personality." These expectations provide motivation for entering treatment, and changes in these expectations may well determine how long treatment will last and how effective it will be. Since expectations are dynamic and subject to change, they must be assessed in juxtaposition with an external referent in order to be of relevance for treatment decisions. Explicitly, we believe that it is useful to consider treatment-relevant expectations within three separate domains: (1) the congruence between patient expectations about the therapist, therapeutic process and outcomes, on one hand, and those experiences that are found in the prospective treatment, on the other; (2) the congruence between social role expectations and the objectives of treatment; and (3) the changes in expectations which occur as initial expectations are confirmed and/or disconfirmed. These three aspects of expectation are presented in Table 4.1 along with general guidelines for their assessment.

Table 4.1
Dimensions of Treatment Expectation

Dimension of Expectation	Assessment Methods
Treatment-Specific	Direct Exploration of:
a. Therapy	Previous treatment;
	Object relations;
b. Therapist	Conscious awareness;
	Hopes, Wishes, Goals;
c. Outcome	Treatment expectation questionnaires.
Social Roles	Direct questioning of:
a. Sexual	Interpersonal relations;
b. Authority	Degree of need
c. Family	fulfillment;
	Indirect review of:
	Family patterns;
	Social functioning;
	Direct family and interpersonal
	questionnaires.
Changes in Expectation	Direct review of subjective change;
During Therapy	Assessment of social patterns.

Treatment Expectations

Patient expectations about the "therapist" and about the therapeutic process establish patient motivation and set the stage for effective involvement in treatment. To some degree it is helpful to distinguish between "expectations" and "preferences." It is notable, for example, that concordance between the therapist behavior that is preferred by the patient and the behavior that is expected appears to be relatively low initially, but increasing correspondence between these dimensions over the course of treatment bodes well for treatment involvement (Tracey & Dundon, 1988). These aspects of patient anticipation thus appear to have motivational properties.

Motivation for treatment is judged to be present if the patient is willing to engage the therapist, if the transaction is free from the interrupting effects of hostility, and if the patient has a felt need to change. As such, motivation is closely linked to preexisting expectations about treatment and to certain enduring personality dimensions which characterize patient responses to information. To a large extent, whether expectations (or preferences) will be confirmed or disconfirmed depends upon the similarity both of patient and clinician expectations about treatment and their understandings of the nature of "mental health."

Treatment-specific expectations usually are expressed as categorical aspects of the patient's conscious experience, hopes, and recollections of prior treatment. Determining the presence of early role models of illness and care seeking also sheds light on less conscious aspects of these current expectations. For example, J.I. reported being resentful as a child of her mother's frequent sickness. In turn, she reported that her parents fought frequently over the mother's incapacity to engage in sexual activities because of headaches and other vague physical complaints. Paradoxically, both parents refused to accept J.I.'s own physical limitations after she was rendered paraplegic, to the point of refusing to discuss the traumatic incident that brought her to that condition. It is no wonder that J.I. experienced such difficulty adjusting to her disability and to the circumstances that initiated it.

Expectations that are subject to direct assessment include expectations relating to treatment length, treatment roles, and treatment outcomes. Direct questions, a review of the patient's treatment history, and a review of prior treatment successes and failures can be supplemented with brief and straightforward questionnaires about one's beliefs in these areas. Obtaining prior treatment records and initiating direct contact with the patient's significant other, his or her primary care physician, and any prior therapists will provide external confirmation of information provided by the patient.

Some evidence suggests that if the expected roles are consistent with those actually encountered in treatment, outcomes may be enhanced, while the clinician's failure to adopt therapeutic postures that are consistent with these generalized expectations may attenuate outcome (Forsyth & Forsyth, 1982).

Other aspects of treatment-specific expectations are found in the patient's global beliefs about the nature of therapist attributes. These role expectations are governed by beliefs in the credibility and expertness of therapists, *qua* therapists, beliefs about the philosophies which govern therapy, beliefs about what issues will be addressed and be relevant in the treatment context, and beliefs about the confidentiality of the proceedings.

Social Role Expectations

Some important role expectations are not readily subject to direct assessment because they are embedded in the patient's history of social roles and functions. These social-demographic-based expectations may be so broad and ill defined that they can only indirectly be captured through a broad review of the patient's background, historical experiences, and social relationships.

In order to capture these expectations, indirect assessment is required. This assessment involves a historical review and a firm understanding of the variations in response that are likely to be associated with different sexual, age, ethnic, religious, socioeconomic, and educational backgrounds. Again, these expectations are expressed as categorical information and are compared to actual treatment qualities and demand characteristics.

The therapist should especially seek information about nuclear family structure and attitudes. This information provides the basis for assessing the development of attitudes about self and others. Of critical importance is knowing what kind of role models were available to the patient and how these roles were reinforced or enforced. How did the patient's parents feel about him/her being born? How did parents deal with patient anger? What were the parents' attitudes about school? What attitudes did the parents have about sex? Did parents show any favoritism among the patient and siblings? How did they convey these attitudes? What were the major problems in childhood? These questions and more like them help define the nature of the patient's role-related attitudes and expectations.

While demographic and social backgrounds, along with their associated expectations, contribute to treatment length, motivation, and effectiveness, we have little indication that they are differentially associated with the value of specific therapeutic procedures, formats, or modalities (Beutler, Crago & Arizmendi, 1986; Garfield, 1986b). The exception to this general rule is in the indication that low socioeconomic status patients respond better to active and time-limited interventions than to either open-ended or nondirective and passive interventions (Goldstein, 1971, 1973; Garfield, 1978).

More importantly, demographic and social characteristics seem to be associated with attitudes that determine the likelihood of seeking mental health treatment, the likelihood of being accepted into such treatment, and the length of time one will remain in treatment (Lorion & Felner, 1986). Lower socioeconomic class patients may have expectations of the therapy relationship and of the treatment process which are so discrepant with those of the treating clinician that they rapidly become discouraged and lose their motivation. Under these conditions, a treating professional has a choice of (1) assuming that the patient will come to acquire roles and expectations which are consistent with those of the treater, (2) take active steps to ensure that productive roles and expectations are learned by the patient, or (3) modify treatment strategies to be consistent with the patient's expectations. Approaches reflecting these various assumptions will be presented in detail in Chapter 10.

There are many indications that the effects of sociodemographic-based expectations on treatment process and outcome exert an impact primarily because of the relationship which such variables bear to the beliefs and philosophies of the therapist (see Chapter 9). When therapists and patients share similar socioeconomic, sexual, and ethnic backgrounds, the likelihood of establishing an understanding relationship and remaining in therapy beyond the first few sessions is enhanced (Beutler, Crago & Arizmendi, 1986).

While similarities of patient and therapist backgrounds enhance treatment commitment and duration, background, ethnic, gender, and age variables have little relationship to treatment response when studied independently of similar characteristics of therapists. There are some exceptions to this general rule, however. For example, being in a high socioeconomic class, being educated, and being female all seem to increase both the likelihood of being accepted for treatment and of developing the motivation to continue treatment (Garfield, 1986b). These issues will be discussed in further detail in Chapters 9 and 10 as they apply to establishing and enhancing therapist-patient compatibility.

Changes in Expectation

It is clear that there are global expectancies that are attached to the role of "therapist" and to the activities of "therapy." To the degree that these global and generalized expectations of treatment roles and benefits are positive, the likelihood of seeking treatment may be enhanced. Moreover, the positiveness of these generalized role expectations may outweigh even very negative therapy experiences or the mistakes of unskilled therapists in the early stages of treatment, preserving satisfactory progress even when treatment is less than optimal (Corrigan et al., 1980).

The benefits of generalized sets can be expected to serve as an angelic shield for the unskilled therapist only for a short time, however. As treatment progresses and as the patient is confronted consistently with a discrepancy between positive, generalized expectations and the specific events occurring in treatment, it is the specific events, therapists, and processes that ultimately determine whether initial benefits will be enhanced, maintained, or lost (Heppner & Dixon, 1981). Even more so, in those cases where patient preferences initially are discrepant with their expectations of therapist behavior, treatment outcome is benefited if patients find that their preferences, rather than their expectations, for therapist direction and support are met (Tracey & Dundon, 1988). Hence, it behooves therapists to prepare patients for the events and happenings of treatment and to assess changes in expectations over time.

In support of the foregoing conclusion, research (Martin & Sterne, 1975; Martin, Moore & Sterne, 1977; Martin, Sterne & Hunter, 1976) has demonstrated that therapist expectations for treatment duration and outcome, when responsive to the expectations and wishes solicited from patients, are more likely to determine treatment change than are patient expectations by themselves. One can conclude from such findings that therapists should be willing to modify treatment formats and durations to fit patient wishes and expectations and, more importantly, that therapists should give careful and close attention to the expressed wishes and desires of those whom they serve.

COPING ABILITY

In order to understand how treatment interventions can alter motivation and compliance, it is useful to differentiate between those qualities of coping behavior that are transitory or changing and those that are relatively stable across a variety of conflict-inducing situations. As we have suggested, transitory expectations and preferences set the range of therapist responses acceptable to the patient and determine how they will view new information and experience. Since established personality characteristics are not accurate predictors of acute responses, an assessment of the patient's behavior within a current stress-provoking environment is necessary in order to select those treatment approaches that will maximize success. It is to the patterns that characterize "current functioning" that we refer with the term "coping ability."

At least two aspects of the patient's coping ability must be considered when selecting interventions. The first of these is the severity of disturbance associated with the patient's efforts to cope. The other is the phase of the behavioral change process that the patient has achieved in seeking resolution to the problems facing them. The first of these dimensions reflects the severity of impairment. The second dimension is expressed as a categorical statement of current problem-solving efforts. These dimensions and the general methods for their assessment are presented in Table 4.2.

Table 4.2
Dimensions of Coping Ability

Dimensions	Assessment Methods
Problem severity	Psychiatric Dysfunction Mental status exam; Review of current assets; Formal psychological assessment.
Problem-solving process	Formal questionnaire; Direct observations of pattern; Historical review.

Problem Severity

Severity of a condition must be assessed in terms of history, symptom complexity, and patient coping styles. J.I., for example had developed a survivor's skill at coping following the incident in which she watched her friend being raped and murdered and was stabbed and left for dead. Without treatment, she learned to survive and take care of herself. She received little parental support for her own pain—either from a mother whose minor illnesses left her helpless, or from a father who was, at the least, emotionally abusive. Hence, when her mother complained of headaches, J.I. developed a bitter resolve to take care of herself and never to be at the mercy of others. She coped, became educated, married, and maintained stable employment in spite of her persistent depression and suicidal thoughts.

Problem severity should be distinguished from the *methods* one utilizes in the coping process. Problem severity speaks only to how well one's coping methods keep anxiety and distress from impairing social and interpersonal functioning. While J.I. coped by denying disability and emotionally distancing herself from others, her mother had coped by becoming helpless and sickly. These different coping styles require different treatments.

In Chapter 3, we observed that in the process of establishing a diagnosis and reviewing the patient's history one also is advised to obtain a description of the behaviors and feelings that are the source of greatest concern. The clinician evaluates the degree of dysfunction associated with each of these problem areas and prioritizes the problems according to the degree to which they interfere with major life functions. Assessment of problem severity enters into decisions about the format and duration of treatment and determines the immediate goals of the interventions selected.

The amount of subjective distress experienced by a patient at any point in time reflects a compromise between the intensity of current stressors and the mitigating influences of various strengths that the patient possesses. These strengths include such attributes as the patient's intellectual level, ego integrity, and available social support systems. Is the patient able to maintain focus on tasks? Can the patient process information in a logical way? Can the patient distance herself from her own needs sufficiently to show empathy for others and/or to anticipate realistic consequences of her actions? Does she anticipate consequences and interpret social cues in a conventional fashion? Is the patient able to develop and benefit from social support systems?

In the case of J.I., problem severity became worse when her place of safety—her car—was destroyed in an accident. Only then did the fragility of her defenses reveal itself. Before then, the severity of her problem was observable only in subtle ways. While she resisted telling others of her suicidal thoughts, the repeated difficulty in establishing intimacy and the frequent conflicts with co-workers and employers were telling, but only to the trained observer.

In DSM-III-R, a global rating scale, the Global Assessment of Functioning (GAF), has been included to help clarify problem severity. This scale is useful and includes anchored ratings to facilitate reliable assessment. In determining problem severity, other dimensions that must be assessed include cognitive level, orientation within one's environment, cognitive efficiency, cognitive control of imaginal processes, affect and affective control, mood, and intensity of experienced conflict. Once the degree of impairment experienced in each problem area is determined, the GAF allows the expression of the degree to which symptoms interfere with optimal or usual functioning across a variety of life activities.

Problem-Solving Process

As we cope with internal discomfort and a world which often interferes with our sense of safety and predictability, we all go through a surprisingly similar set of processes. We exclude certain elements from awareness, we overreact to others, we avoid action, we divert our actions, we assess the effectiveness of our efforts, and we redirect and misdirect our efforts once again. Prochaska (1984) has distilled the consistent aspects of these problem-solving efforts, and has defined four phases through which most people go as they struggle to change: (1) *precontemplation,* (2) *contemplation,* (3) *action* and (4) *maintenance.* These stages ordinarily proceed in an orderly fashion and one moves from one phase to another when attempting to resolve and cope with conflict.

Prochaska and his colleagues (Prochaska & DiClemente, 1982; Prochaska, 1984; Prochaska, Velicer, DiClemente & Fava, 1988) have found that although these problem-solving phases proceed quite orderly and sequentially, one may become stuck at any point when the problem seems unsolvable. While completing any one phase may not be successful at restoring a sense of personal harmony, completing a single step in the process is apparently necessary in order to proceed to the next. Thus, threatening information can be ignored and denied only so long. At the point that awareness of the potential danger is more protective than ignorance, one then becomes aware and begins to inspect the threatening information.

For example, J.I. tended to avoid contemplation of her problems in any systematic way. From her parents, she had learned to avoid disclosure, to distrust those who revealed weakness as well as those who tried to provide support and help, and to "push on" as if the problem weren't there. She was still at a precontemplative phase of problem resolution with respect to her early crisis. The significance of this early crisis and an awareness of needing help became apparent to her only when the later automobile accident robbed her of her ability to deny her vulnerability.

The tendency of therapists often is to view treatment as a uniform process and to terminate therapy at the point the patient moves to the next phase in the cycle rather than adjusting treatment to support the goals of that new phase. Knowledge that there are definable phases in the cycle of problem resolution and that these phases proceed in a more or less common fashion allows therapists to look for the phase represented, to anticipate the next step in the change cycle, and to select aspects of the treatment context that will provide maximal support of the patient's movement.

Fortunately, the assessment of one's status in this process is easily accomplished by a method developed by Prochaska et al. (1988). The procedure involves assessing the patient's awareness of the problem, willingness to identify the behavior as a problem, interest in modifying it, and available alternative solutions. Within this context, knowledge about the patient's prior efforts to cope and what the patient hopes to achieve in the process of coping helps the therapist set the context for effective treatment to occur.

PATIENT PERSONALITY

Personality characteristics both indicate and determine aspects of patients' treatment expectations. We consider the term "personality" to be a description of recurrent but dynamic patterns that are enacted in the face of new and often threatening experience rather than as a collection of static qualities. The implications of "personality" for making treatment decisions thus become apparent. When these personality patterns are viewed in this way, one will first be aware that they are not the equivalent of "problems" unless one's ability to cope with the stressors that evoke these problems becomes compromised. Variability may be observed in the historical significance and generality of the observed patterns, in the degree of personal sensitivity or receptivity that the person maintains to interpersonal sources of influence or support, and in the methods that different people utilize in seeking problem resolution.

These variations among patterns may not only set limits on one's motivation and compliance with treatment, but also serve as indicators for managing the methods and means by which knowledge is transmitted and skills are learned during treatment. For clarity and convenience, we will address the implications of these variabilities under two broad headings: *Motivation and Compliance*, which will include a brief discussion of the limitations of our interventions, and *Response-Specific Personality Styles*, which will take a narrower view of the patient dimensions through which treatments may operate on motivation, compliance, and outcome.

Motivation and Compliance

Much has been written about "nonspecific" or "common" therapist qualities that are assumed to provide the necessary though not sufficient environment for attaining therapeutic change. These common qualities are assumed to set the limits upon therapeutic changes, if not to set the direction of such changes directly. Relatively less has been written about the qualities of patients which serve a similar limit-setting function on motivation and compliance across treatment modes, settings, and formats. Yet, it is commonly assumed that certain patient qualities bode poorly for mental health treatment, while others are seen to be necessary characteristics for benefiting from our services.

For example, most clinicians would consider J.I. to be a better treatment prospect than H.D., the 44-year-old alcoholic patient whose history we reported in Chapter 3. While J.I. experienced anxious arousal to such a degree as to impair effective functioning, H.D. had little arousal (discomfort) and achieved a good deal of secondary gain for his continued social dysfunction. Indeed, he would not have sought treatment except for the social pressure applied by his parents. He was a poor risk for treatment.

While it is useful to distinguish between qualities that are modifiable by treatment and those that are not, this distinction may unnecessarily minimize the effects on patient motivation of tailoring specific therapeutic procedures to specific patient qualities. As helping professionals, we cannot afford to assume that by identifying the limitations of our procedures, subsequent failures are the result of patient qualities over which we have no control. Such an assumption is seductive because it may save the therapist from facing failure, but it also aborts the motivation to create interventions that would be of greatest value to the most needy of our patients.

Recently, some major research groups have begun to address the problem of treating the less than ideally motivated patient (e.g., Goldstein, 1973; Lorion & Felman, 1986; Meichenbaum & Turk, 1987). This trend is positive and indicates a willingness among at least some practitioners to address issues of motivation and compliance as limitations of our knowledge and skill rather than as patient deficits. For example, social persuasion research suggests that motivation and compliance can be enhanced by the establishment of clear expectations, the encouragement of overtly explicit commitments to comply, and the provision of reasonable incentives. Communications and admonitions to change may also arouse anger, fear, or anxiety and these emotions can enhance motivation if the arguments accompanying them are seen as relevant and empowering and when positive or negative incentives are seen as highly likely consequences of behavior (Conn & Crowne, 1964; Burgoon & Miller, 1971; Burgoon, Burgoon & McCroskey, 1974; Boster & Mongeau, 1984).

By the same token, this line of research suggests that new information alone, in the absence of either emotional arousal or response contingencies, does little to facilitate compliance and motivation (Higbee, 1969; Burgoon & Ruffner, 1978). In part, the failure of fear tactics can be attributed to the apparent unlikeliness of the threatened outcome. Hence, legislated sanctions, which instill more readily identifiable fears of apprehension and conviction, facilitate compliance much more readily than information campaigns (cf. Beidel & Turner, 1986; Robertson, 1976).

Compliance research has suggested that the effectiveness of health care admonitions may be enhanced when those who are targeted for change are persuaded to serve as advocates to others for good health care behaviors, when their participation in health care advocacy is made public, and when the behavior to be changed is valued by the patient's reference and support groups (Stuart, 1982; Meichenbaum & Turk, 1987). The Vanderbilt University Psychotherapy Research Program has led the way in attempting to develop interventions for the difficult to treat, characterologically disturbed patient (Strupp, 1980a, 1980b). Likewise, the Langley Porter Center for the Study of Neurosis has explored impediments to effective therapeutic relationships and has proposed procedures that can allay patient resistance to treatment and reverse early treatment failures (Foreman & Marmar, 1984; Gaston, Marmar & Ring, in press).

Often the issue facing mental health professionals is not the absence of motivation among certain patients, but reluctance to use environmental influences for fear that doing so will discount individual initiative and choice. While we must applaud the ethics behind this decision, it is our contention that learning to utilize external resources and to strengthen the persuasiveness of our communications ultimately will enhance freedom rather than limit it. We believe that such knowledge will extend our influence to increasingly large numbers of people whose motivation for treatment and compliance with the requirements of our interventions can be improved.

Response-Specific Personality Styles

While some aspects of patient motivation and compliance are seen as outside of the therapist's domain of influence, there are many patient qualities that bear on their motivation and that are easily accepted by clinicians as grist for the therapeutic mill. Among the qualities over which therapists acknowledge a potential influence, matters of personality structure and defensive styles have always been of interest.

It nonetheless is difficult to obtain a clear consensus regarding the identity of those styles and structures that differentially influence treatment motivation, compliance, and outcomes. Definitions of such variables have been largely determined by one's theoretical preference. Various theories of psychopathology have selected different dimensions of personal functioning and emphasized the worth of these specific dimensions, usually to the exclusion of those valued by other theories.

In the current chapter, we will present descriptive rather than inferential aspects of personality that comprise how one copes and adjusts to new experience. We will be especially reliant on those dimensions that research has suggested may have promise for making treatment decisions. We refer to these personality dimensions as "response-specific" in order to differentiate them from the more general, theoretical aspects of personality to be considered later.

Even avoiding the controversies among theories to the maximal degree, any effort to sort and extract from among the hundreds of characteristics referenced in the literature those which are most relevant to the selection of treatments is a difficult task. In most cases, research simply hasn't addressed the relationship of response-specific personality styles to treatment selection. Our selection of dimensions is based upon a careful review of available literature and at least some evidence that they have empirical, predictive validity (Beutler, 1979a; Beutler & Mitchell, 1981; Beutler, Crago & Arizmendi, 1986; Calvert, Beutler & Crago, 1988).

Our choice of relevant response-specific personality dimensions reflects three aspects of patient functioning: (1) problem complexity, (2) interpersonal reactance/sensitivity, and (3) coping style. These dimensions are interactive and reciprocal; however, convenience and clarity require that we treat them as separate aspects of response for the time being. These dimensions and methods for their assessment are reviewed in Table 4.3.

Table 4.3
Dimensions of Response-Specific Personality Styles

Dimensions	Assessment
Problem complexity	Review of the historical development of the recurrent pattern;
	Assess the role of unconscious processes in the maintenance of the disturbance;
	Assess relative roles of social reinforcements and conflictual needs for the continuation of the symptom pattern.
Interpersonal reactance	Review history of coping with demands and dependency relationships;
	Objective psychological tests;
	Observation of resistance patterns during treatment.
Coping style	Mental status exam;
Internal	Review of interpersonal
Repressive	defenses;
Cyclic	History of stress responses;
External	Dynamic formulation; Direct assessment via personality tests.

Some of the dimensions presented in Table 4.3 are similar to those upon which Axis II personality disorders have been constructed in the *Diagnostic and Statistical Manuals*. For example, two of the three orthogonal dimensions of DSM-III Axis II disorders described by Widiger, Trull, Hurt, Clarkin, and Frances (1987) correspond with those referred to here as "coping style" and "interpersonal reactance," respectively. These two dimensions reflect various aspects of how one deals with discomfort, differing somewhat in situation specificity. "Reactance" refers to one's sensitivity to interpersonal influence and "coping style" refers to the pattern of defenses used to minimize threat to one's self view and sense of internal consistency.

To this list, we have added the dimension of "Problem Complexity," thus extending our consideration to include situational responses and simple habits at one extreme and highly complex and neurotiform behavior on the other.

The dimensions of problem complexity, interpersonal reactance and coping style are all considered to be interactive characteristics that roughly are normally distributed among those who seek assistance for life problems.

Problem Complexity. The Systematic Eclectic Psychotherapy of the first author originally presented problem complexity as an inherent and nested aspect of a patient's problem severity (Beutler, 1983). Both from the standpoint of research on problem severity and on the basis of clinical experience, it now seems quite feasible to separate the two concepts. As we emphasized earlier in this volume, problem severity is an index of acute impairment that is most usefully expressed as a continuous measure.

It is easiest to think of problem complexity as a dichotomous distinction, with one category of the dimension comprising chronic *habits* or *transient responses* whose repetition is maintained either because of inadequate knowledge or by ongoing situational reward (positive reinforcement). We refer to these problems as "habits" to distinguish them from neurotiform or "complex" problems. The latter category is reserved for behaviors that may be repeated as themes across unrelated and dissimilar situations. These complex patterns consist of ritualized but self-defeating efforts to resolve a dynamic or interpersonal conflict whose actual significance is in the past rather than in the present. The symptoms presented are symbolic of an earlier and unrecognized struggle, albeit the form of this struggle seldom bears an obvious relationship to the nature of that forgotten conflict. Such complex and repetitive patterns are maintained by efforts to avoid expected punishments and threats that no longer constitute realistic consequences of behavior in the present situation.

In other words, in comparison to problem severity, problem complexity is a more enduring and less situation-specific quality. Complex problems are represented in behaviors that bear a symbolic, rather than a direct, relationship to initiating events. Complex problems are represented in repetitive enactments of a class of behaviors, the end point of which does not result in gratification but in suffering (cf. Luborsky, 1984; Bond, Hansell & Shevrin, 1987). These problems reflect the classic "neurotic paradox" in that behavioral cycles are repeated in the absence of apparent external reward *and* with the consequence of these behaviors being extreme distress, anxiety, guilt, and negative social consequence. Therapists characteristically consider long-term and insight-oriented treatments to be indicated for such problems (Freebury, 1984; Budman & Gurman, 1983; Thorpe, 1987).

To illustrate, J.I. presented a complex problem in that her fearful response to the automobile accident was overdetermined by earlier experience. The loss of her automobile *symbolized* the loss of power and security, which in turn was a denied aspect of her earlier trauma. Moreover, she did not recognize the relationship between her earlier trauma and her response to the automobile accident—the symbolized origins of her symptoms were unconscious. This is in contrast to H.D., whose alcoholism could be seen as a reinforced and environmentally supported response, augmented by his appetitive enjoyment of the activity.

The fact that a symptom may be a simple habit does not mean that changing is any less difficult than if it represents a dynamic effort to resolve an early mastery struggle with a dominating father. However, it does suggest that the path to change may be different in the two cases.

One clue to problem complexity may be found in the linearity of the relationship between the original instigators of the symptom and the form of the symptom. Elsewhere, the first author (Beutler, 1983) has described two patients, each presenting debilitating symptoms of agoraphobia. One patient's symptoms gradually developed after a harrowing and narrowly averted flying accident. Following this incident, panic attacks began occurring with increasing frequency, and the initial fear of flying gradually extended to a fear of airports, buildings, cars, and people. Finally, the patient, a middle aged, single man, was confined to his house, where he lived with his mother.

The other patient had similar symptoms, but hers arose in a much less direct or linear pattern and with a less specific precipitating event. In a manner that is quite typical of agoraphobia, this young adult woman began experiencing "spontaneous" panic attacks shortly after a series of significant emotional losses. Her boyfriend had just left for the army, her favorite (and agoraphobic) grandmother had just died and been shipped off to burial by train, the patient's parents had just announced their intention to obtain a divorce, and the patient herself had just returned to college where she had few friends. Ultimately, she too was confined to a life in her mother's house. The latter patient's complex phobic symptoms may represent a symbolized struggle to avoid abandonment. Hence, while one patient's symptoms can be considered to be relatively simple and the other's relatively complex, both were severe and debilitating.

A careful assessment of the development of the symptoms and formulation of how the symptoms are supported by the interpersonal patterns which surround their manifestation will ordinarily allow a general determination of how strongly the presenting problems reflect relatively enduring, repetitive, and symbolic manifestations of characterological struggles as opposed to transient, situation-specific, and habitual patterns of behavior. In turn, this determination will provide a focus for the therapeutic interventions, ranging from symptomatic to conflictual, through which these several interventions may be integrated.

Interpersonal Reactance.   Interpersonal sensitivity or vulnerability can be distinguished from the patterns of behavior used for coping with or defending against anxiety. Interpersonal reactance may be categorized along a continuum (high, medium, and low), and describes an individual's likelihood of resisting threatened loss of interpersonal control. Thus, "reactance" defines the stimuli that may excite defensive patterns.

There is more to the concept of interpersonal reactance than simply this, however. The concept of reactance inherently describes the forcefulness of one's efforts to resist external influence. This drive leads the highly reactant patient to become tense when directed to relax (Heide & Borkovec, 1983) or act out when instructed to constrain themselves (Dowd & Pace, in press).

Since all are controlled, at least in part, by external events, punishments, threats, rewards, and limits, freedom is a critical but often false belief. Yet, one's actions are predicated upon how tolerant one is when confronted with experiences which are out of one's control.

J.I. had devoted a lifetime to her early decision to avoid being helpless. To her, this meant avoiding being controlled by others. Hence, she rebelled against becoming like her helpless mother, denied her own physical disability, and resisted any movement of others toward intimacy. All of these things threatened her sense of personal freedom. She was intolerant of even normal situations in which there was implied or actual control by others, and when confronted by her accident with how unrealistic was her belief in personal control, she experienced panic.

Psychotherapy is inherently an experience which threatens one's sense of self control. First, voluntary patients seek help when their confidence in self control and self efficacy are weakest (Bandura, 1977). Second, they seek treatment in an interpersonal context, asking to be controlled even further. Third, there are times when the treatment professional does, in fact, remove all vestiges of personal control by forcing hospitalization or other confinement. Mental health treatment frequently becomes paradoxical in its approach to issues of self control, taking away personal direction in the service of restoring the *feeling* of self efficacy—trading temporary dependence for lasting independence.

The effective therapist is aware of the paradox of treatment control while still valuing the importance of a patient's feelings of control over surroundings. The competent therapist employs treatment procedures which will establish external support and protective control while enhancing subjectively-felt freedom and predictability by reinforcing choice and empowerment. Since reactance can be assessed only within the context of a known environment (i.e., knowledge of what one is reactant to), one can accomplish this complex task only by being sensitive to in-therapy demands.

Another aspect of interpersonal reactivity resides in the need systems which are invoked for a given individual in an interpersonal environment. Needs for nurturance, support, attachment, and regard are all universal social phenomena. However, so are needs for separation, independence, and space. Each person develops a relative balance of needs toward one or the other of these extremes and a different pattern of balancing one with the other.

The particular balance and pattern of enactment defines each person's interpersonal melody and is the driving force which governs interpersonal life. These same needs mark our vulnerabilities to stress and determine if we will find a given situation stressful or not (Lazarus, in press). Concomitantly, symptoms and behaviors are expressions of our successes and failures in this effort. Hence, the pattern of interpersonal, ritualized styles of response mark the targets of our conflict-oriented treatment strategies— the thematic focus. Keeping in mind the interactive role of coping behaviors and interpersonal reactance, we can now expand on this pattern by cataloging the dominant methods by which people cope with threat and conflict.

Coping Style

The Nature of Coping.   Human beings attempt to avoid uncomfortable experiences, but confronting upsetting experiences has pronounced and positive effects on bodily function (e.g., Pennebaker, Kiecolt-Glaser & Glaser, 1988). Defense mechanisms are specific unconscious methods used by a person to avoid anxiety—that discomfort arising from contact with unpleasant experiences. Anxiety is induced as one's beliefs and wants are challenged through actual or anticipated contact with disconfirming external experiences (e.g., J.I.'s resolve to remain in control of her circumstances was challenged by an accident that was out of her control).

Disconfirming events are dissonance-inducing and represent danger to one's view of safety and self. The amount of distress evoked by this cognitive dissonance is a joint function of the seriousness of the stressful event and the method selected for coping with it. Regardless of the seriousness of the event, people construct certain defenses designed to maintain their sense of safety and preserve the stability of their beliefs. The DSM-III-R (American Psychiatric Association, 1987) defines these defense mechanisms as:

> Patterns of feelings, thoughts, or behaviors that are relatively involuntary and arise in response to perceptions of psychic danger. They are designed to hide or to alleviate the conflicts or stressors that give rise to anxiety" (p. 393).

The specific defense mechanisms recognized in DSM-III-R include acting out, autistic fantasy, denial, devaluation, displacement, dissociation, idealization, intellectualization, isolation, passive aggression, projection, rationalization, reaction formation, repression, somatization, splitting, suppression, and undoing. These defenses are somewhat interdependent and fall into characteristic clusters, varying in their degree of adaptability. While any one person may use an infinite variety of specific defense mechanisms, each person tends to rely most heavily on a relatively few interrelated ones, the collection and patterning of which comprises his or her own "Coping Style." These coping styles reflect dominant, stable behaviors which collectively constitute efforts to avoid recognizing and/or confronting the contradictions in one's internal discrepancies—opposing wishes, injunctions, values, impulses, and/or beliefs—or disconfirming information about them. External experiences, including interpersonal interactions, loss, and environmental crises, may serve as the triggering cues to defensive coping patterns if they threaten to reveal the presence of these internal inconsistencies, destroy one's sense of safety, or embody information that would require modification of associated self views. The therapist planfully takes advantage of this fact by evoking and then interpreting defensive patterns by providing information (e.g., interpretations, a model, a homework assignment, etc.) that is discrepant with patient beliefs.

Specific coping styles vary in their ease of activation and extremeness of display as a function of patient reactance (i.e., sensitivity) level. While these concepts are interrelated, we believe that treatment decisions are made easier if we retain a distinction between "coping styles" and "interpersonal reactance."

As we have observed, the term "reactance" describes one's sensitivity to perceived social influence. While such sensitivity may make one vulnerable to anxiety and arouses patterned defensive efforts (i.e., coping styles), it also varies as a function of relationship and situation to a greater degree than do the more enduring, coping styles. The distinction between coping styles and reactance, therefore, recognizes the stability of coping styles relative to reactance. For our discussion, the distinction is further maintained on pragmatic grounds as we will see when we describe more specifically the distinguishing roles of these two concepts in treatment.

Theoretical descriptions of "personality" uniformly attempt to define a finite number of categories by which to describe the dominant ways that one adapts to a changing environment. While they are presented from a variety of philosophical viewpoints and are labeled with diverse descriptors, the various coping styles that have been defined in this way probably reflect a relatively few common dimensions. For example, Folkman and Lazarus (1980) suggest that most people cope either in problem-focused (e.g., externally-directed action) or emotion-focused (e.g., internal action designed to alter emotions without affecting external events) ways. This dimension bears a good deal of similarity to the concepts of Extraversion-Introversion (Eysenck & Eysenck, 1969), Extrapunitive-Intropunitive (Gleser & Ihlevich, 1969), Overcontrolled and Undercontrolled (Megargee,

Cook & Mendelsohn, 1967; Miller & Eisenberg, 1988) and Externalization-Internalization (Welsh, 1952) described by others.

The overlap among measures of various of these constructs (Roessler, 1973) suggests that coping styles vary along a continuum from taking action on or against the environment (i.e., externalized, extrapunitive, extraverted, undercontrolled and/or problem-focused) to taking action toward oneself (i.e., internalized, extrapunitive, extraverted, undercontrolled, and/or problem-focused) to taking action toward oneself (i.e., internalized, intropunitive, introverted, and/or emotion-focused). Both the nature of other dimensions and the identity of subgroupings within the external to internal dimension are subjects of disagreement among investigators. However, at least some of this disagreement can be attributed to differences in methods of observing and measuring coping styles.

Classification of Coping Styles. Ultimately, the test of any conceptual system will be its demonstrated usefulness for shaping treatment decisions. Accordingly, we have attempted to find some of the common dimensions among several such efforts, with an eye to how various coping styles may facilitate treatment (e.g., Beutler, 1979, 1983; Beutler & Mitchell, 1981; Beutler et al., 1986). The reader may find such instruments as the *Defense Mechanism Inventory* (Gleser & Ihlevich, 1969), the *Eysenck Personality Inventory* (Eysenck & Eysenck, 1969), the *Minnesota Multiphasic Personality Inventory* (see especially Welsh, 1952, and Megargee et al., 1967), the *Ways of Coping Questionnaire* (Folkman & Lazarus, 1980) and the *Millon Clinical Multiaxial Inventory* (Millon, 1977) of value for assessing various of the constructs discussed.

The fourfold system by which we classify patients' dominant defensive patterns incorporates many of the divisions of style described by such theoreticians as Eysenck and Eysenck (1969), Millon (1969, 1981), and Welsh (1952), but these four patterns are extended almost infinitely as one factors in concepts of problem complexity, interpersonal reactance, and recurrent needs and anticipations. We have not found it useful to distinguish between "defensive style" (usually thought to reflect unconscious processes) and "coping style" (usually thought to reflect both conscious and unconscious processes).

The specific categories of coping styles that we advocate in selecting treatment orientations focus upon how one processes belief-discrepant information, including the awareness of negative emotions. These categories, along with their reactance level variations (presented parenthetically as low/high qualities), include: (1) *Internalization* (Intropunitive/overcontrolled), (2) *Repression* (Denial/Reversal), (3) *Cyclic* (Rationalization/Sensitization), and (4) *Externalization* (Diversion/Extrapunitiveness).

The cardinal characteristic of an *Internalizing* coping pattern is the redirection of threat toward personally controlled activities. Rather than being denied or transferred to others as blame, sources of anxiety are redirected to one's own failures, sins, or inabilities. One then typically attempts to undo these mistakes through apology or ritual, either of which encounters more self blame. Both high and low reactant groups of internalizers tend to idealize others and to devalue self—they are overly sympathetic or empathic to others' feelings and have little ability to express or recognize their own unwanted anger (Miller & Eisenberg, 1988).

Internalizers rely on constriction of affect, undoing behaviors, and intropunitive cognitions to prevent expression of anger. For example, M.S. was a 25-year-old graduate student in anatomy who developed severe death-related obsessions during a series of required laboratory experiments. She responded by constricting her range of experience, withdrawing from friends, confining herself to her home, and eventually dropping out of graduate school.

As she narrowed her world, M.S. found herself able to keep obsessive thoughts controlled only by the development of ritualistic behaviors. She then blamed herself for being unable to control these rituals.

Internalizing patients like M.S. tend to experience exaggerated levels of anxiety; they are acutely sensitive to self-responsibility and work to contain anxiety when they find they cannot eliminate it. They do this by isolating it internally from its content (i.e., removing the object of the anxiety from the original content of graduate school), engaging in undoing rituals, and/ or restricting the allowable range of emotions to which they will be responsive (e.g., M.S. responded to anxiety but not to anger).

Highly reactant individuals in this group overcontrol their anger to a point that all emotion is submerged behind a sea of intellectualized explanations and misapplied labels. They display brittle defenses against anger, frequently exploding in fits of rage. While they worry, such worry is a cognitive and ruminative experience rather than an emotional one. They tend to report subjectively little distress, but paradoxically often reveal strong physiological responses to environmental stressors (Byrne & Sheffield, 1965). Yet their defenses may rapidly decay when their control is threatened or their stability is challenged.

In Chapter 3 we described the case of A.D., a 57-year-old physician who was interned in the Nazi concentration camps. He overcontrolled emotional expression and retained brittle control by hoarding food and irrelevant scraps of paper—undoing his early deprivation experiences. He managed to keep overt arousal in check by compartmentalizing, intellectualizing, and rationalizing his behavior. However, when confronted by his wife with his hoarding behavior, he became verbally abusive and then apologetic and withdrawn. This brittle overcontrol indexed his high level of reactance to threat.

In contrast to internalizing coping styles, those who rely on externalization reduce or avoid anxiety by transmitting the responsibility for their discomfort to external objects, to others, or to symptoms for which they cannot be blamed. Such individuals are intolerant of minor discomfort, subjectively disown their own actions, and are notoriously unable to reflect either on others' emotional states or on the social impact of their own motives and behaviors (cf., Miller & Eisenberg, 1988). Unlike A.D., whose verbal outbursts occurred when he was confronted with his hoarding, true externalizers do not engage in subsequent self-blame and apology.

Individuals who rely on externalizing defenses tend to be dependent on and overly controlled by environmental stimuli, are active, self dramatizing, or extraverted, and experience anxiety only when deprived of a direct, active method of coping with stress or when blame cannot be transferred.

The high reactant (Extrapunitive) patient may present the defenses described by Gleser and Ihlevich (1969) as "Turning against others," while the less reactant (Diversion) patient is likely to present with a pattern that is characterized by displacement and passive-aggressive behavior. Diversion patterns involve distancing oneself from intense emotions by distraction and displacement. They retreat from distressing thoughts by distracting themselves with physical activities, indirect behaviors, and social gregariousness. H.D., our 44-year-old alcoholic patient, is an example of this pattern. His drinking and unemployment were blamed on his parents (though never to their face) and the lack of good opportunities. High-reactant extrapunitive patients, in contrast to H.D., avoid confronting threatening inconsistencies among wishes and experience by attacking external objects and people (acting out), by projecting blame and unwanted feelings on others, or by controlling others through demanding, somatic symptoms (somatization).

A distinction between Internalization and Externalization patterns may be found in the relative levels of maturity represented by these two extreme classes of coping styles (e.g., Loevinger, 1966; Vaillant, 1971; Cramer, Blatt & Ford, 1988; Cramer, in press). Externalizing patients are relatively immature, their dominant mode of defense becomes fixed at an early point in the developmental process, and these defenses correspondingly are unreliant on and undemanding of intellectual resources. On the other hand, internalizers rely on relatively more cognitively complex defensive styles than their externalizing counterparts. Classical personality diagnoses of characterological, paranoid, and narcissistic patterns capture aspects of an externalizing defensive pattern, while obsessive and avoidant personality diagnoses capture qualities of those with internalizing coping styles.

Between the illustrative extremes of internalization and externalization are at least two other groups of individuals whose distinctive coping styles represent various permutations of internalizing and externalizing defenses. For example, patients with *Repressive* styles are devoted to maintaining their own ignorance—what you don't know can't hurt you. To do this they exercise the principle of transforming threat into its opposite. Low reactant, repressive patients rely principally upon the benign defense of denial and negation to maintain a neutral reaction in the face of threat. The more highly reactant patient is likely to respond in a direction that is opposite (Reversal) to the thrust of impulses and feelings (Gleser & Ihlevich, 1969). This latter pattern reflects the defenses of reaction formation and regression. Among these highly reactant patients, instability is probable and reactive suicidal gestures cannot be discounted.

J.I. is a case in point. Her efforts to deny her own disability, to occlude from awareness her previous traumatic experiences, and her overcompensation for her handicap all suggest a pattern of reversal. Her high reactivity to threatened loss of freedom is noted in the extreme response to her automobile accident and in her devotion to avoiding intimate relationships.

C.A. represents a less reactant version of this denial pattern. C.A., it will be recalled from Chapter 3, presented with depression following a number of significant losses. Her depression represented failure of the denial patterns that she ordinarily constructed to help her cope (quite effectively) with stressors. It was the use of these defenses that helped her minimize the loss of her father, avoid being overwhelmed by her rape experience, and go on after she was disowned by her family. Only when her fiancé was killed did the denial fail her and drive her into treatment.

Finally, *Cyclic* styles are represented both by patients with rationalizing (low reactant) and sensitizing (high reactant) defenses. These cyclic patients tend to be the most unstable and changeable of the four types defined here. M.D. is a case in point (see Chapter 3). This 27-year-old woman exhibited a consistent pattern of extreme response, investing heavily in the development of dependent attachments and then driving the objects of her dependency away through infidelity. As illustrated by M.D., patients with cyclic coping styles vacillate between acting out and withdrawing. The high reactant, cyclic patient manifests very extreme patterns of this type as partially suggested by the diagnoses that characterize this group. In our experience, the high reactant patient may present with Borderline Personality, Paranoid Personality, and Cyclothymic Personality disorders, while the less reactant cyclic patient more often is diagnosed as a Passive Aggressive Personality, with various impulse disorders, Dysthymic disorder, and varieties of symptomatic presentations.

By their nature, cyclic coping patterns are ones of change and instability. Such patients may be blaming and vengeful, then withdrawing into guilt and self blame. They respond to stress with very strong reactions, usually in the form of anxiety, depression, splitting, and agitation, but these reactions are intensified among the more sensitizing, high reactant patients.

Such people are easily hurt, often feel victimized, and have low tolerance for frustration. They often manifest physical symptoms in response to stress and are able only poorly to differentiate among their various feeling states. Because they fail to recognize the nuances of different feelings, their overt responses to a variety of situations also assume a high degree of constancy. Their responses are exaggerated in degree, but the form of these responses is determined more by the intensity of the emotion than by its quality. Hence, virtually any type of stress may induce an extreme response in which anger, fear, and hurt are inseparable.

SUMMARY AND COMMENT

This chapter has presented an overview of the major patient, nondiagnostic factors which we believe are associated with the efficacious assignment of dispositions. These variables are rather arbitrarily divided into those relating to *expectations* which either are brought to or accrue with treatment, *coping ability,* and *personality patterns.*

Research has convinced us of the value of treatment-congruent expectations for predicting and determining the outcome of mental health treatments. This congruence applies both to the mutuality of expectations between the patient and therapist and between patient and the demand characteristics of treatment. That is, mental health treatment embodies certain value systems and beliefs which direct and guide treatment (e.g., Bergin, 1980). These value systems are reflected in the roles that patient and therapist are expected to take, the goals of treatment, the methods employed to change behavior, and type of environment in which treatment takes place.

On top of these role expectations, patients and therapists each have their own value systems and beliefs which guide their participation. Beliefs in the therapist's power, credibility, objectivity, and sensitivity are some of the general expectations which will contribute to treatment involvement. If these latter role expectations are not consistent with the experience of the therapist and the demands of the therapy, treatment may become disappointing. To the degree possible, positive and enhancing expectations should be met. To the degree that the patient's expectations are unrealistic to the problem, to the setting, or to the therapist's own value system, the patient should be taught more conducive and congruent beliefs. Only if adequate congruence exists between what is expected or preferred and what is obtained will treatment realize its maximum effect. Likewise, if patients' expectations change in the direction of congruence, treatment will tend to last sufficiently long to accomplish the objectives and to receive a positive response from patients.

Aside from matters of therapist and patient congruence, we have identified two general aspects of the patient's response that may bear on coping ability and three general personality dimensions which we consider to play a role in treatment selection. The coping ability dimensions include coping adequacy and the problem-solving phase achieved by the patient. Coping adequacy is reflected in the level of patient distress, the stability of interpersonal relationships, and the availability of social resources which facilitate acclimation to stress.

On the other hand, the problem-solving phase achieved by the patient in confronting the problem or conflict at hand may predict the general length and format of desirable treatment. Since problem-solving phases proceed in a relatively consistent and predictable fashion, knowledge of where the patient has become stuck in the process also may help direct the mediating tasks of the interventions across time.

Among the more enduring personality variables described, problem complexity is the most difficult to assess. This dimension reflects the importance of dynamic underpinnings among the presented problems. Complexity is indexed both by the repetitive nature of the associated behaviors, their chronicity, and the presence of etiologically significant, dynamic conflicts that are only symbolically represented in the symptom picture. On the other hand, the patient's level and sensitivity to external demands (reactance) defines, in part, the vulnerability of the patient to engage in this repetitive pattern when under interpersonal threat. One who is reactive against interpersonal control from others tends to resist many forms of therapeutic intervention, even to the point that treatment may induce deterioration.

In concert, the patient's coping style is represented by the nature of the defenses which are constructed against internal discomfort, as arising from intrapsychic threat. The patterns of coping style range from overcontrolled and intropunitive (Internalizing Styles), on the one hand, to diverting and extropunitive (Externalizing Styles), on the other. In between these extremes, individuals are likely to represent variations of instability and reactance levels. Sensitized and rationalizing patients (Cyclic Styles) share a pattern of inconsistency and variability between externalizing and internalizing propensities. They may be unstable and overly sensitive to sources of threat or to react with rationalization and diversion. Other variations include denial and minimization of threat to the actual reversal of its impact (Repressive Styles).

In the latter instances, the patient may approach threat with neutral or even positive affect in order to mask and control unwanted impulses. The pattern of coping adopted correlates with patients' use of available social resources, how psychologically minded and insightful they can be about their difficulties, and how others will perceive and respond to their stress.

SUGGESTED READINGS

Beutler, L. E. (1979a). Toward specific psychological therapies for specific conditions. *Journal of Consulting and Clinical Psychology, 47,* 882–897.

Brehm, S. S. & Brehm, J. W. (1981). *Psychological Reactance: A theory of freedom and control.* New York: Academic Press.

Garfield, S. L. (1986b). Research on client variables in psychotherapy. In S. L. Garfield & A. E. Bergin (Eds.), *Handbook of psychotherapy and behavior change,* 3rd ed. (pp. 213–256). New York: John Wiley and Sons.

Luborsky, L., McLellan, A. T., Woody, G. E., O'Brien, C. P. & Auerbach, A. (1985). Therapist success and its determinants. *Archives of General Psychiatry, 42,* 602–611.

Prochaska, J. O. (1984). *Systems of psychotherapy: A transtheoretical analysis,* 2nd ed. Homewood, IL: Dorsey Press.

5

Environments and Circumstances

Just as diverse theories have very different perspectives about the process of therapeutic change, theories also present sharply contrasting viewpoints about the way that environments both initially shape and subsequently maintain psychological disturbance. Some therapists assign more weight to a patient's past environment than to present ones when speculating about the origin of psychological disturbance. To others, current rather than past environments are conceived as both the principal causes and the reinforcers that maintain psychopathology. Still others place emphasis upon nonenvironmental (e.g., biological and genetic forces) influences in the development of psychological disturbance.

The differences assigned to environmental influences by different theories reflect the historical evolution of theory in the mental health disciplines. Freud minimized the role of current environments, except as applied to the corrective experiences that constituted psychotherapy. Instead, he emphasized the joint roles of biologically based instincts and injunctions derived largely from past environments in the development of psychological disturbance.

Many of Freud's contemporaries and followers were quick to point out that current environments could not be ignored. The decidedly social emphasis that characterized early American psychiatry began as a reaction against Freud's deference to the past and his deemphasis of present environments. The behaviorists, likewise, led by John Watson, reacted to both Freud's emphasis on internal drives as the bases of psychopathology and the technical procedures designed to correct emotional problems. In more contemporary times the pendulum is again swinging back toward biological explanations of disordered behavior.

Between the extremes of Freud and Watson, there have been many people and movements whose influence has been preserved in contemporary views of psychopathology. This is not the place to summarize these many theories nor is it our intention to argue for the importance of the environment in shaping both prosocial behavior and disturbed behavior. Rather, we assume that whether such variables are considered to be of etiological importance or as exacerbating influences on pathological behavior, there are relationships between certain characteristics of current and past environments on the one hand, and one's treatment suitability on the other hand. These relationships must be considered by any integrated theory of psychotherapeutic treatment planning.

Most individuals are members of several related but not necessarily overlapping environments: a specific family environment (often both nuclear family and family of origin), a general social environment (neighborhood, community, friends), and a work-school environment. While these environments often are sources of stress, and certainly are not universally sources of support, they are potential assets in treatment. For example, it will be recalled that J.I. was experiencing marital difficulties in addition to long-term problems associated with her traumatic loss of ambulation and the anxiety associated with her recent accident. Even the stress-evoking spouse of a patient like J.I. may be a resource for treatment by being made co-therapist in a behavioral exposure program to overcome fear of driving arising from her automobile accident.

The environment of the individual includes both the persons in his or her world and the nonpersonal, physical environment (the physical surroundings, availability of food, shelter, clothing, stimulation, etc.), as well. The contributions of both the personal and the physical environment must be considered in understanding individual pathology (does it contribute and in what way, or is it noncontributory to the individual disorder). A knowledge of available reference groups, family ties, friendships, and recreational resources is imperative for the determination of the enabling factors which might support and maintain a patient's adjustment. The absence of social support systems (Schramski, Beutler, Lauver & Arizmendi, 1984) works against both retention in treatment and maintenance of long-term change.

ENVIRONMENTAL STRESSORS

Stressors, both in present and past environments, play a major role in triggering psychopathology. We can see this in the case of J.I., whose accident triggered the influence of denied memories of early loss of environmental control (rape and murder) and thus compounded the extent of her reaction. More positively, the availability of early parental supports contributes to one's ability as an adult to develop supportive networks (Flaherty & Richman, 1986). In turn, severity of psychiatric symptomatology has been found to be related negatively to the closeness of support networks available both to inpatients (Cohen & Sokolovsky, 1978) and outpatients (Horwitz, 1977).

When one is defining the role of patient response to environmental stress, it is helpful to distinguish among stressful events and normal life strains (Billings & Moos, 1985). *Stressful events* are defined as identifiable and relatively major life changes in the areas of health, finances, and interpersonal relationships (e.g., separation, death). On the other hand, *life strains* represent particular stressors that are encountered in the everyday performance of the roles of spouse, parent, and worker.

The accumulation of stressful events and life strains dictate the severity of any given environmental stressor. In turn, this severity is associated with the likelihood that a given event will evoke a pathological response (Parry & Shapiro, 1986). Hence, the same environmental stressor can have quite diverse effects given the context of life strains in which it occurs and the way it is perceived by the individual. Features of stressors like undesirability, magnitude, and time clustering may be potent influences in the development of pathology. At the same time, the extent of a pathological response is mediated by the availability of support networks (e.g., Monroe, Bromet, Connell & Steiner, 1986). Some examples of these environmental influences on treatment considerations are provided in Table 5.1.

Table 5.1
Environment and Treatment Planning

Environmental Factors	Influence on Treatment
Environmental Stressors	
Stressful events	Focus treatment on crisis intervention
Life strains and microstressors	Focus treatment on coping with the strain or stessor
Environmental Resources	
Sociocultural environments	Provide basis for matching with therapist similarity
a. Gender	
b. Ethnicity	
c. Socioeconomic status	

(Continued)

Table 5.1 *(continued)*

Environmental Factors	Influence on Treatment
Social support systems a. The family b. Work environments	Focus on family/marital patterns and support systems Engage systems in treatment

ENVIRONMENTAL RESOURCES

Sociocultural Environments

Gender, ethnicity, and socioeconomic status (SES) have been widely researched as contributors to treatment outcome, but this research has failed to address the role of social support and only inconsistently has sought to understand the role of sociocultural variables in diagnosis and discriminative treatment planning (Lopez & Nuñez, 1987).

A review of the subject index of major textbooks in psychotherapy research reveals few references to socioeconomic class or sociocultural environments aside from ethnicity. The social revolution of the 1970s did not stimulate the amount of research on treatment approaches for the socially disadvantaged that had been hoped (Lorion & Felner, 1986).

A recent review (Beutler, Crago & Arizmendi, 1986) located only 10 adequately controlled studies in which relationships between patient and therapist socioeconomic backgrounds were considered directly in assessing contributors to treatment response. Of these studies, only two specifically applied comparison group methods to the task of defining the relationship between patient and therapist SES. These latter studies (Mitchell & Namenek, 1970; Mitchell & Atkinson, 1983) concluded that treatment and therapist assignments seldom are affected by patient SES. Nonetheless, patient SES relates negatively both to obtaining and remaining in treatment (Garfield, 1986b).

Lorion and Felner (1986) report that the SES of patients negatively influences therapist optimism about treatment outcome and introduces bias into diagnostic decisions. Large scale epidemiological research (e.g., Regier, Myers, Kramer, Robin, Blazer, Haugh, Eaton & Locke, 1984), however, disconfirms the popular views that women, minority group members, and elders have disproportionately high levels of psychopathology.

While differential treatment assignments and outcomes are not widely researched, there are a large number of articles and books that have attempted to define the nature of effective treatment among low SES groups. While these approaches vary in whether they consider social environments to be the causes or consequences of psychopathology, they almost uniformly identify the absence of stable social support systems among low SES groups as a major deterrent to effective change (e.g., Dohrenwend & Dohrenwend, 1981; Caplan & Killilea, 1976).

Programs that attempt to address the needs of the disadvantaged hold in common two basic principles about treating the disadvantaged: (1) there is value in addressing practical and clearly defined problems, and (2) there is a need to provide nurturing social resources and relationships to assist in times of need. Group and family-based treatments may circumvent the problems of disparity between patient and therapist while reducing feelings of isolation and alienation characteristic of these groups (Lorion & Felner, 1986). Moreover, addressing issues within the context of family systems, when these are available, may enhance the skills of naturally defined groups to provide support and assistance to overcome stress.

Well defined, targeted goals and short-term treatments are consistent with the practical mindedness of individuals who are confronted daily with a demanding environment. Demographic similarity may allow therapists to identify with the daily struggles of patients and to suggest applicable, practical suggestions.

Social Support Systems

While social support is an important asset in managing stress, arriving at an understanding about what variables comprise social support has not been uniformly accomplished. To some (Kessler, Price & Wortman, 1985), the important aspects of support networks include living arrangements, frequency of social contact, participation in social activities, and involvement in a social network. Others (Caplan, 1974) add the availability of emotional, cognitive, and tangible assistance to this list, and still others (Cobb, 1976) suggest the equal value of informational feedback.

The desirability of integrating these various aspects of social support into an inclusive definition led Gottlieb (1978) empirically to cluster specific helping behaviors into four superordinate classes of environmental support: (1) emotionally sustaining behavior, (2) problem-solving assistance, (3) unconditional readiness to act in assistance, and (4) environmental action taken on the individual's behalf.

The empirical relationship between social support and successful management of stress has been the focus of a growing body of research (cf. Schradle & Dougher, 1985). Patients who have well established social support systems have been found to respond less pathologically to stressful events than their counterparts who are more socially isolated (Parry & Shapiro, 1986). Likewise, patients with well established support systems tend to have higher self concepts (Ashinger, 1981) and lower incidence rates of psychopathology (Myers, Jacob & Pepper, 1972).

The value of social support is further evidenced in the observation that among urban women those stressed by life events who had an intimate and confiding relationship with a male (either boyfriend or mate) are buffered from depression. Research (Brown & Harris, 1978) on this issue suggests that only 4 percent of women who have an intimate relationship become depressed, whereas nearly 40 percent of women who experience life stress in the absence of an intimate relationship become depressed. The buffering effects of a caring relationship extend to other types of psychological disturbance (Slater & Depue, 1981) and to the nurturing power even of non-intimate friends and acquaintances (Davidson & Packard, 1981).

Interestingly, there are gender differences in the ability to form supportive relationships. For example, women are more effective than men in developing new friendships once support systems are lost (Fischer & Oliker, 1983). Such differences may account for the observation that psychiatric hospitalization and suicide rates among elderly men are over twice as high as among elderly women following the death of a spouse (see review by Yost, Beutler, Corbishley & Allender, 1986).

In their discussion of the interpersonal context of depression, Coyne et al. (1986) extend these findings to suggest that the interaction between stress and social support should predict depression. While it is too early to accept this conclusion definitively, it is relatively clear that a negative correlation exists between depression and one's report of social support (e.g., Andrews, Tennant, Hewson & Vaillant, 1978; Aneshensel & Stone, 1982; Costello, 1982). In particular, marital distress and low levels of social integration have been linked etiologically to the onset and recurrence of depression (Barnett & Gotlib, 1988). Moreover, ambulatory depressed individuals acknowledge making more efforts to obtain social support than nondepressed people, but they also report obtaining less support than others from their environment (Coyne, Aldwin & Lazarus, 1981; Schaefer, Coyne & Lazarus, 1981). On the other hand, friends and relatives of depressed individuals report that their ("supportive") conversations tend to be focused on the depressed person's problems, which in turn makes these supportive others feel depressed and may even drive them away (Arkowitz, Holliday & Hutter, 1982).

We do not yet know the mechanism by which social supports buffer against psychological distress. The interactive roles of social support and life stresses must be considered in assessing patient prognosis, and both may contribute independently to the risk of psychiatric disorder (Parry & Shapiro, 1986). It appears, moreover, that both must be considered in terms of their ability to bolster the success of patient coping strategies.

It has been suggested (e.g., Kessler, Price & Wortman, 1985) that the coping strategies of depressed individuals are characterized by negative self-preoccupations that hamper their ability to cope with confidence, efficiency, and decisiveness. Although the impact of social support systems on these cognitive patterns has not clearly been defined empirically, it is logical to assume that feedback from a supportive environment may draw one away from self to more external considerations, thus lessening the depression. If so, interventions that attempt to bolster the efficiency of coping strategies via social support and feedback may prove to be prophylactic in the treatment of individuals who are prone to affective disorder, and perhaps other disorders as well. Group and family therapies may prove to be critical in at least the prevention and maintenance phases of treatment.

Family Environment and Support. The family is the social system that offers, at once, the greatest potential support and aversive effect. To maximize the supportive potential while minimizing the potential for adverse effect, we must know what factors or variables in the family environment are related to the development or maintenance of disturbed behavior on the part of one or more individuals within that environment. There are a number of lines of evidence that potentially help us clarify the role of different family variables.

Changes in our culture have produced a dramatic shift in the composition, character and function of the family. When therapists work with a family, it is important that they do not respond solely to their own ideal of family structure and function, but from an informed awareness of realistic family patterns.

The most prevalent form of household composition today (23 percent) is one in which two individuals live in a child-free or post-childbearing marriage. The next most common household constellation is not a family at all, but single, widowed, separated, and divorced persons living alone (21 percent). These two family constellations are followed in prevalence by single parent families (16 percent) and dual breadwinner nuclear families (16 percent). The idealized view of the family as a unit led by a father-breadwinner and mother-housewife comprises only 13 percent of the households in North America (Glick, Clarkin & Kessler, 1987).

While the nuclear family involving two generations of adults continues to be a basic family unit in Europe and the United States, only about 7 to 8 percent of American households have ever consisted of more than two adult generations living in the same household. This is true in spite of the fact that life expectancy has increased from an average of 49.2 years in 1900 to 74.6 years in 1983, an increase that might lead us to expect an increase rather than a decrease in the number of multigenerational households.

Another dramatic change in the family system arises from an increase in the status of women, as evidenced by changes in employment and education. At the turn of the century a woman quit working outside the home upon marriage, never to return to the work force. Today, a substantial majority of women work, leaving the work force only temporarily during the childbearing years. This pattern, combined with the fact that the educational status of women has improved dramatically, suggests that women may feel more capable and powerful in modifying unwanted marital relationships today than previously. The increase in the number of single households noted above may partially reflect this new independence of women.

As a corollary of the foregoing, women have assumed increased control over their sexual behavior and reproductive functions in the past few decades. The dramatic increase in the use of birth control procedures means that women need have less fear of unwanted pregnancy than in earlier periods of our history. Concomitantly, the prevalence of premarital intercourse and the number of unmarried couples cohabitating is rising, suggesting that individuals are likely to be more sexually experienced at the time of marriage than in years past.

Given the increasing life expectancy, the change in the work and educational status of women, and the relative sexual freedom and concomitant control over pregnancy experienced by today's women, the life cycle of male-female relationships has been dramatically changed. Thus, it is quite conceivable to think of three phases through which relationships might proceed in the course of one's lifespan: (1) a uniting and friendship phase that may last for an extended period and often includes living together; (2) a family-oriented phase in which children are born and reared; and (3) a post-childrearing relationship based on companionship. In comparison to previous generations, these three phases may be less likely than before to be enacted with the same partner.

While divorce has increased markedly in the United States in this century, the death rate has declined so that the total rate of marital dissolution has remained stable for over 100 years. Yet, the notion of discrete and permanent categories of marital status (e.g., single, married, divorced, widowed) seems no longer accurate in today's society. Rather, the image of a marital cycle in which individuals shift between various marital statuses seems more apt. It is within this changing family scene that family members look to one another for social support.

Several studies have investigated the dimensions of support that operate within the family environment. This research generally confirms that depressive symptoms are most likely to occur when family cohesion is low and willingness to express conflict is high (Billings & Moos, 1982; Billings, Cronkite & Moos, 1983; Barnett & Gotlib, 1988). In fact, level of family support, by itself, effectively discriminates between depressed and nondepressed women (Wetzel, 1978; Wetzel & Redmond, 1980).

Married individuals generally report less depression than unmarried individuals, irrespective of gender, age, and ethnicity (Pearlin & Johnson, 1977). Married individuals are less exposed to various life strains than the unmarried; even when they are subjected to these stressors, married individuals remain less depressed than the unmarried.

Even more importantly, partner stability is a major contributor to maintenance of psychotherapy gains over periods ranging from six months (Schramski et al., 1984) to three years (Riehl, 1986) after treatment termination. In the absence of family supports, self-help groups that are focused upon the provision of support and assistance also have been found to be effective in facilitating the adjustment to loss (Lieberman & Videka-Sherman, 1986).

In turn, previous family relationship patterns have been found to affect one's ability to develop buffering support systems. For example, Flaherty and Richman (1986) studied the independent effects of early parental affectivity and protectiveness on later social relationships. They found that affectivity, particularly from maternal figures, was related to later ability to establish supportive relationships. Parental protectiveness, surprisingly, was not found to be related to this latter ability. This finding, standing as it does in contrast to many well entrenched theoretical concepts, led the authors to emphasize the need for research designed to clarify the relevant subdimensions of social support systems. Studies such as those proposed by these authors would begin the process of specifying the precise aspects of the environment to which interventions may be targeted.

Schizophrenia and the Family Environment. Interestingly, the role of family environment in treatment planning is best illustrated with reference to schizophrenia, a disorder that is severe, overt in its manifestations, and involved with both biological and environmental variables in its etiology and course.

The process of identifying the relative weight of genetic variables and environmental variables in the expression of schizophrenic symptoms and behavior has been a long and complicated one. By the use of a number of research strategies including cross-sectional and longitudinal designs, several conclusions are warranted about the role of family systems in the development of this condition at the present time (Goldstein & Strachan, 1987):

(1) From a cross-sectional point of view (i.e., family interaction once the offspring is manifesting schizophrenic symptoms), parents of schizophrenics are deficient in their ability to focus attention, to empathically take the perspective of another, and to communicate clearly and accurately.

(2) These disturbed family interactions precede the onset of schizophrenia.

(3) Cognitive disturbances and/or cognitive disturbance combined with unusual affective styles reflect and are influenced by family relationships.

(4) Family patterns of expressing emotion are related to the course of schizophrenia. Families high in Expressed Emotion (EE) (high hostility, criticism, overinvolvement) have family members who have more relapses and rehospitalizations than those with low EE.

(5) Across time, there is an interaction between the genetic vulnerability for schizophrenia and the quality of the family environment, such that symptomatic individuals are disproportionately represented among families rated as severely disturbed.

In the early 1960s, a group of British investigators discovered that patients who returned to live with their families following an episode of hospitalization were more likely to be rehospitalized than were those patients discharged to boarding homes and hostels (Brown, Monck, Carstairs & Wing, 1962). In order to further describe the family environmental factors that might be related to this phenomenon, these investigators constructed a semistructured interview called the *Camberwell Family Interview* (CFI).

The CFI requires questioning significant family members concerning their attitudes and opinions about the schizophrenic member of the family. The responses obtained in this process are rated and coded, and scores are calculated to reflect such dimensions of family life as overinvolvement, criticality, and hostility. The combination of these variables has come to be called "Expressed Emotion" or EE.

In subsequent studies, validation has been obtained for the EE construct and its value for defining treatment focus has been emphasized. Among both British and American samples it has been found that the percentage of patients who relapse is much higher among high EE families than in low EE families. Several research groups have now reported that the use of family interventions designed to reduce family EE has been successful in significantly reducing relapse and rehospitalization among schizophrenic family members.

Leff and Vaughn (1985) have provided what are probably the best comparative descriptions of families rated high and low in EE. They observe that high EE relatives are quite intrusive on the interpersonal space of the schizophrenic family member. Very symbolically, these relatives tend to dislike closed bedroom doors and attempt to monitor the patient's daily routine and personal matters. While recognizing that the patient is ill, they often become caught up in the patient's psychotic behavior and confront the patient in an apparent attempt to convince the patient that his/her thinking is delusional. Moreover, high EE relatives tend to be critical of the patient and to make few allowances for the illness in establishing their expectations for the schizophrenic member's functioning.

Low EE families report a belief that the schizophrenic condition is an illness and, in response, these families show empathy in an attempt to understand the patient's condition. This empathy is associated with lowered expectations of the patient's performance both during and after episodes. In the face of bizarre behaviors from the patient, low EE relatives are able to remain emotionally calm and self-contained.

There is no suggestion here that a family environment characterized by high EE is specific only to families in which there is a schizophrenic member. In fact, there is a growing literature to suggest that relationships characterized by high EE are also detrimental for patients with depression (Hooley, 1986). The findings from current research on schizophrenia may indicate, however, that high levels of criticism and overinvolvement interact with a particular vulnerability among schizophrenics, thus leading to detrimental effects on these individuals. The importance of this work is in its delineation of a particular treatment-responsive aspect of the family environment.

J.C., the college student who believed he was Jesus Christ and whose case was described in Chapter 3, lived with his widowed mother, providing an opportunity directly to observe and intervene in the family communication patterns. Explanations of her son's condition along with instruction to shape the mother's response to J.C.'s disturbed behavior resulted in her lowering her expectations of him while at the same time providing support and encouragement for those activities in which he excelled.

Depression and the Marital/Family Environment.   The interaction between a depressed individual and spouse is characterized by a lack of task orientation, a high level of hostility and critical behavior, and a lack of self-disclosure. Depressed women display less problem-solving behavior than do their spouses, and the spouses manifest less self-disclosure. These couples express less facilitative behavior than control couples, and depression tends to reduce aversive behavior in the spouse (Biglan, Hops, et al., 1985).

Among couples seeking marital treatment, subsets of those in which the spouse presents with depression have been compared with nondepressed subsets. Depressed spouses are prone to speak negatively about themselves and positively about their mates. In contrast, nondepressed spouses of depressed individuals have been found rarely to speak of themselves and tend to evaluate their depressed partners negatively (Hautzinger, Linden & Hoffman, 1982).

Hooley (1986) investigated the interaction between depressed individuals and their spouses who were also classified as having high or low EE. In face-to-face interaction, high EE spouses were found to be more negative and less positive toward their depressed partners. They made more critical remarks, disagreed with their partners more frequently, and were less likely to accept what their mate said to them. The depressed mates of high EE spouses exhibited low frequencies of self-disclosure and high levels of neutral nonverbal behavior.

Marital Conflict and Social Support.   The interaction pattern that exists between two marital-sexual partners can be the source of great difficulty and the focus of therapeutic intervention. At these times of marital conflict, other support systems assume great importance. The availability of social networks of support is a significant predictor of depression when life events stress an emotional relationship (Barnett & Gotlib, 1988; Monroe, Bromet, Connell & Steiner, 1986).

Marital conflict is one of the most frequent complaints of those seeking help from mental health practitioners. Cross-sectional and longitudinal emotional interaction research is beginning to clarify the nature and course of marital conflict, revealing that there are clear and consistent interactional differences between nondistressed and distressed couples (Jacob, 1987). Distressed couples, as compared to nondistressed couples, exhibit fewer rewarding and positive exchanges, a relatively frequent occurrence of negative exchanges that occur in sequential, escalating chains of behavior, a general immediate reactivity to events in the relationship, and cognitive and perceptual distortions that result in blaming the other.

These cross-sectional characteristics of the distressed couple are not surprising and, indeed, simply describe the conflicted nature of the relationship. However, while intuitively obvious, they are helpful in their detail and empirical grounding and must receive attention in any treatment geared to reducing marital conflict. These behaviors could serve as either the direct focus of marital intervention or the final goals of other treatments.

Work/School Environments

Freud noted the essence of life and adjustment as involving *lieben and arbeiten*, love and work. In our exploration of clinical research on work and its impact on mental health and psychopathology, as well as its role in assessing the need for and the focus of treatment, we have been impressed with the dearth of attention to and systematic research on the impact of the individual's work and/or school (in the case of children and young adults) life on long-term adjustment. The failure of clinical researchers to attend to the effects of work and school environments on the *development* and *prevention* of emotional disturbance is somewhat astonishing since the number of waking hours that the adult spends in a work setting frequently is greater than that spent at home.

A positive, fruitful work situation affords the individual with many benefits besides money, including activity, variety, temporal structure, social contacts, and identity/status (Warr, 1982). Research on these issues suggests that if one lacks a sense of personal control over immediate work activities (Karasek, 1979), he/she is at risk for losing a sense of emotional well being. Work overload, conflict, role ambiguity, excessive responsibility for people, and troubled interpersonal relationships all contribute to stress from the work environment (Holt, 1982; Kasl, 1978; Fletcher & Payne, 1980).

One of the complaints presented by J.I. at about the midpoint of her treatment was that she had difficulty getting along with her employer. She described him as "authoritarian," "dogmatic," and "uncaring." Her tendency was to rebel against his efforts to control her in a defiant assertion of her own capacity for self-direction. Clearly, her high reactance level made her a ready candidate for work-related stress. Her responses to external directives, particularly from men, easily revealed both her ability to feel victimized and her fear of helplessness, to which she responded with oppositional defenses. Her sensitivity to these directives made working in even the barest dogmatic environment very stressful. A work environment that reinforced her sense of power and self control might be an important contributor to treatment benfit.

The impact of work on the mental health and well being of the individual may be mediated by many variables, including the age of the individual and associated phase of the life cycle, sex, length of unemployment, and work involvement. Changing gender roles may be an especially important consideration, given the number of women who apply for therapy, the changing status of women in society and the role of work in molding self-esteem. Among women in our culture it has been hypothesized that the impact of employment is related to occupational involvement, the quality of the woman's nonoccupational environment, and the quality of her employment relationships (Warr & Parry, 1982). Thus, the salience of work involvement and quality of work success might be expected to be more important to single women than to married women with children.

More obvious in its influence is the lack of work—unwanted unemployment—and its impact on the mental health and emotional well being of the individual and the family. There is little doubt that the impact of unemployment carries in its wake various forms of psychological deterioration (Marsden & Duff, 1975; Warr, 1978; Dooley & Catalano, 1980; Hepworth, 1980; Stafford et al., 1980; Sinfield, 1981; Swinburne, 1981). The negative impact of unemployment increases as the individual's investment in work is greater (Warr, 1978; Stafford et al., 1980).

School occupies a similar role for children and young adults as work does for adults. Events in school can become symbolized as representing larger struggles within the extra-school environment. Thus, family stress is likely to be expressed in the school environment. A move to a residential school, for example, may be seen as parental abandonment even though it is designed by caring parents and by the school itself to provide a comforting and supportive structure. In a similar manner, alterations in the school environment can evoke distress that spreads throughout the family system. Role demands that contradict those established at home, changes in a familiar school's environment, loss of friendships through relocation or conflict, and transitions from elementary to middle school, high school and college all may evoke stress and should be considered in any symptom display within an individual child or family system.

At the same time, school environments can provide stability when family systems are in chaos. As sources of support during transition and stress periods in the family, teachers as well as peers may be incorporated into the treatment program.

SUMMARY AND COMMENT

The patient's environment provides a basis for social support. In this chapter, we have emphasized the role of social support systems in buffering the patient from symptoms, in facilitating treatment outcome, and consolidating treatment gains over time. As we have suggested, these social environments also are relevant to a multitude of treatment planning variables:

(1) In cases of serious disturbance, the family is important in deciding whether or not the patient can be maintained in a non-hospital or special environmental setting. While we believe that hospitalization is to be avoided whenever possible, one of the most frequent reasons for hospitalization is the lack of a stable or sufficient family environment for the patient. Often, if the behavior of the patient (e.g., drug taking, suicidal, psychotic) cannot be contained in the family environment, the hospital is utilized temporarily for a supportive and contained environment.

(2) In cases where the family interaction itself is the focus of difficulty (e.g., marital conflict) or is exacerbating the patient's pathology (e.g., schizophrenia and a high EE family environment), a family/marital format of treatment must be considered as a most efficient way to make inroads into the patient's symptomatology.

(3) Among low SES patients with an intact family, marital and/

or family intervention may bolster coping abilities and provide assistance in times of crisis.

In considering the format of treatment (individual, group, family/marital), the possible utilization of family and/or marital treatment format directly relates to several issues about the family environment of the patient. With individuals (especially the young and the elderly) who depend a great deal on the family environment, a family format of treatment is often the best approach to fostering behavioral change. Likewise, with individuals with low GAF scores, and relatively low-level adjustment with little self-sufficient functioning, the family environment is crucial as a support and sustainer of the patient. In these situations the family may be assessed as contributing to the ill behavior of the patient, or as needing assistance with coping with the patient. In either case, the use of the family treatment format may be seriously considered.

This determination will, in turn, assist in setting the focus of the family intervention (e.g., reduction of toxic family interactions, support of positive family interactions, use of family as co-therapist, etc.). In the absence of a cooperative family, however, group interventions may offer a family substitute. Especially among the economically disadvantaged, group treatments may enhance coping ability by providing a network of resource people who come from similar situations. For these latter groups, paraprofessional group leaders may overcome some of the differences in patients and therapists that are frequently observed to attenuate the development of cohesive groups.

SUGGESTED READINGS

Billings, A. G. & Moos, R. H. (1982). Social support and functioning among community and clinical groups: A panel model. *Journal of Behavioral Medicine, 5*, 295–311.

Coyne, J. C. & Holroyd, K. (1982). Stress, coping, and illness. In T. Millon, C. Green & R. Meagher (Eds.), *Handbook of clinical health psychology* (pp. 103–127). New York: Plenum Press.

Lazarus, R. S. (in press). Constructs of the mind in mental health and psychotherapy. In A. Freeman, H. Arkowitz, L. E. Beutler & K. Simon (Eds.), *Comprehensive handbook of cognitive therapy.* New York: Plenum.

Lorion, R. P. & Felner, R. D. (1986). Research on psychotherapy with the disadvantaged. In S. L. Garfield & A. E. Bergin (Eds.), *Handbook of psychotherapy and behavior change,* 3rd ed. (pp. 739–776). New York: John Wiley and Sons.

PART III

The Treatment Context

Armed with a knowledge of patient diagnosis, environment, and personal characteristics, the clinician is ready to begin planning a meaningful treatment. The first decision to face the clinician is to select the context in which treatment should be offered. Treatment context, as we define it here, refers to the setting, the treatment mode and format, and the frequency and duration of treatment. Options are selected in response to such questions as whether or not to treat the patient at all and, if so, whether the patient should be hospitalized, medicated, or treated with psychotherapy. If hospitalized, in what type of hospital or with what type of medication; or if in psychotherapy, in group, individual, or family therapy?

Figure III.1 outlines the types of decisional options that will be discussed within the three chapters that comprise this section. Alternative treatment contexts are grouped into three domains: those pertaining to the selection of the treatment setting, those relating to the selection of treatment mode and format, and those related to assigning treatment duration and frequency. Following the convention presented both in Figures 2.1 and II.1, heavy arrows draw attention to the primary relationships and dashed arrows to the secondary relationships that we will discuss in this and subsequent sections.

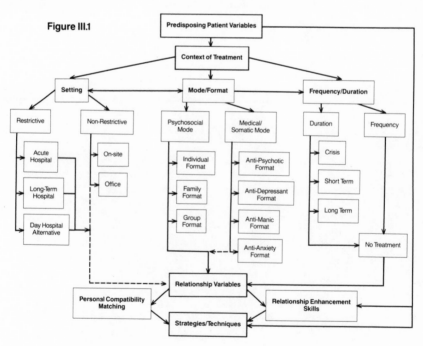

Figure III.1

100

6

The Treatment Setting

There are a number of physical environmental settings within which psychotherapeutic treatment can take place. These settings include the patient's home, feared situations (e.g., neighborhood, airplanes, elevators), private offices, university counseling centers, outpatient clinics, day hospitals, general hospitals, private psychiatric hospitals, and state or federal hospitals. The choice of treatment setting is a major one with far-reaching implications.

The treatment setting itself has certain inherent characteristics which flavor the treatment.

(1) The treatment setting influences whether the consumer of mental health services is called a "client" or a "patient," with all the social and psychological implications of the two terms.

(2) The setting to which an individual applies for assistance may unwittingly determine other specifics of treatment. For example, if one applies for evaluation in a family clinic, one is likely to have family treatment.

(3) The choice of treatment setting, made by either the consumer or the clinician doing the evaluation, determines the financial cost of treatment.

(4) The setting determines who will ultimately be in charge of the treatment. In psychiatric hospital settings, physicians typically assume this role; in other settings, it is frequently assigned to psychologists.

(5) The setting has an impact on the range of treatment planning

options typically used by the clinicians working in that setting. Clinicians in HMOs, for example, are probably more inclined to recommend planned brief therapy than is the private practitioner.

While consumers of mental health services unwittingly determine major aspects of their treatment plan by the location in which they choose to apply for assistance, in this chapter we will address the question, "What are the clinical indications and contraindications recommending a particular treatment setting to an individual or family?"

It is useful for treatment planning purposes to classify treatment settings according to the goals of acute care, rehabilitation, and maintenance care (Frances, Clarkin & Perry, 1984). The goal of acute care is appropriate when an individual is in a crisis situation and needs assistance in regaining psychic equilibrium. This care is usually provided in outpatient crisis intervention, intensive care partial hospitals, and acute care, short-term psychiatric inpatient units.

The goal of rehabilitation involves the extinction of self-defeating behavior patterns, the resolution of conflict, and the learning of new, more effective behavior patterns. These goals are furthered in settings such as outpatient offices and clinics, partial care rehabilitation hospitals, day treatment centers, halfway houses, and longer-term inpatient settings.

Finally, maintenance goals involve an attempt to assist a vulnerable individual to maintain current functioning that appears to be optimal given the condition and its history. Such support of vulnerable individuals takes place in outpatient settings, chronic care partial hospitals, and chronic care inpatient hospitals.

Another way to conceptualize treatment settings is on a continuum of least restrictive (e.g., private or clinic office, patient's home) to most restrictive environments (e.g., hospitalization) (Newman & Howard, 1986). In this conceptualization, the optimum situation is one in which the patient has the most personal control and the least restrictive treatment possible.

LEAST RESTRICTIVE TREATMENT SETTINGS

Treatment at the Site of Difficulty

There are practical and theoretical reasons why one might want either to assess and/or treat certain behavioral conditions at the site in which the problematic behaviors occur. For assessment, the clinician may want to observe the troubled behaviors as they occur, rather than depend upon the verbal account of such behaviors by the patient in the clinician's office. The patient may have limited powers of self-observation, either through anxiety while in the troubled situation or because of general limited sense of self and the difficulties involved. The patient may be too young or mentally impaired, and thus may not have sufficient verbal capacity to report accurately. Or, the patient may have a keen internal sense of what happens but is not articulate in reporting to the clinician.

The prototypic case of treatment at the site of difficulty is *in vivo* desensitization for phobic responses to objects and situations. For example, G.B. was a single, 24-year-old woman who developed a severe phobia of buildings greater than one story in height after falling 23 floors in a faulty elevator. She was unable to come to the treatment clinic which was on the third floor of a major university hospital. Therefore, treatment began by meeting the patient in a grassy area adjacent to the hospital. On-site treatment concentrated on approaching and entering buildings. At first these buildings were one floor, unfamiliar residences, but later treatment sites extended to large, open shopping centers and, finally, to multistory buildings.

Family therapists are the ones who most frequently provide assessment and treatment on site—in this case, in the home. In devising a family treatment for acting out adolescents, Patterson (1982) and colleagues spent hours in the home observing sequential interactions, and developing a contingency model for the occurrence of deviant adolescent behavior. Falloon and colleagues (1985) also have argued that behavioral family intervention with families having a schizophrenic member should be conducted in the home. The probability of cancellations is lessened when treatment is done in the home, and there is an increased likelihood of all family members being present. Since the behaviors that are the target of modification occur in the home setting, and since desired new behaviors must take place there, treatment at the home site increases transfer of learning.

Office Treatment

If there is no compelling reason to treat the patient at the site of difficulty or in the home, the clinician will typically see the patient in his office, either privately or in a clinic. This setting is arranged to provide privacy for the disclosure needed to work on personal difficulties.

In the now familiar case of J.I., for example, an office setting was selected for treatment both because of the convenience that this setting provided for the therapist and because this environment was conducive for ensuring the patient's sense of safety. In the beginning, the objective was to reduce the patient's anxiety sufficiently that she could learn a relaxation response and cognitive coping strategies, and an environment that was removed from the objects of her fear was conducive to this task.

THE PSYCHIATRIC HOSPITAL

Patient's level of functioning, available social support systems, prior psychiatric hospitalization history, and level of cooperativeness with therapy determine the level of treatment restrictiveness (Newman, Heverly, Rosen, Kopta & Bedell, 1983). In general, there are two types of patient populations that alert the clinician to the need for restrictive treatment settings: (1) patients who experience an acute exacerbation of symptoms; and (2) chronic patients of whatever diagnosis (Bachrach, 1988) who are characterized by a long-standing need for support and maintenance.

The Psychiatric Hospital as a Treatment Setting

It is a gross oversimplification to refer generically to the psychiatric hospital, since these hospitals and their individual units are quite diverse in the diagnostic and social class characteristics of the patients, policies, and staffing patterns. However, the descriptions of psychiatric hospitals as environments are at primitive levels. Furthermore, there is little useful information available on the role of the hospital environment in enhancing patient outcome.

The overall goal of hospitalization for acutely disturbed patients is to control and contain behavior that has not been so managed in the community. Thus, numerous authors (Gunderson, 1978; Leeman, 1986) have emphasized the role of the hospital milieu in providing a structured environment with limit setting, support, and nurturance while the patient regains control. Gunderson (1978) has articulated the five crucial milieu functions of containment, support, structure, involvement, and validation. The milieu contains patient activity by preventing assaults, homicides, and suicides. The staff provides a supportive network by attempts to encourage the patient and bolster self-esteem. Structure is inherent in the milieu's organization through predictable schedules and staff. Involvement between patient and others is provided through unit meetings and participation in milieu activities. Validation of the patient's individuality is provided through individual treatment and individual contact between the patient and therapist.

There have been some attempts to measure the atmosphere created by staff, patients, and the physical setting of the hospital ward. The Ward Atmosphere Scale (WAS) (Moos, 1969, 1973) is a self-report instrument that can be completed by both patient and staff concerning their perceptions of the ward environment. It measures dimensions of spontaneity, support, practicality, order, insight, involvement, aggression, clarity, submission, autonomy, and control. For example, wards in VA hospitals characterized by high staff control have been found to be predictive of good community tenure among discharged, unmarried schizophrenics (Moos & Schwartz, 1972).

By these and other methods, it appears that hospital units characterized by relatively small size, high staff-to-patient ratio, low staff turnover, broad delegation of responsibility with clarity of authority and decision making, low levels of anger and aggression combined with high levels of support, a practical orientation, order, organization, and consistency are optimal for good patient care and outcome (Ellsworth, 1983; McGlashan, 1986).

It is possible, of course, that patients with different problem areas and diagnoses may require different environmental supports (Leeman, 1986). The movement to create specialized units for patients with specific problem areas such as anorexia and bulimia, and substance abuse, or for specific age groups such as the elderly and adolescents are a move in this direction. It seems quite plausible that anorexics, for example, would need specialized structuring around food intake and exercise. Borderline patients may need an emphasis on structure and limit setting and focus on their interpersonal issues (Gunderson, 1985).

Beyond the control and protection functions and the institution of medication when appropriate, the picture becomes less clear. We believe that role induction of the patient and family into the acceptance of need for aftercare may be crucial for long-term outcome, as suggested by Glick and Hargreaves (1979). In this regard, education of the patient and family about the condition and need for treatment, as well as careful discharge planning, are essential aspects and functions of the hospital environment.

RESTRICTIVE SETTINGS FOR THE ACUTE PATIENT

Acute Psychiatric Hospitalization

There are situations either at the time of initial assessment or during the course of a treatment when patients' behaviors are out of their own control and/or when the environment cannot contain behavior that is potentially self-destructive or destructive to others. It is at clinical crises like these that the clinician considers a change of setting—the most available of which is usually an acute psychiatric hospital—in order to stabilize the patient's life.

Indications for Hospitalization. The indications and events giving rise to the option of acute hospitalization (Flynn & Henisz, 1975; Spencer & Mattson, 1979) are as follows:

(1) The individual poses an immediate danger to self or others (e.g., acutely suicidal, homicidal, violent behavior, loss of control due to prolonged alcohol and/or drug abuse).

(2) The individual is experiencing symptoms and/or exhibiting deviant behavior that is not tolerable to him or those around him.

(3) The individual's behavior is a serious threat to his/her adaptation to life, and the patient must be placed in a protective environment so that this destructive behavior ceases.

Three of the diagnostic examples that we provided in Chapter 3 might warrant hospitalization, albeit for different reasons. J.C., the young schizophrenic man who believed he was Jesus Christ, may warrant hospitalization, especially if he becomes acutely suicidal as he approaches his 33rd birthday; H.D., the 44-year-old, unemployed alcoholic with several professional degrees, may warrant hospitalization to withdraw him from alcohol intoxication and to initiate a comprehensive treatment program; and M.D., the 27-year-old borderline woman, who has established a pattern of erratic and often destructive behavior, may warrant hospitalization for self-protection and to establish predictable levels of supportive structure.

Part of the problem both in knowing when to recommend hospitalization and in evaluating its effectiveness is the lack of a precise knowledge of the particular hospital setting in which patients are to be placed. The clinician must ask: "What is the interpersonal nature of the hospital environment?" "What are the treatment goals and strategies?"

Kiesler (1982) reviewed the effects of hospitalization compared to alternative treatments. This review suggests that patients with more focal symptoms or with a less chronic or pervasive condition might respond favorably to acute hospitalization. The treatment of alcoholism is a case in point. Alcoholism is a prevalent condition which the average clinician is bound to encounter and which is often sufficiently focal to respond to acute inpatient care, at least as an initial step in treatment.

Miller and Hester (1986) concluded from controlled comparison treatment studies that there is no advantage for residential over nonresidential treatment settings in treating alcohol abuse. The outcome of the intervention was more influenced by the content of the program than by the setting in which the program was executed. The one possible differential treatment indicator was that intensive treatment may be more beneficial for more severely deteriorated and less socially stable individuals, while less intensive treatment may benefit individuals who are less disturbed, more changeable, and at an earlier stage of their condition. Hence, chronic and long-term treatment may be more clearly indicated for J.C. (our 24-year-old schizophrenic) than for M.D. (our 27-year-old borderline) because his condition relatively is more entrenched and stable. However, even in the case of J.C., there are probably alternative treatments that will be preferable to chronic care hospitalization.

Acute Day Hospital Treatment

Probably the most available alternative care to acute hospitalization is the so-called day or partial hospital. This treatment setting can be utilized as an alternative to hospitalization or as a treatment setting in its own right.

Partial hospitalization emerged in the early 1960s as an important component in the array of community-based treatment services. In 1963 there were only 141 partial hospital programs serving 3,680 patients. Within 10 years there were 1,280 programs serving 186,000 patients. While there is evidence for the efficacy of partial hospitalization, partial hospitals have in general been poorly designed and do not target specific diagnostic groups and treatment problems. In this array of day hospital programs, however, one can schematically discern three types of partial hospitals: intensive care partial hospitals, chronic care partial hospitals, and rehabilitation programs (Klar, Frances & Clarkin, 1982). These programs vary in terms of goals, methods, and expected length of treatment, and an unstable, periodically suicidal patient like M.D. (our 27-year-old borderline), as well as J.C., might better benefit from an intensive care partial hospital program than from a chronic care, residential facility except during times of acute suicidal crises.

Like the acute hospital unit, the intensive care partial hospital provides rapid assessment and stabilization of acute symptomatology for those patients in acute distress. The goals of acute care correlate with a short-term focus of from one to four months. Acute care partial hospitals can serve as an alternative to acute hospitalization. There is some debate about the number and type of patients that can use the intensive care partial hospital as an alternative to chronic residential care and rehabilitation programs. Wilder and colleagues (Wilder, Levin & Zwerling, 1966) suggested that two-thirds of patients deemed appropriate for hospitalization were also suited for partial hospitalization. Intensive care partial hospitals can also be used to shorten inpatient stays. Herz, Endicott and Spitzer (1976) reported that for patients who reside with their families brief hospitalization followed by partial hospitalization is superior to lengthy inpatient treatment.

RESTRICTIVE SETTINGS FOR THE CHRONIC PATIENT

Bachrach (1988) has pointed out that, prior to the recent deinstitutionalization policies, it was easy to define the chronic patient. In those not so distant days, the chronic patient was the one who spent most of his life in a state mental hospital. Since illness and hospitalization are not necessarily synonymous nor coterminous, chronicity cannot be defined only in terms of a diagnosis or functional disability. There is growing consensus that diagnosis, duration, and disability are all needed to define the chronic patient, though there is some difficulty in operationalizing these terms.

Long-Term Hospitalization

There are still some hospitals (e.g., state facilities) and some hospital units (e.g., long-term units in private hospitals) that have a length of stay (LOS) of one to two years for selected patients. The burden of the proof for the necessity of such care clearly rests with proponents of long-term hospitalization to show differential effectiveness, given the cost and restrictive environment. There are no data to date that show the differential effectiveness of long-term hospital stay (see Glick & Hargreaves, 1979).

ALTERNATIVES TO HOSPITALIZATION

Kiesler (1982) has concluded that alternative care is superior to hospitalization in a number of ways: cost/benefit ratio; hospitalization reinforces further hospitalization; greater socialization in alternative care settings. In not one instance reviewed did hospitalization have a positive impact on the average patient which exceeded that of the alternative care investigated. Indeed, in most cases, the alternative care had more positive effects than hospitalization.

It does not follow that one should do away with psychiatric hospitals. Individuals who are suicidal, homicidal, etc., will continue to need hospitalization. Often the alternative care facilities are not available for these patients, and they need a more structured environment than the ones available. Nonetheless, Kiesler's findings suggest that relatively few patients actually require hospitalization, and when alternative care is available it should be tried first.

The foregoing recommendations certainly apply in the cases of J.C., our schizophrenic; M.D., our unstable, borderline woman; and even H.D., our family-dependent alcoholic. In these cases, the alternatives that demand serious consideration include: community living programs (Stein & Test, 1980); Soteria homelike setting (Mosher & Menn, 1978); day-care treatment with the same activities as the inpatient care (Herz, Endicott, Spitzer & Mesnikoff, 1971); visits from public health care nurses and medication (Pasamanick, Scarpitti & Dinitz, 1967); and specially designed outpatient care (Levenson, Lord, Sermas, Thornby, Sullender & Comstock, 1977).

The foregoing care programs have several features in common. They provide basic support that is not limited to scheduled sessions each week; most provide constant availability of staff (e.g., day care) during the day; all employ social systems interventions; and there is emphasis on behavioral skill building.

Several cautionary and practical clinical notes must be added, however. First of all, alternative care programs are intensive ones that demand active and enthusiastic personnel who are available on an emergency basis. It is difficult to retain such people in positions, in part due to deficiencies in funding for mental health programs and the current ethos of supporting hospitalization (third-party carriers) over the alternatives. This predilection for inpatient settings may reflect a social view that inpatient care is medical treatment while alternatives are social intervention, and not to be covered by medical policies.

Chronic Care Partial Hospitals. The chronic care, partial hospital program provides a setting with humble expectations, high symptom tolerance, and a low-key environment that offers concrete and practical treatment approaches for the chronic patient. Attendance requirements are flexible: Patients are not ordinarily required to spend the entire day in the program and often take leaves of absence if they find work. Chronic schizophrenic patients, especially those without families, frequently fare better in a chronic care partial hospital than those treated in the outpatient setting (Guy, Gross, Hogarty & Dennis, 1969; Linn, Caffey, Klett, et al., 1979). Good patient outcome has been associated with program settings that offered relatively more occupational therapy, lower patient turnover, and relatively longer stays (Linn et al., 1979).

Rehabilitation Programs. In contrast to the low-key environment for the chronic patient in partial care, the rehabilitation day hospital aims to engender the development or reacquisition of skills to facilitate return to work and resumption of family role. Patients generally require four to eight months of treatment in a five-day week schedule.

TREATMENT SETTINGS VS. TREATMENT PROGRAMS

We agree with Paul (1978), who asserts that the essential element in the care of the chronic patient is not the *setting* in which the work is done but the *nature of the treatment.* Paul's comments take the focus off the physical setting of the treatment and emphasize that the "setting" is less the physical location and more the organizational structure created by the treatment personnel. Ultimately, one does not select to place a patient in a hospital or a day treatment program, but rather in the hands of treatment personnel who are united and systematic in their maintenance of a particular treatment focus.

Paul and Lentz (1977) demonstrated the effectiveness of a social learning approach to the care of the chronic patient in a well-designed multimodal community-based setting. Eighty-four patients were drawn from a larger pool of chronic patients in four state hospitals in Illinois. They were between 18 and 55 years of age, with a primary diagnosis of schizophrenia and with a history of two or more years of continuing hospitalization. All the patients were of low socioeconomic status and on the average had spent 17 years in mental institutions. The majority could not handle basic life support functions of feeding themselves, clothing or bathing themselves, or carrying out a normal conversation.

The research design employed in this study allowed a systematic comparison of the efficacy of two psychosocial programs (milieu and social learning) as well as a traditional hospital treatment for returning chronic patients to the community. A large regional state hospital was used as the site of the traditional treatment, while the psychosocial programs were located in a regional mental health center. Treatment effects were assessed in four areas: (1) the development of personal and interpersonal skills; (2) enhancement of instrumental role performance skills such as vocational and housekeeping skills; (3) reduction of bizarre behavior; and (4) provision of aftercare, including contact with at least one supportive person in the community. Patient and staff behaviors were tracked over a three-year period.

The two psychosocial programs were designed so that 85 percent of the patient's waking hours was devoted to acquiring social and self-care skills. In addition, there were formal classes in reading, writing, and arithmetic, homemaking, and grooming. As social skills accrued, patients were given increasing exposure to the outside world.

While similar in nature, the social learning program emphasized the establishment of reinforcing contingencies while the milieu program simply offered opportunities and exposure. In contrast to both of the psychosocial programs, the traditional hospital program consisted primarily of a large percent of unstructured time and relatively little time devoted to classes, meetings, and focused activities.

By all measures of therapeutic outcome, the social learning program was more efficient and effective than either the milieu or the hospital program. The social learning program treated and improved more patients and released more to independent living and community placement than either of the other two programs. In addition, the social learning program was effective in creating a greater impact on a wider range of behavioral problems than either of the other treatments.

While the social learning program had positive results on both adaptive and maladaptive functioning, the milieu procedures influenced only maladaptive behavior. The social learning program produced behavioral improvement and release to community living equally across the range of patient demographics, regardless of previous type and length of treatment, or the nature or level of initial disability. In terms of actual cost, the direct dollar savings by the social learning program over the six-year period of the study was two-and-a-half times greater than the hospital program and 28 percent greater than the milieu program.

Such findings as this not only lend an optimistic view to the care of the chronically mentally ill, but also emphasize the importance of fitting the treatment environment to the needs of patients rather than to the comfort needs of staff. While social stimulation and reinforcing activities require more time and effort on the part of staff than more traditional chronic care environments, they are also more rewarding in the long run as patients begin to change and grow.

SUMMARY AND COMMENT

Research (Ellsworth, 1983) has found the following hospital setting characteristics to be optimal for maximal outcome: small units, short stays, high staff-to-patient ratio and interaction, low staff turnover, low percentage of psychotic patients, maintenance of clear lines of authority and decision-making in the context of broad delegation of responsibility, high levels of support, practical orientation, order and organization, consistency, expectation of patient participation and interaction, and focus on generalizing inpatient results to after-care settings.

Two large VA studies (Gurel, 1964; Ullmann, 1967) found small wards to be associated with more improvement than large wards. Some find a positive relationship between high staffing levels and positive treatment outcome (Dickey, 1964; Gurel, 1964; Ullmann, 1967; Linn, 1970). However, others (e.g., Ellsworth et al., 1972) have pointed out that high staff turnover rates and high staff-to-patient ratios exert an indirect effect on outcome, being mediated by the role played by the success achieved in placing chronic patients in the community.

Some researchers (e.g., Fairweather, 1964; Schulberg & Baker, 1969) have suggested that a wide range of patients on a ward is therapeutic, whereas others (cf. Ellsworth et al., 1972) have noted the recent trend towards setting up specialized wards for homogeneous patient groups. These latter procedures are questionable in view of such evidence as that provided by Ellsworth et al. (1979) indicating that unclassified and mixed wards are linked to larger and more rapid gains.

A major contributor to treatment benefit in the institutional atmosphere involves the attitudes of staff and patients. Lawton and Cohen (1975) have summarized the following ward atmosphere dimensions: (1) staff involvement; (2) patient autonomy; (3) staff control; (4) patient mutuality; (5) ward morale; (6) order and organization; and (7) activity level. Staff involvement was the only factor that they found consistently predicted positive outcome, however. Moos and Schwartz (1972) observed that wards in VA hospitals characterized by both staff and patient report of high staff control were predictive of good in-community tenure among discharged, unmarried schizophrenics.

With so few studies in this area, it still remains unclear what aspects of the hospital environment are therapeutic. The most obvious function of the acute hospital unit is to control the patient's behavior during an episode of acute upset often involving suicidal behavior, thought disorder, and lack of concern for personal care. Beyond the control and protection functions and the institution of medication when appropriate, the picture becomes less clear.

With the majority of individuals who present for psychological help, the desirable treatment setting is a relatively unrestricted one, usually consisting of the psychotherapist's office or the natural environment in which the difficulties occur. It is with the more seriously disturbed patient who exhibits acute symptoms that are out of control and that pose a danger to self and others, or the patient with chronic disability and major areas of dysfunction that the treatment setting must be restrictive. Hospitalization for acute and serious symptoms such as suicidal behavior and psychotic symptoms may be indicated for a brief period of time, especially if crisis intervention is not adequate to the task, in order to bring the patient back to pre-acute levels of adjustment. Patients with longstanding symptomatic behavior and extremely low levels of social functioning may need a treatment program involving a restricted environment with intense focus by coordinated staff. Such intense programs are probably most successful when they focus on the reduction of bizarre behavior and the learning of social skills, and when comparatively less attention is given to psychodynamics. These programs can be located in a variety of settings such as state hospitals or community mental health centers, and the important element in their effectiveness is the learning experience itself rather than the physical setting.

SUGGESTED READINGS

Ellsworth, R. (1983). Characteristics of effective treatment milieu. In J. Gunderson, O. Will & L. Mosher (Eds.), *Principles and practice of milieu therapy* (pp. 87–123). New York: Jason Aronson.

Kiesler, C. (1982). Mental hospitals and alternative care: Non-institutionalization as potential public policy for mental patients. *American Psychologist, 37,* 349–360.

Paul, G. L. & Lentz, R. J. (1977). *Psychosocial treatment of chronic mental patients.* Cambridge, MA: Harvard University Press.

7

Treatment Mode and Format

Two modes of treatment are defined by the avenue through which a therapeutic effect is sought—psychosocial and medical/somatic—and both modalities must be considered in treatment planning for the majority of patients. In contrast to the modes of treatment, the formats of treatment describe a more specific system of delivering the treatment mode. Among medical treatments, the formats reflect drug groupings and electroconvulsive shock therapy (ECT). Among the psychosocial treatments, formats reflect individual, group, marital, and family service delivery systems.

Within the domain of a given mode and format, there are varieties of more specific procedures. By the same token, the medical/somatic treatments include a very large number of psychoactive medications, psychosurgery, and electroconvulsive therapy (ECT), each of which may vary in combinations and dosage levels.

For the present, we will limit our discussion to the dominant forms of psychotherapy, including in this term dynamic, experiential, interpersonal, behavioral, and cognitive therapies. At a later point, we will address these approaches in much more specific terms. Similarly, our presentation of the medical/somatic mode of treatment will be restricted largely to a description of the most frequently used psychoactive medications.

The authors wish to thank Ms. Martha Frankhauser for her comments and suggestions for the section of this chapter on medical management.

PSYCHOSOCIAL MODES AND FORMATS

The psychosocial mode of treatment is usually delivered in some combination of three typical formats: (1) individual (one patient and one therapist), (2) family/marital (nuclear family or marital couple and therapist), and (3) group (group of unrelated patients and therapist). The treatment format refers to the person or social unit that serves as the vehicle of intervention and is present for all or most of the therapy sessions. In this chapter, we will review the indications for the selection of each of these three formats of treatment.

Treatment strategies (e.g., behavioral, psychodynamic, etc.) and treatment format are often confused even in professional writings. For example, many writers (e.g., Lewis & Usdin, 1982) refer to "family therapy" (a format of treatment) as if it connotes specific techniques of intervention. Such authors also are inclined to refer to behavior therapy (a set of procedures) without due regard to whether the behavioral strategies are applied in an individual, family, or group format. In fact, most strategies of intervention can be used in a variety of treatment formats.

Not only does making a distinction between treatment strategies and formats make sense on logical and conceptual grounds, but such a distinction is important because it may be reflected in the nature of the mediating treatment goals selected. Being clear in this distinction also may help accurately to predict both the speed of effects and the types of outcomes that will be affected by interventions. Thus, a given treatment strategy may have a different impact and outcome depending upon which treatment format is selected to implement it. For example, an interpretation given to an individual alone or in front of spouse either may help the spouse empathize with the individual or be used as a weapon against the other, depending on both how and to whom it is presented.

A Historical Perspective

We briefly will review the historical perspectives that have given rise to the three distinct psychosocial treatment formats that are prominent today in order to yield clues as to the distinct therapeutic advantages of each. In this process we will develop guidelines for the use of each format. Later in the chapter, we will discuss research that provides support for and comparisons among the three formats.

Individual Treatment Format.   In the Western culture in which psychotherapy has arisen, the individual typically has been considered to be the site of the problem or difficulty. Therefore, the individual rather than the family or support group was usually the focus of the intervention. From the traditional perspective of health and illness, it has always been the individual who needed to see the doctor in order to be treated. Breuer's and Freud's pioneering work (1955) and subsequent development of the psychoanalytic method had a profound impact on the practice and development of psychotherapy in the United States. Their work focused exclusively on an individual treatment format and established this as the primary, if not exclusive, context in which to explore the intrapsychic conflicts of an individual.

The individual therapy format constitutes a significant proportion of the practice of 95 percent of clinicians (Norcross, 1988). Individual therapy has firmly established its effectiveness, and at least some evidence suggests that it may be more effective than a group format in altering individual clinical symptoms (e.g., Nietzel, Russell, Hemmings & Gretter, 1987).

In our culture, an individual format appeals to both the patient and the therapist for a number of reasons. It is, for example, the format that provides the most confidentiality and is most conducive to revealing embarrassing wishes, fears, and obsessions. There also is an implicit clarity of roles in the individual treatment format. This familiarity with and clarity about patient role definition and the complementary role assumed by the therapist are not as clear nor can they be as easily anticipated in reference to family and group treatment.

Family Treatment Format. A shift from an individual treatment paradigm to a family treatment format historically occurred during the mental hygiene movement of the 1930s. Social service agencies and child guidance clinics, in particular, perceived a need for more efficient and economical ways of providing mental health services to the community. Family sessions were instituted initially to gather necessary information about the patient and to establish the treatment alliance with the family as a whole.

John Bell, a professor of psychology at Clark University, is credited as the first to utilize the family interview format in working with children and their parents circa 1951. Ironically, Bell's use of the family format was based upon his misunderstanding of the frequency with which John Bowlby at the Tavistock Child Guidance Clinic in London used this procedure. At the time, Bowlby, frustrated in a treatment impasse with a male adolescent patient, brought in the mother, father, and patient as an extraordinary, not a typical, move. Bell interpreted Bowlby's description of this event as representing usual and conventional treatment in London.

At approximately the same time period, Nathan Ackerman, a child psychiatrist, began to work with the entire family in regular family therapy sessions. Ackerman was not only an energetic therapist but also a prolific writer (e.g., Ackerman, 1958), and his articles and books are revealing of his early attempts to articulate a theoretical rationale for the strategies of family treatment, a rationale that was firmly identified with earlier psychoanalytic training.

The introduction of the marital treatment format took place quite separately from the introduction of the family treatment format. Both the rise of the marital counseling profession and a movement within the field of psychoanalysis to investigate the dynamics of married partners contributed to the evolution of this format of treatment (Broderick & Schrader, 1981). By the late 1920s and early 1930s there were two marriage counseling centers in the United States. By 1942, a professional association for marriage counselors had been formed. Conjoint treatment, the treatment of both spouses together, gradually grew in popularity so that by 1960 15 percent of all treatment sessions were conjoint and by the mid 1980s, 50 percent of all clinical practitioners used this format of treatment regularly (Norcross, 1988).

In parallel with the marriage counseling movement, psychoanalysts independently became interested in the psychodynamics of spousal relationships. Oberndorf (1938) was the first to report on the sequential analysis of five married couples. From this work, he constructed a theory of interactive neuroses in marriage. Somewhat later, Mittelman (1948) reported on his concurrent but separate psychoanalytic treatment of a series of marital partners. In 1949, Henry Dicks, a British psychiatrist, began his psychoanalytic investigations of marital couples which resulted in a psychodynamic theory of faulty marital interactions (Dicks, 1967).

Historically, then, the use of family and marital formats derived in large part from an emphasis on the contextual origins of the presenting problems of the individual patient. At the present time, both marital and family therapy have been accepted well within the armamentarium of the mental health practitioner (Norcross, 1988). Their long-term as well as immediate effectiveness is well established, even in comparison to group and individual therapies (e.g., Haas & Clarkin, 1987; Hazelrigg, Cooper & Borduin, 1987).

The development of family/marital treatment formats served several adaptive functions in the evolution of treatment approaches: (1) they came to be recognized as important adjuncts to individual interventions with problematic children and adolescents because they acknowledged that the family environment contributed to the origin and maintenance of individual difficulties (cf. Gadow, 1985); (2) these family formats were found to be helpful in establishing a treatment alliance with the entire family so as to diminish treatment dropouts with children and adolescents; and (3) they were well suited to the relatively brief treatment of specific problems that have assumed such importance in an age of health cost consciousness.

Group Treatment Format. Joseph Pratt (1907) is usually credited with the first application of group treatment in the United States. Pratt was a Boston internist who used a supportive and didactic group format to assist patients to cope with tuberculosis. Pratt used these groups to educate patients in the treatment of their condition and to provide a context for mutual support in the form of testimonials and weekly reports of progress.

During World War II, the use of group therapy grew because of its potential efficiency and the lack of available psychiatric personnel to respond to the increasing need for services. However, beyond this practical consideration, there was a growing conception of man as an interpersonal being whose psychological disturbances were directly related to faulty ways of interacting with others. The group treatment format soon came to be seen as a way to approach these interpersonal issues.

In the 1940s, Kurt Lewin (1947) began to study group climate, leadership styles, and intergroup conflicts. Stimulated by his ideas, a movement developed in which behavioral scientists used the small group as a microcosm for studying interpersonal forces. In 1947, the National Training Laboratory (NTL) was initiated under the auspices of the National Education Association. The goal of the NTL was to conduct research on group behavior and to improve the capacity of professional individuals to utilize effective group management skills within their organizations. The famous T(raining)-group was utilized as a method to facilitate personal learning and change. Interpersonal honesty, self-disclosure, and group feedback became the core techniques of these T-group experiences.

During the 1960s and early 70s, the small group experience became an expansive commercial enterprise as so-called "growth centers" proliferated. But, with their rapid expansion and commercial motivation, there was little emphasis placed on defining the standards for leaders or selection criteria for participants.

During the 1960s and 70s, encounter groups arose in great numbers, including Gestalt groups, EST groups, Rolfing groups, sensory awareness groups, Transactional Analysis groups, etc. These groups originally were not designated as "therapy" groups, and concomitantly neither identified the leaders as "therapists" nor the participants as "patients." They touted egalitarianism of leader and participant with the goal being to enhance personal growth through face-to-face interaction, a here-and-now focus, self-disclosure, and intense emotional expression.

Parallel with the encounter group movement, more traditional group psychotherapy was evolving. S. R. Slavson, a leading group theoretician, founded the American Group Psychotherapy Association (AGPA) in 1942, which expanded dramatically during the 1960s and 1970s. The AGPA has had enormous impact in encouraging and fostering theory, training, and research in the field of group psychotherapy. Most notably, the AGPA worked successfully to develop standards for practitioners that included both theoretical and experiential training in group methods, while bringing the human growth movement into closer alliance with psychotherapeutic aims and procedures.

The historical origins of the group treatment format suggest that it was based in part on the functional advantages that it afforded: (1) an efficient mode of conveying information to individuals suffering from medical and psychological difficulties; (2) support and encouragement from individuals with similar difficulties; (3) a means of reducing or circumventing the resistances frequently encountered in an individual treatment format; (4) an interpersonal setting in which interactional patterns could be played out and systematically examined.

The group format provides the advantages that accrue when a troubled individual takes the risk of expressing and sharing within a social world. Yalom (1975) emphasizes the curative value of the group format based upon this principle of controlled socialization. The interaction of a number of individuals with somewhat similar difficulties can bring about the installation of hope and a sense of universality. It can impart information, convey a sense of altruism, enhance interpersonal learning, facilitate group cohesiveness, promote catharsis, and encourage the development of socialization skills.

Factors in the Selection of Format

There are a number of factors that guide the clinician in the choice of treatment format. Unfortunately, there is little research evidence upon which to base choices of treatment format. While research literature indicates that group can be an effective treatment format (e.g., Beutler et al., 1987; Budman & Springer, 1987), the research in this area is relatively disappointing in its volume and failure to establish the effective differential mechanisms of group treatment (Kaul & Bednar, 1986).

Family therapy outcome literature has begun to be more successful than group therapy literature, both in establishing a high level of clinical efficacy and in delineating the nature of the problems for which it is effective (Gurman, Kniskern & Pinsof, 1986; Jacobson, Follette & Pagel, 1986). However, this literature provides little information about the mechanisms of change or the circumstances under which this treatment format works best (Hazelrigg et al., 1987; Bednar, Burlingame & Masters, 1988).

The bulk of outcome literature is, of course, based on observations of individual therapy (Smith, Glass & Miller, 1980; Steinbrueck, Maxwell & Howard, 1983). Meta-analysis suggests that the individual therapy format is more effective than group (Nietzel et al., 1987) and more conventional reviews suggest somewhat tentatively that family and marital therapy may be at least as effective as group format (Haas & Clarkin, 1987).

A recent study by Pilkonis et al. (1984) investigated the relative outcomes of the three formats. Some differential treatment effects emerged that have implications for selective treatment planning. There was an advantage in favor of individual therapy in heightening self-awareness among lower-class patients, an advantage in favor of group and conjoint therapy in lessening interpersonal problems among chronically ill patients, and an advantage in favor of conjoint treatments among the satisfaction ratings of older patients' significant others.

Another clinically meaningful finding of this study was the observation that higher dropout rates occurred among individual patients whose significant others exhibited symptomatic behaviors.

Related research (Jacobson, Follette & Pagel, 1986) suggests that those marital partners who maintain a traditional role preference that emphasizes the husband's independence and the wife's dependence produce relatively poorer responses to treatment than couples with less traditional value systems. This finding not only emphasizes the importance of treatment of the dependence-independence value system to be discussed in Chapter 9, but extends this concept both to interactional patterns among couples and to specific treatment interventions. Such specific effects—clinically related to specific mediating goals for a specific individual and/or family—can serve as a model for future controlled research.

With the foregoing as background, we can now consider several variables that are important in the selection of treatment format: (1) the symptomatic or conflictual complexity of the chief complaint, (2) differential mediating goals of treatment, (3) life-stage context, (4) phase of disorder, (5) treatment efficiency, and (6) patient preferences.

Problem Complexity.   The nature of the symptom or conflict may indicate a positive response to one or another treatment format. In general, if the symptom or conflict reflects a transient or uncomplicated pattern that is under the control or direction of the individual patient, with little confounding from the current family environment, then it can be dealt with in either individual or group therapy. If, however, the symptom or conflict is significantly confounded by the current marital/family interpersonal environment, then family/marital therapy format may be the format of choice. Likewise, if the symptom or conflict is interpersonal in nature, extends beyond the home environment, is easily observed to be destructive in group interactions, and is largely ego syntonic, group therapy may be the format of choice. If the pattern is less easily observed in routine social involvements and is ego dystonic, individual treatment is frequently advantageous.

For example, in relationships between parents and an adolescent who emits delinquent behavior, the presence of a coercive interaction with the parents is a controlling influence that may require family intervention (Patterson & Forgatch, 1985). While they may have had little influence in the generation of the problem, the family may be adversely influenced by it and react to it poorly, only to then assist in maintaining the problem. To be more specific, reconsider the case of J.C., the 24-year-old student who believed he was Jesus Christ and who encountered treatment resources by happenstance while he was looking for the machines that he believed were controlling his mind. This case represents an illustration of how incorporating the patient's mother into the treatment transferred her concern and isolation into productive channels. Instead of feeling blamed for his condition, she could be a productive force in his treatment.

Similarly, if the problem directly reflects a marital conflict—a disturbed relationship between husband and wife—the conjoint treatment of the marital pair will likely be most efficient. If one member of a marital dyad is symptomatic, the selection between an individual and a marital format is more complicated (see agoraphobia as a paradigm below). Moreover, the research briefly reviewed above (e.g., Jacobson, Follette & Pagel, 1986) suggests that the selection of treatment format may be complicated by both the nature of the balance of the dependence and independence strivings between the marital partners and the orientation of the treatment model. Very traditional couples with well entrenched wife dependency-husband autonomy roles may do so poorly in conjoint marital therapy that individual formats of treatment may be indicated. Likewise, such a pattern may suggest use of a treatment method that focuses upon systems conflicts rather than on overt behaviors.

Agoraphobia as a Symptom Illustration. Research suggests the example of agoraphobia to illustrate the decisional process in selecting between individual and marital treatment formats when one individual in a marital pair is symptomatic. Agoraphobia represents an overt, behavioral, and measurable symptom that is clearly manifested by one individual and that is amenable (at least, in many situations) to treatment intervention. As such, agoraphobia is a wonderful experiment in nature for investigating the interplay between an individual symptom and the interactional context, and allows us to explore how symptoms like this respond to intervention. An investigation of this situation may provide some leads as to the genesis, course, and treatment outcome of an individual symptom that occurs in an interpersonal context.

The prevalence of agoraphobia among married women has generated several types of investigations: (1) those that seek to define patterns of interaction between an agoraphobic woman and her husband; (2) those that seek to determine the influence of the husband on the woman's treatment outcome; (3) those that assess the influence of the marriage on the outcome of treatments for the phobia; and (4) those that explore the use of the husband as a co-therapist.

In one sample, Buglass, Clarke, Henderson, Kreitman, and Presley (1977) found that the personalities of husbands of agoraphobic women were not distinguishable from those of the husbands of nonagoraphobic women. Moreover, the marriages of individuals in both groups were described in similar terms before the onset of symptoms. However, there are subgroups of agoraphobic women whose husbands are not so well adjusted. Out of a total of 36 cases involving the treatment of married agoraphobic women, Hafner (1979) found a subgroup of seven cases in which the husband displayed abnormal jealousy that adversely influenced the wife's response to treatment. In these cases, as the woman's symptoms improved, the husband's jealousy increased. Hafner and Ross (1984) suggest that wives' increased independence and autonomy may have caused these husbands to distance themselves emotionally from their spouses, leaving them confused and uncertain.

The foregoing point is well illustrated in the case of M.S., the young graduate student discussed in Chapter 4, who had to discontinue her education when she became obsessively preoccupied with germs and phobic of dirt. This young woman had elected to rise above the rather modest academic achievements represented both by her husband and by her parents. When she did so—and in spite of his best efforts—her husband became threatened by her autonomy, and her parents began placing great demands on her. Her position as "rescuer" in the family became overburdening and her husband began to lose the important role of provider.

For a patient whose symptoms express such a specific interpersonal dynamic as those of M.S., involvement of her husband in treatment may be considered to be crucial. While geography prevented direct involvement of M.S.'s parents in the treatment process, training both the patient and her husband in exposure procedures allowed the patient to respond to her parents more assertively when she visited them, while at the same time restoring a valued role of helper to her husband.

The effects of the sequential use of marital and exposure therapy for coexisting marital and phobic-obsessive problems in a manner similar to that used with M.S. have been reported by Cobb, McDonald, Marks, and Stern (1980). During the first phase of this reported treatment, 11 couples were seen conjointly in either a 10-session *in vivo* exposure treatment with the spouse as a co-therapist or behavioral marital therapy to reduce marital discord. Following a three-month break from treatment, each couple received the alternative treatment. At the completion of the two treatment phases, the couples given exposure treatment showed significant improvement in both phobic-obsessive and marital problems. In contrast, the couples given marital treatment showed improvement only of marital problems, suggesting the potential value of combined treatments.

In a manner that illustrates this latter point further, Munby and Johnston (1980) contacted 66 agoraphobic patients five to nine years after behavioral treatment for the phobia. Three different treatment trials were represented in the original treatment conditions. Trial 1 included patients who had been treated individually in conventional psychotherapy. Trial 2 included patients who had been treated with various behavioral strategies in an individual format. Trial 3 included married agoraphobic women who had been treated in a home-based treatment with the husband as a co-therapist, utilizing procedures similar to those in Trial 2. Patients in Trial 3 responded slightly better to treatment initially and made less recourse to other therapies during the follow-up period than those treated by the other methods. The authors note that this apparent superiority of conjoint treatment may result from the intended aim of this approach, i.e., to teach the patient and the spouse to deal with the agoraphobic symptom themselves, with a consequently lessened need for professional intervention.

There are several therapeutic implications arising from this accumulated set of data relative to the prescriptive treatment of a spouse with a well-defined symptom complex. First of all, phobic symptoms can be successfully treated with behavioral strategies such as desensitization and *in vivo* exposure whether in a individual, group, or marital/group format.

An important secondary consideration, however, involves the interpersonal context (i.e., the marital relationship) in which the symptomatic individual resides. In addition to the consideration of a marital treatment format for those cases in which systems issues are prevalent, a marital therapy format has been used sometimes simply to enlist the spouse as an ancillary therapist who helps to foster the exposure treatment of the spouse. Such a role also seems to lead to beneficial therapeutic outcome.

It appears that in a *minority* of cases, the clinical hypothesis that the symptom plays a functional role in sustaining a homeostatic marital relationship is true. Therefore, the clinician evaluating such cases must be alert to the need for marital treatment either concomitant with or prior to the treatment of the individual with the phobia.

Mediating Goals of Treatment. There is some evidence of a direct relationship between the format of treatment and the mediating goals of the treatment (Table 7.1). The various formats foster different kinds of therapeutic relationships, and different kinds of problem-solving styles. They may also appeal to different coping styles of the patients.

Table 7.1
Treatment Format and Mediating Goals of Treatment

Treatment Format	Mediating Goals of Treatment
Individual format	Extensive self-disclosure in private atmosphere; Development of intimacy and sharing with another; Development of intense identification, modeling, transference with therapist; Individualized attention during crisis.
Marital format	Direct observation of intensive spouse interdependence and conflict; Assessment of "both sides" of the conflict; Access to both sides of a collusive process; Development of mutual communication and problem-solving skills; Elicitation of support for symptomatic spouse from mate.
Family format	Observation and change in family communication and problem-solving skills; Increase in parenting skills with children.
Group format	Identification and modeling with other patients in the group; Use of advice and support from peers.

The individual format is the most private and leads to the most intensive attention toward the patient. This probably also leads to the more intense identification and modeling of the individual patient with the therapist. This modeling may be beneficial in some circumstances and potentially harmful in others. For example, functional individuals with subtle and conflicted intimate relationships will probably play them out in individual therapy where they can be examined and changed. The familiar case of J.I. is illustrative of this point. This 34-year-old woman experienced considerable difficulty with intimate relationships following her own stabbing and the rape and murder of her childhood friend. In individual therapy with a male therapist, J.I. initially presented as gregarious and nurturing. As the treatment intensified, however, she began to withdraw and to exhibit the angry core that one would expect, given her history. This portrayal, then, served as the means by which her pattern of denial and minimization could be approached.

With less functional, borderline patients, on the other hand, the intensity of an individual treatment format may lead to destructive acting out. An unstable, cyclic patient like M.D., whom we described in Chapter 3, may be quite unable to appreciate her own social stimulus value in individual therapy and the intensity of individual therapy may provoke the same type of acting out that occurs in other intimate relationships. To the degree that such acting out is not conducive to her developing either awareness or control, a group treatment format may be useful either as a supplement to individual treatment or as the primary treatment mode. A group format may reduce the intensity of treatment, thus posing less of a threat to the highly reactant patient's limits of tolerance. At the same time it may provide supportive control for externalizing and cyclic patients whose acting out may be destructive (Linehan, 1987).

Life-Stage Context.   Individuals who are especially dependent upon family support systems may benefit from a family treatment format. This group of patients includes children and young adolescents, as well as the elderly who reside with family. This group also includes individuals of all ages whose severity of illness is such that they depend upon others for support and direction (e.g., individuals with schizophrenia).

The case of J.C., the 24-year-old schizophrenic who believed he was Jesus Christ, comes to mind in support of this point. Given his dependency upon his mother for financial support, room, and board while attending school, it would make little sense to attempt to lessen his tie to the maternal bond. Indeed, by incorporating his mother as a key figure in the treatment program, one can bring to bear the power of the maternal bond as a reinforcer of appropriate responses.

Phase of Treatment and Course of Disorder.   There are some (usually quite serious) conditions which have a predictable course which can be matched with a planned treatment course. These conditions, such as schizophrenia and bipolar affective disorder, entail acute episodes interspersed with maintenance phases of the condition. Treatment must be planned and sequenced in concert with these phases.

Wynne (1983) has pointed out that given the condition we call schizophrenia the patient must be treated for the problem areas that are salient within the context of the different phases of the condition. The goal is not to treat schizophrenia *per se,* but to treat the problems that are prevalent at any given point in time. Phases of this condition that are noted include crisis points followed by acute psychosis, a subacute phase, and a subchronic phase. Wynne suggests matching these phases with a flexible approach always geared to the problems at hand. He suggests matching the problem phases with the use of family contacts (first-crisis contact) and medication, and then gradually beginning conjoint family meetings (acute psychosis) and psychoeducational approaches to the patient and family (subchronic phase).

Like schizophrenia, bipolar disorder has quite discernible acute and nonacute phases which should be countered with different treatment parameters, always depending upon the problems that are the foci of intervention (Clarkin, Haas & Glick, 1988). In general, crisis periods involving exacerbation of patient symptoms often require medication, acute hospitalization, or crisis intervention, and involve the social networks of the patient, especially the spouse and/or family. In between episodes, one must assess the problem areas and set the treatment for the mediating goals accordingly.

The phase of problem resolution achieved by the patient may also set the stage for treatment format. The further the patient has progressed along the phases of problem resolution (e.g., precontemplation, contemplation, action, and maintenance), the more clear the potential advantage of multi-person treatments. Group or family treatments for individuals who have achieved the action and maintenance phases are particularly pertinent. Individual treatments, on the other hand, are more clearly indicated in the precontemplation and contemplation phases of problem resolution.

Similarly, the complexity of the problem presented by the patient may have some bearing upon the nature of the format selected, as well. Group and family treatments may be particularly advantageous for providing the support and assistance needed in the resolution of symptomatic complaints. On the other hand, complex problems, representing recurrent, neurotic themes may at least initially benefit from individual therapy. Of course, the complexity of the problem must be weighted against the patient's stage of problem resolution in making these latter determinations.

Treatment Efficiency.   In general, an individual treatment format is the least economical of those considered here, since it requires the equal time of one patient and one therapist. The group format is more cost efficient than individual treatment in distributing therapist time among many patients. The efficiency of this format is made even greater, potentially, by the presence of group members as sources of advice and support. Likewise, the family format is efficient in that it approaches the difficulties of everyone in the family as they interlock with each other.

There are situations where treatment format may be chosen specifically because of its efficiency. Group exposure *in vivo* for agoraphobics is as effective as individually conducted exposure programs (Emmelkamp, 1986). For the alteration of such external symptomatic behaviors, the group not only saves therapist time, but also may provide the patient with coping models and lead to fewer dropouts.

In addition, spouses of patients may be included in the treatment in order to increase the efficiency of the learning and retention of learning. Barlow and Waddell (1985) have found that including the spouse in the behavioral treatment of agoraphobics leads to more utilization of desensitization in the follow-up period, for example.

Another form of efficiency is when the treatment will assist in spreading benefits to others. For example, Patterson (1982) has found that on follow up, after treating acting-out adolescents in a family treatment format, not only the identified patient but also siblings of the patient were less likely to exhibit problem behaviors than either matched controls or their siblings who did not receive the treatment.

Patient Preference.   In clinic settings, patients often strongly prefer individual treatment and see group treatment as a poor second choice even though similar benefits might be achieved by both formats (Budman et al., 1988). In the same way, couples come wanting conjoint treatment for what they clearly perceive as a relationship difficulty. Families sometimes seek out a family-oriented clinic when asking for help in dealing with a teenage member; at other times, they target the teenager as the "problem" and systematically avoid the implications of shared responsibility embodied in family therapy.

As we will note in later chapters, the establishment of the therapeutic alliance contributes as much variance, if not more, to good outcomes than the issues of treatment format and technique. Therefore, if a patient has a strong preference for a particular treatment format, resisting such a request may jeopardize the treatment alliance. Serious consideration should be given to the request for a certain treatment format, at least in the beginning phases of treatment.

Relative Indications

While research literature is still unclear on the subject, clinical wisdom suggests a number of relative indicators for differentiating among the probable benefits for individual, group, and family psychotherapy.

Individual Format.   The relative indications for the individual format of treatment include the following:

(1) The patient's symptoms or problematic ways of relating interpersonally are based on internal conflict and a coping style that manifests itself in repetitive life patterns that transcend the particulars of the current interpersonal environment.

(2) The patient is an adolescent or young adult who is striving for autonomy from family of origin.

(3) Problems or difficulties are of such an embarrassing nature that the privacy of individual treatment is required for the patient to feel safe.

Early in the treatment of J.I., for example, individual treatment was initiated. This decision initially was based upon the disruptive nature of the patient's anxiety responses following the automobile accident from which her symptoms of distress were reactivated. However, even after these symptoms came under some control, individual treatment continued for some time, based upon the assumption that J.I.'s anxiety and her inability to establish intimacy both were reflections of internal conflicts arising from her early trauma that extended beyond specific situations and people.

Family Format.   An individual patient is a member of a family. In systems oriented terms, the problem does not reside in the individual but in the family/social system.

This central tenet or hypothesis of the family movement has received some research support, but through time the hypothesis has been questioned, reshaped, and modified as it has been tested directly in research programs. It is no longer tenable to think that *all* individual pathology is under the control of the family system. However, even when the symptom bearer is schizophrenic and there is a major biological component in the development and manifestation of the condition, the family has an impact on the development of symptoms and on the short-term course of the individual's symptoms.

Before recommending family or marital treatment, we presuppose that the clinician will have evaluated the family/marital unit. In contrast to the evaluation of the patient for individual or group treatment format, the family/marital treatment must be preceded by a family/marital evaluation. Consequently, the clinician needs indications for when to include the family/marital unit in an evaluation.

Family/marital evaluation is almost always essential in recommending appropriate treatment in the following circumstances:

(1) A child or adolescent living in the home is the identified patient and focus of intervention.

(2) The presenting problem is sexual difficulty or dissatisfaction.

(3) The presenting problem is a family/marital difficulty that is serious enough to jeopardize the marital relationship, family stability, parenting ability of the couple, health, or job stability (e.g.,

child neglect or abuse, disruptive extramarital affairs, spouse battering, preoccupation with job problems, or instability).

(4) Recent stress and emotional disruption to the family (e.g., serious illness, injury, job loss, death) or a family milestone that has been experienced as disrupting (e.g., young adult leaving home, marriage, birth).

Following a family evaluation, the indications for a family treatment format include:

(1) Family problems are presented as such without any one family member designated as the identified patient; problems are predominantly within the relationship patterns.

(2) Family presents with current structured difficulties in intrafamilial relationships, with each person contributing collusively or openly to the reciprocal interaction problems.

(3) Adolescent acting-out behavior.

(4) Improvement of one family member has led to symptoms or signs of deterioration in another.

(5) Chronic mental disorder (e.g., schizophrenia) in one family member; there is a need for the family to cope with the condition.

Even short-term marital treatments within the context of any of several treatment models can be expected to achieve significant benefits. Yet, there may be some advantage favoring those treatments that attend to emotionally laden experiences that underlie interaction patterns rather than those that simply attend to the development of problem-solving skills (e.g., Johnson & Greenberg, 1985). Such findings serve to remind us that format alone is not a sufficient recommendation when we design differential treatments.

The case of J.C. again comes to mind as an example of a situation indicating the need for family intervention. In this case, the patient's chronic symptoms of schizophrenia and sole reliance on his mother highlight the need to provide support to established systems. Family intervention promised to provide both rejuvenation to the waning energies of J.C.'s mother and a method of enhancing productive mother-son communication that is likely to help the patient avoid hospitalization. In this latter case, a program that focused on training J.C.'s mother in how to communicate effectively and when to withdraw from rescuing efforts was selected.

This example of skill training can be contrasted with the usual marital therapy format in which the objectives may focus more on uncovering the highly charged issues that characterize the relationship and allow emotional expression than on building communication skills (cf. Johnson & Greenberg, 1985). Several related factors indicate the potential value of a marital format of treatment:

(1) Marital couple is committed to each other and presents with symptoms/conflicts that occur almost exclusively within the marriage.

(2) One marital partner has an individual symptom, e.g., agoraphobia or depression, that is maintained or exacerbated by the marital interaction patterns.

(3) Need to involve a spouse in an effective treatment program for the mate (e.g., spouse suffers from anorexia or obesity, or from phobias, and the mate is needed to assist in behavioral treatment, increase treatment compliance, and provide general support).

(4) The couple's relationships suggest the presence of some role flexibility.

Our obsessive-compulsive graduate student, M.S., for example, responded well to marital treatment. This format provided an opportunity for her husband to play an effective role in the treatment process, and thereby reduced his fear that he would be displaced if she were effectively treated and completed her education. This format also provided some needed nurturance to M.S. herself, who feared that she would lose important sources of comfort if she became self-sufficient and others came to depend too heavily on her.

Because the marital treatment format has so much face validity for marital problems presented as such, there is very little research but some clinical literature on when one would use the individual format for marital discord, including the not uncommon situation in which one partner wants treatment and the other does not (Bennun, 1984).

In the case of J.I., who suffered from post traumatic stress, for example, marital therapy served as an appropriate format late in treatment, after initial driving phobias were reduced and after the thematic pattern that characterized her resistence to intimacy was clarified in the course of individual treatment. At that point, the marital conflict could be approached as an example of her difficulty in establishing intimacy and as an opportunity to learn alternative interpersonal patterns.

Group Format. In developing treatment indicators for a group treatment format, we will distinguish homogeneous groups from heterogeneous groups, since this is a clinically and conventionally useful distinction (Frances, Clarkin & Marachi, 1980; Yalom, 1985). It is also a distinction that reflects an implicit predilection to focus treatment on either symptomatic behaviors as in homogeneous groups or on interpersonal conflict as addressed in heterogeneous groups.

Heterogeneous Group.   Group members in a heterogeneous group format present different symptoms, but frequently are found to be quite homogeneous with respect to interpersonal difficulties. While heterogeneous groups use a number of strategies and techniques, they are more likely than homogeneous groups to use experiential/gestalt and dynamic techniques.

The indications for heterogeneous group are:

(1) Patient's most pressing problems occur in current interpersonal relationships, both outside and inside family situations. Examples would include:

(a) patient is lonely and wishes to get closer to others; social and work inhibitions; excessive shyness;

(b) patient has an inability to share; manifests a cyclic coping style, including selfishness and exhibitionism; needs excessive admiration; has difficulty perceiving and responding to the needs of others;

(c) patient is excessively argumentative; oppositional toward authority; shows passive-aggressive traits;

(d) patient is excessively dependent; relatively unable to individuate from family of origin; difficulties with self-assertion;

(e) patient has an externalizing coping style in interpersonal situations; tends to act immediately on feelings.

(2) While the patient does not have predominant interpersonal problems, there may be other reasons to refer to heterogeneous group, such as:

(a) becomes intensely involved with individual therapist and cannot maintain self-observation;

(b) is extremely intellectualized and may benefit by being confronted about this defensive style.

The clinical example that comes to mind to illustrate these principles is that of M.D., the borderline patient presented in Chapter 3, whose cyclic instability led her to self-destructive acts of promiscuity and suicidal behavior. As we suggested earlier in this chapter, heterogeneous group treatment may provide support and control while limiting the degree of intensity to a level with which M.D. can cope.

Homogeneous Group.   Homogeneous groups are targeted for a specific symptom complex such as phobias, schizophrenia, alcoholism, etc. While these patients are homogeneous with reference to a specific symptom, they are, of course, heterogeneous on most nondiagnostic dimensions. The strategies and techniques of these groups tend to be educational, supportive, and behavioral.

The primary indication for a homogeneous group is when the patient presents with problems that are significantly attributable to a specific symptom complex for which a specialized group is available. These would include:

(1) specific impulse problems such as obesity, alcoholism, addictions, gambling, violence;

(2) problems adapting to and coping with acute, environmental stressors such as cardiac ailments, divorce, iliostomy, terminal illness;

(3) problems associated with a specific but transient developmental phase of life such as child-rearing, geriatrics;

(4) specific symptom constellations such as phobias, schizophrenia, bipolar disorder.

In contrast to M.D., whose borderline instability would not be expected to respond in a group environment in which all participants exhibited a similar cyclic coping pattern, H.D.—our 44-year-old, family-dependent but highly educated alcoholic—might respond to a homogeneous group intervention. The group format may provide needed confrontation and feedback and could solicit a commitment to a course of treatment and behavior that may exert greater force than that achieved in individual treatment. Such a group may also provide a laboratory for exposing family interactions that contribute to H.D.'s destructive behaviors, as well as a substitute support system for his absent family.

Typical Treatment Format Issues

While the indications and contraindications for the various treatment formats are helpful, they are somewhat abstract and need to be applied with flexibility in any individual situation. In order to add some figure and ground to the issues, we will briefly enumerate some of the typical clinical situations that force the issue of which format might be the most beneficial.

Symptomatic Spouse: Individual vs. Marital Format. It is not uncommon for a married adult to present to a clinic or therapist with mild to moderate symptomatic complaints, along with some degree of marital conflict or dissatisfaction. These individuals often come for treatment alone, and then during the initial evaluation interview they focus on their complaints and difficulties with their spouse and, at times, their children. Sometimes they have reached the point of "action" in their problem resolution efforts, and are openly entertaining (or threatening!) separation and/or divorce. Some individuals may conceive of all their difficulties as being due to the marriage and assume that divorce would be the solution. Often they do not want the spouse to know they are seeking help.

The obvious questions arise: What is the spouse like? Does the spouse contribute to the individual's symptoms and conflicts? Or is the individual the main focus of difficulty? Can the individual obtain symptom relief without involvement of the spouse in treatment? How are the individual's symptoms and interpersonal difficulties affecting his/her parenting skills and the adjustment of the children?

In the case of J.I., initially the intensely disruptive nature of her post-traumatic symptoms argued in favor of an individually oriented treatment. Later, however, introducing her husband to the treatment sessions allowed an opportunity for her to practice emotional sharing, provided support for him, and helped her observe the methods she used for maintaining distance. Had a marital treatment format been introduced earlier, it would have been very easy for the patient to lose sight of the recurrent nature of her interpersonal pattern and to treat the marital interaction as the problem rather than as either a source of support or an example of the problem.

A marital or family evaluation is useful in situations such as that presented by J.I. in order to help answer some of the questions that might influence which format of treatment will be the most efficient one with which to begin treatment.

YAVIS Patient: Group vs. Individual Format. The YAVIS patient (young, attractive, verbal, intelligent, single) is functional, minimally symptomatic, and presents with difficulties in interpersonal relationships, but is positively motivated for treatment. Will such a patient benefit more from individual or group therapy? The research is not clear in providing an answer to this question. There are no clear differences favoring one or the other format across patients and situations (e.g., Budman et al., 1988), and probably at this time the issue can be settled only by assessing the specific issues in the individual case. Some patients are shy and want the privacy of individual treatment, and place overriding value on its status and methods.

As a general rule, group treatment is an efficient procedure with YAVIS patients who have an overall good adjustment and relatively mild or situationally induced symptoms. Symptoms such as this are likely to respond to a variety of interventions, as long as these interventions embody the caring and supportive qualities that we consider to be the nonspecific, core ingredients of effective treatment.

We observed earlier in this chapter that there is an additional consideration that may also differentiate between selecting an individual and group format. This consideration bears upon the stage of problem resolution achieved by the patient. To reiterate, YAVIS patients who have achieved the problem resolution stage of action or maintenance may be especially good candidates for group therapy. Among these high functioning patients, however, a failure to have achieved this level of problem resolution probably does not contraindicate the use of group therapy, and we would still consider the option of individual therapy first in the case of individuals who are at the stage of precontemplation or contemplation.

The Individuating Adolescent.   The adolescent living at home who is attempting to gain some degree of independence but who still regresses to power struggles and acting-out behavior can serve to illustrate the indicators both for family and individual therapy formats. In general, the older the adolescent/young adult and the more well adjusted, the more likely the individual can benefit from individual or group treatment. This implies that the growing adolescent who is still living in the family of origin already must have established some degree of independence from the family environment and be motivated for personal change in order to profit from individual therapy. In contrast, the younger the adolescent and the more he/she is enmeshed and existing in a conflicted state of dependence-conflict with the parents, the more likely that some family intervention will be needed until individual treatment is possible.

THE TREATMENT MODE OF MEDICAL MANAGEMENT

Medical modes of treatment have been found to be beneficial in their own right not only for the alleviation of certain symptoms but also for preparing the patient for psychosocial intervention. The major medical modes of intervention include the use of psychotropic medications (oral administration or by intramuscular or intravenous injections) and electroconvulsive therapy (ECT). We believe that while psychoactive medications can alleviate biological abnormalities and help to relieve certain symptoms, patients learn little from the use of the medication, which is best used to alleviate the pain of psychological and physical symptoms and prepare the patient for learning more adaptive coping strategies. At their worst, some psychotropic medications mask problems and entail harmful, albeit rarely lasting, side effects.

For differential treatment planning, the clinician needs to know the general classes of psychotropic medications and the indications for their possible use. It should be noted that many medical illnesses, as well as the drugs used for their treatment, can cause changes in mood and thought. These physical changes can be associated with behaviors that are mistaken for functional psychiatric symptoms. Evaluation of the role of physical and iatrogenic effects in symptom development is necessary before medications are prescribed. Non-physician practitioners have found it helpful to have a working relationship with a physician (general practitioner, internist, psychiatrist) who can evaluate and prescribe medications if needed in conjunction with psychotherapy.

History and Classes of Medications

There are a number of ways to classify medications: (1) by chemical structure (e.g., phenothiazines, tricyclics, benzodiazepines); (2) by their neurochemical mode of action (e.g., monoamine oxidase inhibitors); (3) by their psychological mode of action (e.g., central nervous system stimulants or depressants); (4) by their dominant clinical effect (e.g., antipsychotics, antidepressants, antianxiety agents, antimanic medications). In this presentation we will use the latter classification system, both because it is closer than the other systems to the clinical reality of treatment selection and because it is more easily communicable to the clinician who does not have current knowledge about chemical structure and neurochemical action.

Antipsychotic Medications. The antipsychotic or neuroleptic medications include but are not limited to the phenothiazines (Thorazine, Mellaril, and Stelazine), the thioxanthenes (Taractan, Nayane) and the butyrophenones (Haldol).

The efficacy of antipsychotic medications has been most clearly established with schizophrenia (see Klein et al., 1980, for a review), both during hospitalization for a symptomatic phase and during aftercare following hospitalization. Schooler et al. (1980) found that while over 70 percent of the patients in a placebo group relapsed and were rehospitalized within one year, this rate was significantly reduced by maintenance on fluphenazine. While a combination of fluphenazine and role-training procedures was apparently deleterious for some patients, in general the combination treatment produced additive benefits.

One of the most exciting and promising developments in the treatment of individuals with schizophrenia via a combination of medication and psychosocial intervention derives from research on "expressed emotion" (EE) (Brown, Birley & Wing, 1972). As previously noted, these investigations have revealed that high EE families, characterized by the presence of critical comments, hostility, and overinvolvement with the schizophrenic member, precipitate higher relapse rates than low EE families. Subsequent treatment studies involving the combination of family management and antipsychotic medication have consistently found beneficial effects in the form of comparatively fewer relapses and rehospitalizations for combination treatments over unitary ones (Falloon et al., 1982; Leff et al., 1982). The 24-year-old J.C., whom we have described periodically throughout this volume and who believed he was "Jesus," would certainly be a candidate for such a combination treatment as that suggested by this research.

NIMH (Schooler & Keith, 1984) currently is undertaking a multisite study of the combined effects of fluphenazine and a version of behavioral family management, which includes psychoeducation, communication training, and problem-solving skills (Falloon et al., 1985). Since the side effects of antipsychotic medication are serious and lasting when they occur (e.g., tardive dyskinesia) and since a substantial number of schizophrenics on medication alone relapse, it is anticipated that this multisite investigation will shed light on the interaction of various medication delivery formats (time of ingestion, dosage, blood level monitoring, etc.) and different family management strategies.

It should be emphasized that the nonmedical clinician who provides psychosocial intervention should be knowledgeable of, and alert to, the signs of adverse side effects of antipsychotic medications. If family management is included in the treatment plan, family members also can be taught about these side effects and they, too, can be helpful in detecting them. When educated about typical side effects, family members usually provide information about early signs of negative drug reactions that they have noticed with their family member, and this information can be incorporated into treatment education.

Antidepressant Medications. The most common antidepressant medications include tricyclic antidepressants (TCAs) (e.g., Elavil, Tofranil, Sinequan), second generation antidepressants (e.g., Trazodone, Ludiomil, Prozac), and monoamine oxidase inhibitors (MAOIs) (e.g., Nardil, Parnate, Marplan). The effectiveness of antidepressants on the symptoms of depression during acute depressive episodes has been documented in numerous clinical trials (Klein et al., 1980). It is with serious depression, as noted by anhedonia, mutism, etc., that these medications are most clearly indicated.

The value of antidepressant medication among outpatient, nonpsychotic depressed individuals remains controversial. In a recent review, Klerman (1986) notes that the majority of studies have shown the equivalence or superiority of brief psychotherapy compared to antidepressant medication (usually a tricyclic). This conclusion is supported by studies by McLean and Hakstian (1979); Blackburn, Bishop, Glen, Whalley, and Christie (1981); Bellack, Hersen, and Himmelhoch (1983); Gadow (1985) and Beutler et al. (1987). Studies comparing medication with social-skills training (Bellack, Hersen & Himmelhoch, 1983), response prevention for obsessive-compulsive disorder (Christensen, Hadzi-Pavlovic, Andrews & Mattick, 1987), and interpersonal psychotherapy (Weissman et al., 1981) have found drug and psychotherapy modes to be equivalent. Other studies, especially those employing cognitive and behavioral therapies, have found some superiority in favor of the psychosocial treatments relative to medication alone among certain groups of depressed adults (Steinbrueck et al., 1983; Beutler et al., 1987), hyperactive children (Gadow, 1985), and patients with phobic disorder (Mavissakalian, 1986).

While neither medication nor psychotherapy shows a clear superiority among most studies of moderately depressed, outpatient groups, it is often assumed that the combination of the two modalities of treatment will be synergistic (i.e., the combined effect is greater than the sum of the two component treatment effects). The data, however, are inconsistent. For example, Blackburn et al. (1981) found the combination of tricyclics and cognitive therapy superior to either alone among depressed outpatients, but not among patients in a general practice. Bellack et al. (1980) found no combination effect of antidepressants and social-skills therapy; and Gadow (1985) found no additive effects for behavior therapy and antihyperactive medications among children.

Psychopharmacologists have often held that patients with endogenous depression (RDC criteria or DSM-III Melancholia) usually respond better to either tricyclics or ECT than to psychosocial treatments alone. However, efficacy studies of psychotherapy for endogenous patients have challenged this conventional wisdom (Klerman, 1986). While medications do appear to do best among those with endogenous depression, Blackburn et al. (1981) found that both endogenous and nonendogenous patients responded to cognitive therapy to equal degrees. Likewise, Kovacs (1980) did not find a correlation between the presence of endogenous symptoms and poor response to cognitive therapy.

Similar issues have been raised with respect to the maintenance of treatment gains. Tricyclic medications have demonstrated effectiveness in preventing relapse among those with recurrent unipolar depression (Davis, 1976). In several studies of maintenance treatment with combined medication and psychosocial therapy (Klerman et al., 1974; Covi, Lipman, Derogatis, Smith & Pattison, 1974), antidepressants were shown to be relatively effective in symptom reduction while the psychosocial treatments (IPT, group therapy, marital therapy) were advantageously effective in producing changes in interpersonal functioning.

Translating these findings to clinical practice, we would probably not consider antidepressant medications seriously in the case of C.A., the 36-year-old woman described in Chapter 3, whose depression was recurrent secondary to her father's death and the subsequent death of her fiancé. In a patient with similar vegetative signs and recurrent depressions, however, and in which there was less indication of situationally induced onsets, a medication trial would be indicated. The intensity and instability of the depressions noted by M.D., our borderline patient with a history of recurrent affairs and suicidal behaviors, may warrant medication consultation to determine if the severity and cyclic nature of these depressions would be responsive to pharmacotherapy. The constraining factor in this decision, of course, would be the concern that the patient would abuse the medication and use it in her suicidal acts.

Antimanic Medications. A diagnostic distinction between Bipolar Disorders and Unipolar Depressive Disorders is central for medication management. In the assessment of patients with mood irregularities (depressed or elated), it is important to assess the history of one or more periods of elevated, expansive, or irritable mood (see Decision tree for Differential Diagnosis of Mood Disturbances, page 380, DSM-III-R). Bipolar Disorder is characterized by one or more manic or hypomanic episodes, usually with an accompanying history of depressive episodes.

The major prophylactic antimanic medications are lithium (Eskalith) and carbamazepine (Tegretol). Lithium and antipsychotics such as chlorpromazine and haloperidol have well-established efficacy in the management of acute manic episodes (Klerman, 1986). Carbamazepine (Tegretol), as well as benzodiazepines such as Lovazepam and Clonazepam, also have been used effectively in the treatment of acute manic episodes. However, there are only a few investigations of the combined effects of medication and psychotherapy in the long-term treatment of bipolar patients. It is noteworthy, however, that Shakir et al. (1979) effectively have utilized a combination of lithium treatment and group therapy, while Davenport and colleagues (Davenport, Ebert, Adland & Goodwin, 1976; Davenport & Adland, 1988) have utilized successfully a combination of lithium and couples group treatment in treating bipolar patients and their spouses. Since the bipolar patient has recurring episodes which disrupt family life, couples groups may be a particularly reasonable vehicle for enhancing the marital dyad's ability to cope with the instability of the patient's condition.

Antianxiety Agents. The most used antianxiety agents are benzodiazepines (Librium, Valium, Tranxene, Serax, Activan, Xanax). Nonbenzodiazepines (e.g., Buspar), propanediol carbamates (e.g., Miltown) and barbiturates (e.g., Ludimil) are older anxiolytics and are rarely used today.

Klerman (1986) notes a growing consensus that alprazolam (Xanax) and clonazepam (Klonopin) reduce panic attacks. For example, panic attacks (patients with diagnoses of Panic disorder with agoraphobia, or Panic disorder without agoraphobia) have been successfully reduced with alprazolam (Xanax) (Carr & Sheehan, 1984) as well as with several antidepressant medications (TCAs and MAOIs). Klerman observes, however, that there currently are no studies on the effects of drugs on the avoidant behaviors that are often associated with anxiety.

A review of studies on the combined effects of exposure therapy and imiprimine (Mavissakalian, 1988) suggests that these two modalities of treatment have mutual potentiating effects on phobic symptoms. That is, the combined effects are superior to the sum of the individually administered treatments. Moreover, both treatments exert an effect on panic symptoms, although whether or not these latter effects are synergystic (i.e., mutually potentiating) remains open to question. Behavioral exposure, moreover, appears to positively affect avoidant as well as panic behaviors, making the combined treatments advantageous in those cases where breadth of effect is a significant consideration. In spite of these positive findings, however, there is little evidence as to which specific behavior therapy techniques affect panic attacks in any way analogous with the way exposure affects avoidant behaviors.

Two examples come to mind to illustrate differential response to medications among patients with anxiety disorders. The reader will recall the case of M.S. from our earlier discussions. This young female graduate student was forced to terminate her academic pursuits when she became obsessed with thoughts of germs and dirt. She subsequently developed stereotypic cleaning rituals and phobias of dirty dishes and clothes. Neither tricyclic antidepressants nor anxiolytics were successful in providing significant relief from her rituals, but a benzodiazepine was helpful in reducing the intensity of her agitation and allowed continued psychosocial intervention that did eventually produce moderate success.

As a point of contrast, chlorimiprimine, a tricyclic that has been used with increasing success for the treatment of obsessive-compulsive rituals, was used successfully with A.D., the 57-year-old college professor who engaged in ritualized hoarding behaviors. In this latter case, the lack of motivation rendered individual psychotherapy of little value, but somatic treatment, nonetheless, exerted a direct effect on the intensity of his compulsive symptoms.

Referring Patients for Medication

DSM-III-R diagnoses are probably most helpful in medication treatments, but even here the same DSM-III-R diagnosis among several patients does *not* assure the same etiology, pathogenesis, neurochemistry, course, or drug treatment response (Frances, Clarkin & Perry, 1984). Furthermore, many patients present with a clinical picture that does not meet the clear, clean boundaries represented in DSM-III-R diagnostic labels, and many patients present with "multiple diagnoses" (meeting criteria for one or more diagnoses, such as Schizophrenia and Major Depression and/ or Schizoaffective Disorder). While diagnoses based upon syndromes (a categorical way of thinking) are helpful in determining who requires treatment, *dimensional* assessment of target symptom severity will better assist in referral for medication management and for continued assessment of the patient's response to medical treatment.

Before initiating a medication regime, the psychotherapist should take a careful history of what medications and doses were used in the past, and the nature of the patient's particular response. If the patient has responded positively to an antidepressant in previous treatments, it may be an argument for using it again. Moreover, a major problem with any somatic treatment regimen is patient compliance. If a patient is treated medically, the psychotherapist needs to initiate frequently some discussion with the patient about the medication, its rationale, compliance with the regime, and effects.

SUMMARY AND COMMENT

We have described two major modalities of mental health treatment: Psychosocial and Medical. Within the psychosocial modality of intervention, formats typically used include individual treatment, group treatment, and family treatment. While these modalities have different indicators and enabling factors, they can also be used in combination. The principal aims of these treatments are different. Family and marital therapies are designed to view systems rather than symptoms and individual problems. Hence, they are of greatest advantage in reducing interpersonal conflict or enhancing separation efforts among patients with cyclic or externalized defenses, or when patients have achieved the state of "action" in problem-solving efforts. Conversely, individual therapy is most clearly indicated when problem complexity suggests neurotiform patterns and when problem-solving efforts are in preactivating phases.

Medical modes of therapy include a variety of medications. The specific uses of these medications are primarily determined by the nature of the symptom picture presented. The major areas of intervention include psychotic confusion, anxiety, depression, and mania. Since medications typically affect the primary symptoms and universally include side effects, psychosocial interventions may be useful for maintenance and for the correction of interpersonal difficulties.

In this chapter, we have described some of the conditions and indicators for the various modes and formats of treatment. However, the nature of mode and format will also be affected by factors which we will describe in greater detail in later chapters. The defensive style of the patient may also have important implications for the selection of psychosocial formats.

We will see the nature of these decisions as we begin to describe the nature of psychosocial treatments in greater detail.

SUGGESTED READINGS

American Medical Association, Department of Drugs, Division of Drugs and Technology. (1986). *Drug evaluations,* 6th ed. (Chapters 5–8). Chicago, IL: American Medical Association.

Falloon, I. R. H., Boyd, J. L. & McGill, C. W. (1985). *Family management of schizophrenia.* New York: Guilford.

Gurman, A. S., Kniskern, D. P. & Pinsof, W. M. (1986). Research on marital and family therapies. In S. L. Garfield & A. E. Bergin (Eds.), *Handbook of psychotherapy and behavior change* (pp. 565–624). New York: John Wiley.

Jacobson, N. S. & Margolin, G. (1979). *Marital therapy: Strategies based on several learning and behavior exchange principles.* New York: Brunner/Mazel.

Klein, D. F., Gittelman, R., Quitkin, F. & Rifkin, A. (1980). *Diagnosis and drug treatment of psychiatric disorders: Adults and children,* 2nd ed. Baltimore, MD: Williams & Wilkins.

Klerman, G. L. (1986). Drugs and psychotherapy. In S. L. Garfield & A. E. Bergin (Eds.), *Handbook of psychotherapy and behavior change,* 3rd ed. (pp. 777–818). New York: John Wiley and Sons.

Linehan, M. M. (1981). A social-behavioral analysis of suicide and parasuicide: Implications for clinical assessment and treatment. In J. F. Clarkin & H. I. Glazer (Eds.), *Depression: Behavioral and directive intervention strategies* (pp. 229–294). New York: Garland STPM Press.

Yalom, I. D. (1985). *The theory and practice of group psychotherapy,* 3rd ed. New York: Basic Books, Inc.

8

Treatment Frequency and Duration

Treatment intensity reflects the integration of treatment duration with the frequency and timing of treatment visits. In this chapter, special attention will be given to the indicators for time-limited treatments and to those conditions that indicate variations in the frequency and spacing of treatments. We will end this chapter with a rarely discussed topic: the conditions under which one might select a treatment of zero duration and frequency—that is, the indicators for not treating a given patient.

TREATMENT DURATION

Logically, treatment terminates when the goals negotiated between patient and therapist throughout treatment have been accomplished. It is clear that if the goals of the treatment are crisply conceptualized, clearly articulated in the therapist's mind, negotiated and renegotiated between therapist and patient, and measurable, then the duration of the treatment can be specified within reasonable parameters. However, there are complications to this formula. Sometimes the goals of the treatment are not agreed upon by therapist and patient, and the therapist may utilize therapeutic time to get the patient to adopt what he or she considers to be more reasonable goals. At other times, the duration of the treatment is one of the key elements in getting the goals of the treatment accomplished (e.g., time-limited treatment may use the brevity of treatment to keep the patient motivated). And, unfortunately too often, it is not clear how long it will take to achieve the treatment goals even if they are acceptable both to patient and therapist and are appropriate to the treatment selected.

Treatment duration is, in one very real sense, an outcome of whatever occurs in the treatment process and progress. If the patient does not get into the process of treatment (e.g., responds to the treatment and the therapist with hostility, does not do therapy homework, does not talk in group therapy sessions), then the treatment will either take longer or be aborted early. If the patient, on the other hand, works appropriately but still does not respond with symptomatic improvement, some therapists may recommend that the length of treatment be extended in hopes that further work will yield results. Other therapists may refer the patient. Similarly, if the patient responds to the initial stages of therapy, the therapist and patient may recognize this accomplishment as either a call to quit or a call for longer treatment and readjusted goals, again depending upon a variety of factors.

Finally, there are certain patient and treatment matches that, themselves, dictate the duration of treatment. For example, some symptoms (e.g., simple phobias, situational somatic stress reactions) and even a more complex problem like major depression can be attacked successfully and cost efficiently in brief therapy (Budman, 1981; Beutler & Crago, 1987; VandenBos & DeLeon, 1988). There are other more chronic situations, e.g., a patient with a number of clear manic episodes, that need a treatment involving many treatment episodes over a long—if not interminable— period of time.

History of Therapy Duration

In an interesting discussion of the history of psychodynamic therapy since its beginnings with Freud and his followers, Malan (1963) has elucidated the factors that have lengthened therapy from its initial and intended brief duration. In his exploration of effective therapeutic techniques, Freud proceeded from hypnosis through suggestion to free association; all the while the therapist was becoming more passive. It is a story, in Malan's eyes, of patient resistances to recognizing the overdetermination of symptoms, the necessity for working through the roots of neurosis in early childhood, the nature of transference and dependence, and the inevitability of negative transference in the termination phase of treatment. In each instance, recognition of what the patient was resisting was met with therapists' increasing passivity, as reflected in the therapist's willingness to follow the lead of the patient, a sense of timelessness being conveyed to the patient, and increasing therapist preoccupation with even deeper and earlier experiences of the patient.

The history of behavior therapy stands in some contrast to that of psychodynamic therapy. Like psychoanalysis, behavior therapy was initially designed to be brief, and to some extent behavior therapy has remained so (Wilson, 1981). This brevity is largely due to the specificity of behavioral goals in this treatment orientation. Behavior therapy lasting between 25 to 50 sessions is commonplace, and rarely exceeds 100 sessions (Wilson, 1981). For example, the average treatment at a metropolitan behavioral therapy center was found to be 50 weekly, one-hour sessions. Like its dynamic therapy counterpart, there are a number of important patient characteristics that tend to lengthen the treatment, including poor or variable patient motivation, problem severity and complexity, failure to accomplish therapy assignments, and lack of social and family support.

Dose-Effect Relationships in Outpatient Psychotherapy

In general, the greater the total amount of treatment (in numbers of sessions) and the longer the duration of treatment, the greater the benefit to the patient. In 20 of 33 studies reviewed, Orlinsky and Howard (1978) found a positive relationship between the therapeutic benefit and the total number of therapy sessions. In another 22 studies which specified the total time (duration) spent in therapy, 12 found a positive relationship between outcome and duration while nine demonstrated a near zero magnitude relationship.

These general conclusions about the relationship between duration, frequency, and outcome are too broad to be clinically useful in the specific case. However, more recently Howard, Kopta, Krause, and Orlinsky (1986) have demonstrated a dose-effect relationship based upon a narrow review of well-controlled studies of individual therapy. Data from 15 samples on 2,431 outpatients in individual (nonbehavioral) therapies were analyzed. The results were in the form of estimates (based on the best-fit lines produced by a probit analysis of each set of raw data) of the expected percentage improved for the selected number of sessions. Expressed in this way, the results indicated that 10 to 18 percent of patients can be expected to show some improvement before the first session, and by eight sessions 48 to 58 percent can be expected to have measurably improved. About 75 percent of the patients showed measurable improvement after 26 sessions.

In order further to refine the dosage-effect relationship, the authors divided the patients into three rough "diagnostic" categories: depression, anxiety, and borderline-psychotic. For those patients with anxiety and depression, 50 percent improved by 13 sessions of treatment. In contrast, for the borderline-psychotic group, treatment effects took longer to produce—a comparable 50 percent of the patients did not improve by self-ratings until sometime between the 13th and 26th sessions, and by clinical ratings not until the interval between 26 and 52 sessions.

As the authors point out, the dosage-effect curve could be used as a guide for peer and clinical review, and for setting reasonable treatment time limits. The use of the specific dosage-effect curve generated by these authors is limited by the sample they used (outpatients in nonbehavioral individual-format treatments), and methodological limitations (crude and narrow measures of patient improvement, gross diagnostic assignment made by the reviewers). Nevertheless, the methodology has tremendous value for more precise delineation of treatment duration in differential therapeutic treatment planning.

Indications for Duration of Least Restrictive Treatments

Having suggested that treatment duration is in many ways the outcome of the treatment process, we can now specify some of the relative indications for varying treatment duration among the least restrictive treatments available, as they derive from the clinical and research literature.

Indications for Crisis Intervention. Butcher and Koss (1978) note that it is quite difficult to investigate the effectiveness of crisis intervention because of the wide range and diversity of individuals and problems that present for a rapid intervention. It is an easier research task to describe the characteristics of individuals who present in crisis, and to identify what happens to the affected person during and following intervention. Some of the relative indications for crisis intervention can be identified in this way, as can patient-enabling factors that allow outpatient crisis intervention to be helpful.

Diagnostically, patients who come for crisis intervention run the spectrum from transient situational disorders, to neurotic and personality disorders, to psychotic episodes (Jacobson et al., 1965). The triggering event for requesting crisis help may range from exacerbations of severe symptoms, drug-induced symptoms, eruption of family violence, responses to death and loss, and diagnosis of serious medical conditions. Whatever the specific symptoms and the precipitating events, there is a sense of urgency that is conveyed by the patient and often the patient's support system (family or intimate others) to which the mental health worker resonates. This urgency may be conveyed by patient's symptoms, level of distress, suicidal threats or behavior, psychotic behavior that is dangerous to self or others, disruptions to the family environment, severe depression, aggressive behavior that is out of control, etc. All of these patterns may be severe enough to warrant urgent and intense treatment attention.

Almost always, crisis events are accompanied by an eruption of symptoms. Indeed, if manifest symptoms predate the crisis events, crisis intervention probably will not be a sufficient treatment alone. In this case, more intensive treatment is indicated. To the degree that symptoms are *initiated* by the crisis rather than simply exacerbated by it, the precipitating stress can become the focus of the intervention (e.g., serious injury or illness, death of family member or loved one, job loss, extramarital affair). On the other hand, if symptoms exist before the crisis, then treatment is focused more broadly and in concert with the principles of the continuing treatment regimen. More suggestions for focusing treatment in this latter case will be presented in Chapter 11.

Indications for Time-Limited Therapy. One way for the clinician to organize his/her thinking is to evaluate the patient for the possibility of planned brief (i.e., time-limited) treatment. Only if the patient does not meet the criteria for brief therapy should one consider open-ended intervention or planned long-term therapy as an alternative.

In the current clinical climate, the enthusiasm for brief therapy is so high that it is considered by many to be the treatment to be tried first for every patient suitable for psychotherapy (Wolberg, 1965; Budman & Gurman, 1983). We take exception to this conclusion and believe that there are many clinical situations in which time-limited treatment would be inappropriate, even as a first trial. Most psychotherapy research has been done on brief and time-limited therapy. In fact, there is a concern among those in the psychotherapy research community that the investigation of manualized, long-term therapies is technically beyond our grasp at this point in time. Consequently, literature comparing brief and longer-term therapy is sparse. On the other hand, clinically there is a growing consensus about the nature of the indications for time-limited treatment.

For any treatment to be effective, time limited or not, the patient must be willing to remain in the process long enough to receive a therapeutic dose. Hence, a first consideration in defining the indicators for time-limited treatment must be to understand what factors contribute to premature termination. Even a cursory review of this literature will reveal that there are a number of patient characteristics that are indicators of dropout risk. These include low education and income, minority status (Baekeland & Lundwall, 1975; Garfield, 1986b), and the presence of externalized and somatic symptoms (DuBrin & Zastowny, 1988). All of these factors indicate that maintaining patient investment and motivation will be problematic.

Clearly, therapist communication and sensitivity also contribute to early dropout (e.g., Goldstein, 1973; Tracey, 1987). Hence, patient factors must be considered in concert with therapist-controlled aspects of treatment. In later chapters we will address methods of preparing poorly motivated patients for treatment and developing communication styles that enhance treatment progress. However, since time-limited treatment tends to keep poorly motivated patients in treatment somewhat longer than open-ended treatment (cf. Goldstein, 1973), one also might conclude that patients who are at high risk for premature termination may be candidates for time-limited treatment. Thus, some potential indicators for planned, time-lim-

ited treatment may include characteristics that weigh against the motivation for long-term, time-unlimited treatment.

It also is clear that one cannot consider the duration of a treatment
without at the same time considering the breadth or complexity of the
patient's problem. Therapists as a group tend to consider short-term treatment as most appropriate for patients with situational reactions, narrow
band and unidimensional problems (Budman & Gurman, 1983; Burlingame & Behrman, 1987). We accept this attitude in asserting that the
more complex the problem, the more the treatment objectives should be
focused on the driving, underlying conflicts, and the longer it probably
will be. Conversely, the less complex the problem, the more the focus and
goals can be restricted to changing symptomatic presentations. The authors
of the various brief therapy models (e.g., behavioral, cognitive, interpersonal, psychodynamic) have specified the various patient indications and
contraindications for the time-limited approach.

As Tables 8.1 and 8.2 indicate, the rather stringent enabling factors
articulated by the dynamic therapist's approach to conflict resolution in
brief therapy are in contrast to the few enabling factors articulated by the
more cognitive and cognitive/behavioral approaches whose focal aims are
symptomatic change. Some of these enabling factors will be noted in our
discussion of the investigations of the brief treatments of depression later
in this chapter. In this sense, the symptom-oriented brief therapies are
probably more versatile than the conflict-resolving brief therapies.

Tables 8.1 and 8.2 are less a list of indications and more a list of
occasions (the types of problems) for which there are detailed treatment
packages that can be applied to these problems. Many of these brief treatment packages, utilizing a mixture of treatment strategies and techniques,
have been validated by research. Hence, the accompanying tables do not
contain an exhaustive list of indications for brief therapy, but rather present examples of the current range of problem areas that have been successfully approached in brief therapy packages.

Generalizing from two representative models—the psychodynamic
model, representing conflict-oriented approaches and the cognitive/behav-
ioral model, representing symptom-oriented treatment—one gets a sense
of the qualities of the patient and the kinds of problems that are suited
for a brief or focused intervention.

The Example of Time-Limited Therapies for Depression. Over the last 15
years there has been a great deal of research on time-limited treatments of
individuals who complain of mild to moderate depressions. Brief treatment
packages, usually conducted in an individual treatment format, utilizing
behavioral, cognitive-behavioral, and interpersonal therapy models and
treatment strategies, have been researched and found helpful. This effort

Table 8.1

Indications for the Brief Conflict-Focused Therapies

Indications

(1) Focal intrapsychic conflict involving separation (Mann, 1973), Oedipal issues (Sifneos, 1972), narcissistic injury (Goldberg, 1973), or stress response syndromes (Goldberg, 1973; Horowitz, 1976).

(2) Goal is character change in one focal area.

Enabling factors

(1) Patient has had at least one significant relationship in early childhood.

(2) Patient relates quickly, flexibly, and openly to consultant.

(3) Patient can focus on a central conflict in the evaluation.

(4) Patient is willing to examine feelings and behavior, including those that occur during the evaluation toward the evaluator.

(5) Patient has relatively high ego strength as evidenced by educational, work, and sexual performance.

(6) Patient is motivated to change behavior and understand self better.

(7) Patient is intelligent and able to communicate verbally thoughts, feelings, and fantasies.

Table 8.2

Indications for the Brief Symptom-Focused Therapies

Indications

(1) Anxiety disorders: agoraphobia (Gelder, Marks, Wolff & Clarke, 1967), panic disorder, generalized anxiety, hyperventilation, examination anxiety, interpersonal anxiety.

(2) Depression of mild to moderate severity (Lewinsohn, Biglan & Zeiss, 1976; Rush, Beck, Kovacs & Hollon, 1977; McLean & Hakstian, 1979; Klerman, Weissman, Rounsaville & Chevron, 1984).

(3) Deficits in social skills (Argyle, Bryant & Trower, 1974; Percell, Berwick & Beigel, 1974; Meichenbaum & Turk, 1976).

(4) Sexual dysfunctions (LoPiccolo & Lobitz, 1973; Kaplan, 1974).

(5) Compulsive rituals (Rachman, Hodgson & Marks, 1971).

Enabling factors

(1) Concrete problem orientation suited for lower class patients (Lorion, 1973).

recently has been capped and furthered by an NIMH multisite study of the treatment of depression.

In the following paragraphs, we will briefly survey the research that has been done on the topic of differential, time-limited treatment effects in depression, and use it as an example of the principles of treatment selection. In the course of this discussion, we will emphasize treatment duration, but we will also begin to illustrate the strategies and techniques of psychotherapy to be presented in greater detail later.

Many authors (Kovacs, 1983; Bellack, 1985) suggest that the relative equivalence of cognitive (Beck, Rush, Shaw & Emery, 1979), behavioral (Bellack, Hersen & Himmelhoch, 1981), and interpersonal (Klerman, Weissman, Rounsaville & Chevron, 1984) treatments for depression may be parsimoniously explained as being the result of their common elements: a clear rationale, time-limited contracts, a planned and focused theme, etc.

On the other hand, the conclusion that all of the brief treatment approaches, with their different treatment foci and strategies/techniques, are equally effective for most patients is neither intuitively satisfying nor congruent with most clinicians' experiences (e.g., Bellack, 1985). Another interpretation of these findings, and one that relates to the central thesis of this book, is that the preponderance of current studies were performed on a heterogeneous group of patients (homogeneous only on the relatively unproductive dimension of Axis I diagnosis) and that factors other than level of depression are important for revealing a differential treatment response. As an example of a more refined approach to the general problem of depression, Jacobson et al. (1987) is completing clinical trials of cognitive-behavioral marital versus individual cognitive-behavioral therapy with depressed individuals. He reports that when patient depression is considered alone, the individual format of treatment is just as effective, if not more so, as marital therapy. When marital conflict also is present, however, a marital format is more effective than an individual format for alleviating both depression and marital conflict.

In an extensive review of the research studies of the brief treatment of depression, often combined with medication, Jarrett and Rush (1987) have begun to clarify the specific nondiagnostic patient indications for the various time-limited therapies for depression. They suggest the following conclusions and generalizations:

(1) Patients with high levels of self control respond especially well to behavioral treatments (Rehm, 1984; Simons et al., 1984).

(2) Neuroticism is associated with relatively poor response to interpersonal therapy (Weissman et al., 1978).

(3) The endogenous-nonendogenous distinction may be important in predicting immediacy of response (Prusoff et al., 1980). Among those with endogenous depression, the clinician should consider medication referral if time-limited treatment does not yield a relatively quick response.

(4) Matching patient problem areas with treatment focus is productive. If the patient lacks social skills, behavioral training is beneficial (Bellack et al., 1983).

(5) Treatment must be based upon a model of symptom generation that is consistent with the patient's history. In a sense, these are not treatments for depression, but multifaceted treatments for social skill deficiencies, cognitive distortions, and interpersonal conflicts, all of which can result in the appearance of depressive symptoms. The treatments are not so much "diagnosis"-driven as driven by a multifaceted model of conflict and symptom development that provides an approach to changing personal and psychosocial variables that relate to current symptoms and possible future ones.

Indications for Long-Term Therapies. We have implied above that patients who do not fit criteria for brief therapy should be considered for therapy of unlimited duration. In and of itself, this is probably true, but there are other more positive indications for long-term intervention as well.

Malan (1963) has indicated that patients with many conflicts (i.e., those with "complex" problems in our terminology) and those with several different focal conflicts are suited for long-term therapy. Psychoanalytic treatment is targeted at the achievement of self-knowledge by the process of working through relationship themes (transference and transference analysis), and incorporates the ambitious goal of character change. These methods and goals demand a lengthy therapeutic endeavor. These goals especially are consistent with the treatment of severe character disorders, such as borderline personality disorder (Kernberg, 1984).

In behavioral and cognitive-behavioral treatment paradigms, treatment may extend beyond the initial time limit of 15 or 20 sessions if the outcome goals are not accomplished in the designated period of time. This lack of goal attainment usually reflects patient resistances of various sorts (see Wilson, 1981). Similarly, in the behavioral tradition there are specific patient groups and problem areas that demand longer therapeutic effort because of the severity and complexity of the problem presented (e.g., the treatment descriptions provided by Linehan (1987) for the behavioral treatment of parasuicidal females). Similarly, the reader may recall M.D., the 27-year-old borderline woman whose repeated suicidal behavior usually followed the termination of an affair with a married man. This patient's instability is typical of the patterns observed by Linehan for which she recommends behaviorally oriented, long-term, group treatment.

In all treatment orientations, there are patients who have complex, chronic, or recurring conditions that require an extended treatment relationship. We say "treatment relationship," not "treatment duration," because the therapy may go for a period of time, be ended, and then start again when needed. These chronic conditions may fit more or less clearly into a diagnostic category (e.g., schizophrenia, bipolar disorder) or they may be more difficult to categorize (a chronically depressed but functioning individual, with intermittent suicidal ideation).

Duration of Restrictive Treatments

To this point, this chapter has been concerned almost exclusively with the duration and frequency of outpatient therapies which cover the majority of patient treatment episodes in the United States. However, it is important to note that the duration of treatments is also an important issue in restrictive treatment environments, such as hospitals, day hospitals, and alternate care facilities, even though little is known about efficacy as related to duration of these treatments.

Length of Hospitalization.   The research literature now contains a number of investigations which have compared the benefits of short versus long-term hospitalization (Rosen, Katzoff, Carrillo & Klein, 1976; Mattes, Klein, Millan & Rosen, 1979; Herz, Endicott & Spitzer, 1976; Glick & Hargreaves, 1979). Most of these studies can be questioned on some methodological grounds. However, the data to date suggest little additional benefits for long (i.e., greater than four weeks) hospital stays over shorter ones.

The Glick and Hargreaves (1979) study illustrates some of the foregoing issues. Patients admitted to the same clinical research unit were randomly assigned to either short-term (21 to 28 days) or long-term (90–120 days) hospitalization which included milieu, individual, group, and family format treatments, as well as somatic therapy. While there were no differences at follow-up between the short-term and the long-term groups with affective and personality disordered patients, there were significant differences among the schizophrenic patients. At one-year follow-up there was a modest but statistically significant difference in global outcome favoring the long-term schizophrenic group. At two years post-discharge, global outcome scores favored the long-term treatment group for those schizophrenic patients having good premorbid functioning, but not for those having a relatively poor premorbid state. The differential effect of short-term and long-term hospitalization was most pronounced for women.

The most parsimonious explanation for the more beneficial effect of long-term hospitalization noted in this study among good premorbid schizophrenics is found in the extent of their participation in post-discharge psychotherapy. Long-term patients continued in outpatient therapy at about two visits per month regardless of good or poor prehospital functioning. On the other hand, short-term hospital patients showed declining psychotherapy participation with time, at least among the good premorbid group.

As a result of such research, there is a growing consensus (e.g., Klerman,

1986) that hospital stays should be brief, and that the burden of proof for added benefit is on the proponents of long-term hospitalization. These proponents point out that the studies done to date pit short stay against even shorter stay, so the value of truly long-term (one year or more) hospitalization has not been tested.

Long-term hospitalization continues to be the norm, especially among state hospitals, selected units of some private hospitals, and some smaller private hospitals that specialize in long-term care. In state hospitals, the patients retained for long-term care are chronic patients, often without a family, who need lifelong custodial care. For these patients, there is no adequate alternative to the hospital milieu.

On the other hand, long-term patients treated in private hospitals are relatively affluent, have caring families, and have been placed in long-term hospitalization in the hope of facilitating substantial therapeutic change. A study of some 9,000 patients across 32 hospitals, all members of the National Association of Private Psychiatric Hospitals, provides additional data on the kinds of patients and variables that are related to length of stay (NAPPH, 1985). Demographically, these patients are almost exclusively caucasian, the majority between the ages of 20 to 64. Almost half have never married. The large majority are students or employed, with a high school education or better. Hospitalization costs are paid by private insurance.

Allen and colleagues (1987) have devised a clinically useful and potentially researchable method of thinking about which patients might utilize long-term hospitalization. They asked experienced clinicians at the Menninger Foundation, a prestigious private psychiatric hospital having units of varying lengths of stay, to compose vignettes describing patients whom they considered to be ideal candidates for brief, intermediate, and long-term hospitalization. Factors most frequently mentioned by the clinicians in their vignettes included such *patient* factors as diagnosis, course of condition, premorbid functioning, treatment alliance; *environmental* factors that included stressors and family roles; and *treatment* factors such as the amount of prior treatment, nature and breadth of current treatment goals, and the posthospital treatment plan.

Aspects of patients identified by clinicians as determiners of longer hospital stays included the presence of a severe personality disorder diagnosis, chronically poor adjustment, poor treatment alliance, pathogenic family background, the amount of prior treatment, and the ambitiousness of treatment goals. The prototypic long-term hospital patient defined in this latter study was a severely depressed individual who had made multiple suicide attempts, responded poorly to a previous short-term hospitalization, and had both a nonsupportive family and severe character pathology. Of course, it remains for research to show what specific effects long-term hospitalization as opposed to alternative treatments has on such patients, and what the outcome is. At the moment, it seems logical to consider long-term hospital treatment for this latter patient.

INTERRELATIONSHIPS OF FREQUENCY AND DURATION

Even less is known about treatment frequency than about treatment duration. Many therapies arrive at an arbitrarily defined frequency of one session per week, but ideally the frequency should be related to the treatment model and mediating or outcome goals. If the model and mediating goals are dependent on the development of a transference neurosis, for example, three to four sessions per week are appropriate. If the model is based on the mediating goals of learning new behaviors, the issue becomes one of massed versus distributed learning. If the model is aimed at crisis intervention, then frequent sessions are indicated for support and guidance during the time period that precedes restabilization.

Wilson (1981) chides his behavioral colleagues for being so noncreative in the effective utilization and variation of therapy session frequency. He points out that it is commonplace for behavior therapists to utilize spacing of sessions at the termination of treatment in order to avoid abrupt termination and to foster generalization and maintenance of change. While there are some problems that respond equally to massed and distributed learning, such as female organismic dysfunction (Ersner-Herschfeld & Kopel, 1979), there may be others (e.g., obesity) that require a program of effective maintenance strategies following inital change. In general, those problem situations and behaviors that have high relapse rates call for booster or follow-up sessions to help maintain initial gains. Such a program might include a variable frequency of therapy sessions, beginning with massed sessions followed by sessions of decreasing frequency. We will discuss this issue in greater length in Chapter 12.

Differential Treatment Considerations

As explicated in our model of differential treatment assignment (see Chapter 2), there are a number of crucial, interactive variables that determine appropriate treatment selection. Many of these variables have been described in Chapters 3 through 5. We will summarize here the interactive effects of these variables with treatment duration and frequency.

Nondiagnostic Patient Variables. While problem severity, if defined solely by symptom intensity, has little relationship to treatment duration, it does relate to treatment frequency. Often, the more intense the symptoms, the greater the need for support during the early phases of treatment and until symptom intensity abates.

The complexity of the problem and the coping ability of the patient probably have a more direct bearing on treatment frequency and duration than does problem severity, as we have defined it here. The ability of the patient to focus on one or several central issues in treatment will tend to shorten the duration of treatment. On the other hand, patients who are motivated for change but who have multiple problems and/or cannot focus on a reasonable number of treatment objectives will tend to require extended treatment (Malan, 1963). Likewise, poor motivation for treatment and/or change will tend to lengthen treatment and reactive patients, who have difficulty accepting therapist influence, support, and interpretation may need longer treatments than those who can more readily accept information and advice from the outside.

The stage of problem resolution achieved by the patient when therapy begins will also logically affect the duration of treatment—the further along the patient in problem resolution, the shorter the treatment. In general, the more problem areas the patient has, the longer the prescribed treatment. However, it may be necessary to make a decision to address only one or several of an array of problems, thus shortening the treatment somewhat.

Relationship Variables. Matching of therapist and patient potentially affects the duration and frequency of treatment in a number of ways. In general, an optimal match between therapist and patient on a number of demographic and personality variables potentially shortens the treatment, since two well matched and compatible participants can be expected to quickly achieve a focus for treatment.

Likewise, preparation of the patient for treatment is crucial in determining treatment duration. There is evidence to suggest that when patient and therapist negotiate goals, and when there is discussion of role responsibility between therapist and patient, the treatment proceeds to its work more efficiently, thus effectively shortening the length of treatment. In the so-called "brief" treatments, part of treatment preparation may include specifying, from the beginning, the duration of the treatment, and doing so tends to speed the process.

Diagnostic Variables. Diagnoses that involve a serious, chronic, or recurring condition suggest treatments of longer duration than those conditions that are less chronic and severe. Diagnoses such as schizophrenia, bipolar disorder, and recurring depressions are examples of this conclusion. These conditions require increasing the intensity of treatment, either on an ongoing basis or at least when needed during recurrent episodes. In contrast, diagnoses which reflect simpler symptom descriptions, such as agoraphobia and depression, are treatable in relatively short periods.

Following this logic, we can contrast the probable treatment intensity of several patients whose cases we have reviewed in previous chapters. For example, J.C., the young man who believed he was Jesus Christ, would be expected to require a longer course of treatment than J.I., whose car accident reactivated a trauma-induced response from years before.

In these examples, one can see why we have suggested that symptom severity (i.e., intensity) does not bear a strong relationship to treatment duration, even though it might bear such a relationship to treatment frequency. Thus, severity of distress was noticeably lower for J.C. than for J.I., who will not be likely to require the long-term, ongoing care and periodic hospitalizations that are likely to typify the treatment of J.C. At least initially, however, J.I. is likely to require two or three sessions of psychotherapy (or behavior therapy) per week while J.C., if he is not hospitalized, may require less frequent contact. A treatment session each week will probably be as valuable as more frequent sessions in this latter instance.

Format and Setting of Treatment. Individual, group, and family/marital treatment formats can all be brief or longer-term in duration (see Budman, 1981), depending upon factors such as the breadth and complexity of the problem. While there is nothing inherent in the treatment formats that necessitates brief or long treatments, there are some considerations that bear attention.

Group treatment, because of the logistics of organizing a group into a cohesive unit, tends to be longer than individual brief treatments. However, even here there are specific time-limited formats for treating depression (e.g., Sank & Schaffer, 1984; Yost et al., 1986), and conditions arising from inhibited emotional expression (e.g., Daldrup et al., 1988). By its nature of sharing time with a group of patients, the length of the treatment may interact with the format in such a way as to result in different outcomes. For example, in one study, outpatients with neurotic and characterological problems were assigned to psychodynamic treatments in either an individual or group format, each conducted within the context of either brief (mean of 22 sessions) or longer (mean of 76 sessions) duration therapy (Piper, Debbane, Bienvenu & Garant, 1984). The best outcomes were obtained among patients in brief individual and longer-term group therapies. The results of the brief group treatment were significantly less positive. These results suggest an interesting interaction between format and duration as related to outcome.

Marital and family treatments also tend to be brief (Gurman, 1981), in comparison to many individual treatments. Gurman has suggested a number of reasons for this phenomenon, including the fact that marital and family involvement selects for healthier individuals, and those for whom both transference reactions and dependency on the therapist normally will be less intense. These reactions are further diluted and contained in a marital and or family therapy format, allowing treatment to involve a shorter course.

Once again, we can use the case of J.I., our patient with PTSD, as an example. J.I. was treated in a combination of individual and marital formats and the treatment was of relatively short duration—approximately one year—largely because she had family support systems available to her and she exhibited stable behavior. Had she been less stable, with more chronic symptoms, she may have been assigned to a group treatment format with an indefinite duration.

It should be mentioned at this point that treatment settings tend to weave an average expectable treatment duration into their fabric. Short-term hospital settings, long-term hospital settings, day hospitals with a moderate-length rehabilitation, and supportive programs are all examples of this assertion. Likewise, funding mechanisms build treatment duration and/or frequency directly into their coverages. For example, managed health care alternatives (e.g., HMOs) place emphasis almost exclusively on brief therapies for obvious financial reasons.

In each of these cases, treatment duration usually is assigned in a way that is quite independent of those dimensions that logically would dictate treatment intensity—i.e., the nature, severity, and complexity of patient problems. Except for the demands of Diagnostic Related Groupings (DRGs), treatment duration is even more dependent on treatment setting and funding mechanisms than on patient diagnosis, an interesting observation given the medical rationale underlying both DRGs and traditional diagnosis. Given this relative inattention to patient needs and presenting problems, developing an effective treatment program frequently requires some mixing of treatment settings in order to be responsive to a patient's presentation.

THE DECISION NOT TO TREAT

While this volume concentrates on the use of psychotherapy, it is not restricted to these considerations. The decision to delay or not give mental health treatment more generally is an important dispositional decision. Knowledge of the contraindications to treatment as well as the indicators for specific types of treatment are important in the clinician's armamentarium.

Clinician Reluctance to Recommend No Treatment

It is interesting to note that prospective patients are much more reluctant to proceed with intensive psychotherapy than the professional providers of psychotherapy are to recommend it. A survey of a busy Manhattan medical school clinic investigated the incidence of the disposition of no treatment as made by the clinicians (Frances & Clarkin, 1981). Of 500 consecutive evaluations, only four were not recommended to treatment by the evaluators. In contrast, fully 10 percent of the clients refused to continue the evaluation or to accept the clinician's recommended treatment. There are other data to suggest that patients are not reluctant to self-select short treatment. The modal treatment is approximately one session (Koss & Butcher, 1986), and of those who stay longer than one session, many drop out before absorption of the procedures. Furthermore, most people for whom clinicians recommend formal treatment do not get it, but instead obtain assistance informally from their own support systems of ministers, friends, etc. Both patients and circumstances often dictate that people with clinical problems get very brief treatments. However, the common assumption may be that the doctor knows best, and that reluctant clients are not as knowledgeable and wise as the clinicians. However, we should pause and examine this assumption. A case in point may be appropriate.

M.V. was a 54-year-old married woman who had been seen in a university outpatient clinic for six years, rotating to a new therapist-in-training each July. A review of her history indicated that she initially had been hospitalized briefly with a diagnosis of Postpartum Depression. Her depression was described as including psychotic features and she was started in long-term psychotherapy and antipsychotic medication.

When one of the authors was assigned as the supervisor at the beginning of yet another training year, a review of the medical chart and patient history failed to reveal either a single instance of psychotic symptoms or of vegetative signs of Major Depression during the prior six years. Nonetheless, she had been maintained on Stelazine throughout the intervening six-year-period, and had been seen one or two times per week for psychotherapy. She continued to carry the diagnosis of Major Depression with Psychotic Symptoms, although the diagnosis had lost its provisional status. When asked, the patient did not know why she was coming for treatment except that "I get depressed sometimes." Charting her depression over a four-week period indicated that it was closely correlated with struggles with her husband and that it was of only mild severity at its most severe point.

M.V. was a dependent and compliant woman who may easily have stayed in treatment because it fit the needs and perception of her many therapists. Interestingly, the idea that the patient might not need treatment had occurred to the trainee therapist, but he was reluctant to say anything either to the supervisor or to the patient, laboring under the belief that he was simply not sophisticated enough to see her complex problem. The options of discontinuing treatment and referring her back to her own social support group, retaining her in medication clinic only, or entering her into marital therapy had not occurred either to six sequential therapists or their supervisors.

There are probably a number of reasons why clinicians are reluctant to recommend against entering treatment. From an economic point of view, it is not in the interests of the clinician to recommend no treatment to a potential paying customer. Insurance companies are certainly concerned about the financial incentive to treat when treatment is not needed, and they are increasing their efforts to get detailed and specific treatment goals and to obtain notes indicating progress toward achieving these goals.

While it seems clear that economics could play a role, this does not seem to be either the exclusive or even a major reason for referring all willing patients into some form of treatment. The survey noted in the preceding paragraphs, for example, was done in a low-cost clinic in which the evaluators' and therapists' incomes were not affected by the number of patients seen. Perhaps, like the trainee therapist of M.V., we all fear that we will miss something important and covertly assume that by recommending treatment for all who are interested that we will both minimize our losses and probably help the patient as well. This assumption may be correlated with the belief that treatment can help everyone and does no one harm.

This empathic feeling for those who present with emotional discomfort and the felt need to give assistance may be some of the most compelling reasons for rarely prescribing no treatment. Driven by the motivation to assist others who are in psychological pain, the clinician is in a situation where he or she may overlook or deny the limitations inherent in the psychotherapeutic enterprise, including both those arising from his/her own limitations and those arising from the field and its current treatment armamentarium. In our calmer moments, we all recognize data that indicate we do not have successful treatments for some conditions and problems. There is, of course, always a gap between the research literature and the one individual being assessed at the moment. But the wise clinician will at least compare the group data with the individual in question, and raise the possibility that there are times when no treatment may be the best choice at the moment.

If one goes for a physical checkup because of a vague but clear pain in the chest and the physician reports nothing wrong and no need of treatment, there may be immediate relief and joy. One may even enjoy instantaneous warm feelings toward the physician who is simply reporting the good news, as if he is giving you good protection during the year. The human situation may be quite different if someone with a problem goes to a therapist and is told that no treatment is recommended. One can feel that the clinician does not appreciate the problem or the pain, that he is simply rejecting *me*. There is no "objective" evidence that the pain does not need treatment nor that there is no treatment for it. Under these circumstances, the clinician may be motivated simply to offer treatment and, when it does not work (or, if it makes things worse), to then leave it to the patient to decide to discontinue.

The clinician may, of course, experience a strong dislike for a patient during an initial evaluation and may not be interested in developing a helping relationship with the patient. One might decide against treatment on this basis or, conversely, the idea of recommending against treatment may arise, but may be countered by the thought that one should control countertransference feelings and treat the patient anyway. Faced with the negative implications, one may resolve this dilemma by treating the patient in spite of negative feelings. One must learn to identify the objective indications for recommending no treatment in order to prevent negative feelings toward the patients from dictating important treatment decisions.

Relative Indications for No Treatment

In general, the relative indications for considering no treatment include the following: (1) treatment may not be necessary, (2) treatment may have no effect, (3) treatment may be a factor in worsening the patient's condition, or (4) the prescription of no treatment may be a therapeutic move (Frances & Clarkin, 1981).

Treatment Is Not Necessary.   The success of Bob Newhart's television role as a clinical psychologist and therapist paradoxically provides at once a statement about the general acceptance of psychotherapy in our culture, a derisive comment on its power, an indication of public interest in its workings, and revelations of misconceptions about its application and goals. By its very acceptance and pervasive influence in the culture, psychotherapy can be overutilized. In this atmosphere, it is quite conceivable that relatively healthy individuals will seek psychotherapy when faced with common life crises: marital disputes, problems with normal adolescents, disappointment at occupational failures, reactions following health crises, etc.

Research on spontaneous remission provides some indication of the problems and the kinds of individuals who are likely to experience recovery without treatment. In 1952 Eysenck claimed that two-thirds of neurotic patients improved over a two-year period whether they received psychotherapy or not. His challenge to the effectiveness of therapy brought intense and extensive responses. However, current analyses (Lambert, Shapiro & Bergin, 1986) suggest that Eysenck overestimated the spontaneous remission rate.

Furthermore, and more importantly for treatment planning, these analyses suggest that we can probably be more precise than we usually are as to which patients are likely to show remission without intervention. For example, Endicott and Endicott (1963) found that only 9 percent of borderline and schizophrenic patients improved spontaneously, whereas up to 54 percent of patients with less severe diagnoses showed untreated improvement. Overall, it appears clear that spontaneous recovery rates vary for different symptom patterns, as follows (from highest remission to lowest): anxiety and depressive disorders, followed by hysterical, phobic, obsessive-compulsive, and hypochondriacal disorders (Bergin & Lambert, 1978).

Bergin and Lambert point out that future research on this issue should note prior duration of disturbance, degree of disturbance, and environmental stresses and supports, all of which are likely to have more impact on prognosis than the patient's diagnosis alone.

For what individuals, then, is treatment not necessary? Individuals with a history of good adjustment (relatively few or no symptoms, good vocational and interpersonal adjustment, low symptom severity and complexity), who are currently under stress because of common difficulties in life, may not need direct, professional assistance. The evaluation feedback itself, assuring the individual of his/her relatively healthy adjustment and ability to handle the crisis, is probably helpful for many of these people. However, this group of individuals must be distinguished from: (1) those who are healthy but undergoing stress response syndrome (Horowitz, 1976) with its symptoms of repetitive, disturbing fantasies of the stressful event, and (2) those less well-adjusted individuals who need more assistance in managing stress.

Treatment Is Likely to Have No Effect. With accumulating data on the outcomes of psychotherapy with different patient groups, we are currently in a reasonably good position to single out patient groups that are not likely to benefit from treatment. A patient may not benefit from treatment for a number of reasons, including two basic ones: (1) the patient does not or cannot become involved in the basic process of the treatment and, therefore, does not profit from it; and (2) an effective treatment for the specific problems that the patient presents has not yet been developed.

The former group includes poorly motivated patients without incapacitating symptoms, and patients with malingering or factitious illness. The latter group includes antisocial or criminal behavior, and the iatrogenically infantilized patient.

Treatment Is Likely to Have Negative Effect. Some patients become worse during mental health treatment, whether because of the treatment itself or because of treatment-related variables (Lambert, Shapiro & Bergin, 1986). Negative outcomes or deterioration effects of psychotherapy have been estimated at between 9 percent (Smith et al., 1980) and 11.3 percent (Shapiro & Shapiro, 1982). Patient variables, therapist variables, and patient and therapist interactions all are possible contributors to negative effects. For example, impatient, authoritarian therapists who demand immediate change have been implicated in negative effects of group treatment

(Lieberman, Yalom & Miles, 1973). Sachs (1983) found that technical errors of procedure, such as failure to focus the session, failure to address the patient's negative attitudes about the therapist and/or therapy, passivity in the face of patient resistance, and use of ill-timed or inappropriate interpretations are associated with negative outcome. The combination of serious patient disturbance and counterproductive therapeutic techniques such as those designed to challenge and break down patient defenses are among the interactive qualities that may be related to worsening of patient conditions (e.g., Fairweather et al., 1960; Horwitz, 1977; Strupp, Hadley & Gomes-Schwartz, 1977; Sachs, 1983).

The term "Negative therapeutic reaction" (Freud, 1955; Sandler, Holder & Dave, 1973) has been used to describe patients who become worse in response to presumably correct analytic interpretations. It is hypothesized that this occurs in patients who have a need to remain disturbed or become worse as a form of self punishment, or among oppositional patients who are motivated to defeat the therapist. Patients with histories of negative therapeutic reactions in long-term individual dynamic therapies may require the use of other strategies, the use of briefer treatments, or the support of minimal treatment.

In evaluating seriously disturbed patients, clinicians must take care to consider the possibility of negative effects accruing from treatment. That possibility can be curtailed in some instances by taking particular care to assign the patient to a therapist who has experience with and is skilled in the use of effective approaches for such individuals. Clinically, the patients most at risk for a negative response to treatment include those high-reactant individuals who are noncompliant and who fail to develop an investment in the treatment. These may include borderline patients with a history of treatment failures, patients who enter treatment to support a lawsuit or to justify a claim for compensation or disability, and those whose expectations are so discrepant from the demand characteristics of treatment environment as to predestine frustration and lack of gratification.

Given that the DSM-III-R criteria for Borderline Personality Disorder (BPD) include intense anger, idealization and devaluation of others, the development of unusually conflicted and unstable relationships, and self-destructive behavior, it is not surprising that many efforts to sustain long-term treatment with borderline patients fall on rocky times. Suicide attempts made by these patients apparently are related to the intensity of the relationship with the therapist, and there are some instances of psychotic reactions to the intense therapeutic relationship.

Some (e.g., Linehan, 1987) have suggested that in order to diffuse the intense one-to-one relationship with the borderline patient, a group treatment format should be used. Outcome data are needed to indicate the effectiveness of this approach. In the meantime, it remains clear that bor-

derline patients with prior treatment histories involving intensely conflicted relationships with therapists, accompanied by destructive acting-
out behavior, should be assigned to another intense treatment only after
much circumspection. Brief, supportive treatments during times of situational stress, group treatments, or periodic reevaluation only may be utilized in these situations.

There also are those occasional patients who seek treatment in the context of a court case (e.g., physical symptoms and psychological symptoms
following a work accident), the results of which would be support for a
claim for compensation or disability. While the patient may need medical
and paramedical support for physical recovery, a psychological treatment
which encourages the patient to explore the felt need for regressive disability may be threatening and counterproductive.

No Treatment as a Therapeutic Move.   There are some occasions when the
clinical evaluator may prescribe a no treatment option for a patient as a
therapeutic move. That is, doing so may constitute an attempt to get
the patient to undergo therapeutic change in reaction to the behavioral
prescription itself. For example, the recommendation of no treatment may
be used as a paradoxical injunction with oppositional or highly reactant
patients who are prone to refuse the treatment if offered by a mental health
professional (e.g., Seltzer, 1986; Shoham-Salomon & Rosenthal, 1987). A
highly reactant patient may counter the therapist's recommendation of no
treatment by developing an investment in the process itself. In this case,
the evaluator can "give in" and suggest a trial of treatment "against my
better judgment."

There are other patients who, far from being oppositional to treatment,
seem to be addicted to psychotherapy and to drift from one treatment to
the next. Such individuals may even regress while in treatment, developing
a dependency upon the therapist rather than using the treatment to improve their own resources. When such patients are between therapists and
apply for yet another treatment, they may be encouraged to take a "vaca-
tion" from treatment and to attempt to handle things on their own for at
least a while.

SUMMARY AND COMMENT

While therapists tend to emphasize and remember long-term treatments,
most patients seek and ensure only short-term treatments. They do this by
dropping out of treatment prematurely or finding alternative resources.
It behooves mental health practioners, therefore, to plan for short-term
durations and seek interventions that will work within the time frames
that most patients will allot to resolving their personal distresses.

In this chapter we have emphasized that treatment duration is positively related to such patient predisposing variables as problem severity, problem complexity, and the absence of social resources. We have also emphasized that the setting in which treatment takes place, the format selected for treatment, and such nebulous qualities as patient attachment to the therapist all influence treatment duration as well. As a general rule, longer-term treatments are required for addressing the conflicts that underlie complex problems, while short-term treatments, of necessity, are symptom-focused. Likewise, the more protected and controlled the treatment setting and the more highly reactant the patient, the greater the necessity of long-term treatments to allow the focus and closeness necessary to resolve conflictual issues. On the other hand, individualized treatments, symptomatic treatments, and treatments taking place within the patient's home environment and social systems augur against long-term treatments.

Collectively, treatment intensity reflects some interaction of treatment duration and frequency. Highly intense treatments promise to be both long-term and frequent, while low-intensity treatments lack both qualities of duration and frequency. The least intense treatment, for example, is the prescriptive recommendation against treatment altogether. Far from being a simple matter, however, the decision to recommend against treatment should carefully be considered in cases where the condition is itself transitory and time-limited, where dependency attachments are likely to provoke negative reactions, where the presence of secondary gains work against treatment effects, and where alternative support systems are available.

Overall, the clinician should consider the no-treatment option first and require the burden of proof to rest with demonstrating the need *for* treatment rather than the lack of such need. In a similar way, the clinician is obligated by current knowledge to consider time-limited, brief treatments before long-term and expensive treatments. Only if there are clear indications for long-term treatments can one justify them over briefer intervention models. Patient preferences and financial status are important considerations, but even when the patient desires long-term interventions and has the resources to support this desire, options should be presented and discussed.

SUGGESTED READINGS

Budman, S. H. (Ed.) (1981). *Forms of brief therapy.* New York: Guilford.

Endicott, N. A. & Endicott, J. (1963). "Improvement" in untreated psychiatric patients. *Archives of General Psychiatry, 9,* 575–585.

Herz, M., Endicott, J. & Spitzer, R. (1976). Brief versus standard hospitalization: The families. *American Journal of Psychiatry, 133,* 795–801.

Koss, M. P. & Butcher, J. N. (1986). Research on brief psychotherapy. In S. L. Garfield & A. E. Bergin (Eds.), *Handbook of psychotherapy and behavior change,* 3rd ed. (pp. 627–670). New York: John Wiley and Sons.

Malan, D. H. (1963). *A study of brief psychotherapy.* New York: Plenum.
Orlinsky, D. E. & Howard, K. I. (1986). Process and outcome in psychotherapy. In S. L. Garfield & A. E. Bergin (Eds.), *Handbook of psychotherapy and behavior change,* 3rd ed. (pp. 311–384). New York: John Wiley and Sons.

PART IV

Relationship Variables

There are two general considerations that must be addressed in understanding the role of the therapeutic relationship in treatment outcome. The first of these is that of patient and therapist compatibility. Those attributes that therapist and patient bring with them to the relationship may enhance the connection between them. To the degree that we can define those characteristics that constitute a "fit" between a patient and a therapist, we may be able to empower the therapeutic process and selectively assign patients to therapists.

On the other hand, one must also consider carefully those things that the therapist can do to facilitate the development of a compatible relationship. This issue bears both upon overcoming resistances within the session and establishing a collaborative contract that maintains both participants' motivation and commitment.

Section IV consists of two chapters that respectively explore these aspects of the helping relationship and their roles in treatment selection. Figure IV.1 outlines the concepts to be addressed in our consideration of these relationship issues. Note, for example, that the figure reflects our belief that both demographic and interpersonal variables contribute selectively but differently to decisions designed to enhance the compatibility of treatment relationships and to the selection of outcome goals.

Activities that are conducted in order to prepare the patient for treatment differ from those designed to adjust the in-therapy environment to the patient's needs and expectancies. On the one hand, pretherapy preparation seeks to bring the patient's view of the treatment experience closer to that of the therapist. On the other hand, managing the in-therapy environment is designed to make the therapy fit the patient's preexisting expectations. In turn, both are precursors for the development of specific strategies. This connection, as portrayed in the accompanying figure, emphasizes that therapeutic strategies, however well conceived, lose their power in the absence of a collaborative alliance with a benign and helpful therapist.

Figure IV.1

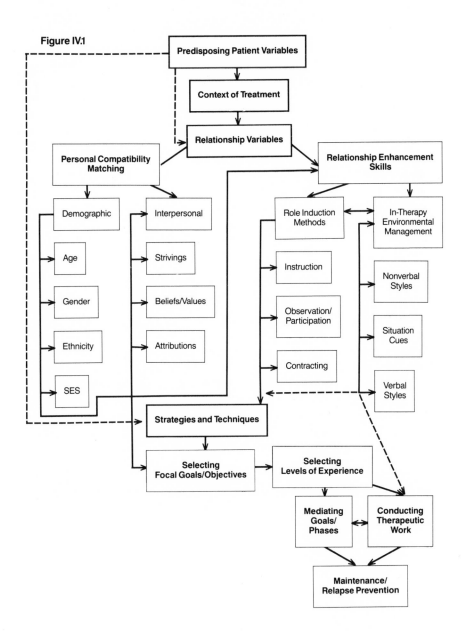

9

Therapist-Patient Personal Compatibility

What enables two people to form a collaborative relationship—boss and subordinate, physician and patient, therapist and client? Does this compatibility, or "psychotherapeutic resonance" as some (cf. Larson, 1987) have called it, derive from the ability to identify, within ourselves, a similarity with the experiences of the other? Or is it the intrigue of our differences; the press to see the world from a different vantage point? Is it as simple as being understood, or is it that we perceive that the other person *struggles* to understand us? The chemistry of personal compatibility is poorly understood. Yet, it is the essence of much of what we do.

The importance of the patient-therapist relationship to somatic therapies is frequently underemphasized (e.g., Martelli, Auerbach, Alexander & Mercuri, 1987; Snyder & Forsyth, in press). Therapeutic alliance and personal compatibility variables usually are considered to be incidental or even irrelevant to the outcomes of somatic treatments. This viewpoint contrasts with the place these factors are accorded in psychotherapy, where they generally are recognized as important contributors to improvement. Even among psychotherapists, however, contradictory views are held with respect to the degree of importance to place on aspects of the treatment relationship. For a significant minority of theorists and therapists, such variables are the essence of treatment. For most theorists, however, relationship variables and interpersonal compatibility, while considered to be very important, are accorded a secondary role in accounting for treatment effects; they are separated from the "specific" contributors to outcome by the labels, "common" or "nonspecific."

The matters of identifying and distinguishing the specific and common (i.e., nonspecific) contributors to treatment effectiveness are not simply resolved. The common and even many of the particular ingredients that are presented as unique elements of different psychotherapy models (and manuals) are elements integral to the delivery of any mental health treatment. Nonetheless, relationship and expectancy effects are called "placebo effects" when somatic treatments are empirically investigated; thereby, they are excluded from serious consideration when it comes to evaluating the effectiveness of a specific treatment.

The contributors to placebo responses in somatic treatments are among the active ingredients of psychosocial therapies. It is curious that ingredients of such importance to the effects that we attempt to achieve with any mental health treatment are written off as "noise" variables in one modality and accepted as central in another.

We take the position that all effective mental health treatment consists of systematically encouraging, building upon, and managing a patient's expectations, perceptual judgments, and evaluations of self and others. This influence is accomplished through the interpersonal forces to which we collectively refer as the "collaborative treatment relationship." The assumption that psychotherapy is a process of impression, perception, and expectation management holds no less for somatic treatments than it does for psychosocial ones. Perceptions and judgments formed within an interpersonal relationship are the processes by which people succumb to and overcome demoralization. Out of positive interpersonal contacts with a therapist, the cognitive elements are constructed that form the foundations of faith, hope, and the range of emotions that are important in psychopathology, mental health, and psychotherapy.

To call the variables from which these benefits are constructed "nonspecific" is to minimize both their predictability and the control which can be established over them. To call them "common" or "placebo" is to imply incorrectly that they operate in the same way in all treatments and among all patients. For example, Rounsaville et al. (1987), reporting results from the NIMH collaborative study of psychotherapy and depression, conclude that therapists' technical skill in Interpersonal Psychotherapy (IPT) increases with the presence of general, facilitative characteristics of the treatment. They suggest that even "nonspecific" therapeutic qualities are functions of therapist technical skill in specific modalities. Hence, their role and effects may change with the type of therapeutic procedures utilized and the competence with which these procedures are employed.

It is more nearly accurate to refer to these general treatment qualities as "potentiating" factors which catalyze the more discrete and distinctive interventions used in the change process than as "nonspecific" or "common" factors (cf. Rounsaville, Chevron, Prusoff, Elkin, Imber, Sotsky & Watkins, 1987; Jones, Cumming & Horowitz, 1988). If one accepts the potentiating role of the setting and of the relationship in which treatment occurs, it readily becomes apparent that psychotherapy cannot be considered to represent a set of activities that can be contrasted to and considered discretely different from those forces which promote change in somatic treatments. The study of psychotherapy is the study of rhetoric and hermeneutics (Frank, 1987)—the study of how therapists and treatment environments induce transformations of meanings and beliefs; of how these transformations alter patient feelings and problems. Treatment, in other words, is the study of persuasion and influence in the process of healing, behavior change, and skill enhancement.

PERSUASION AND THE THERAPEUTIC ALLIANCE

While the forces of persuasion are important processes in all mental health treatment, they can be most clearly understood when studied directly, and it is this study that constitutes both psychotherapy practice and research. Rather than being a distinct class of treatments, therefore, psychotherapy is the supraordinate treatment under which all specific mental health interventions occur.

The specific applications of designated procedures, ranging from chemical agents to selected interpretations, cannot be extracted arbitrarily from the psychotherapy process. They can be investigated, however, as ingredients within the broader framework which that process implies. That broader process is composed of the meanings and attributions which accrue within the relationship between the identified patient and the identified source of influence, in most cases a therapist. To study this relationship necessitates identifying the forces of persuasion and exploring how and under what conditions these forces facilitate or impede the effects of specific interventions.

While some, including such pioneers of the foregoing position as Strong (1987), have questioned how many innovative applications have accrued to clinical practice from a perspective of social persuasion, others have suggested that such a viewpoint has had a far reaching impact on current perspectives. Weary (1987) asserts that recent years have seen a significant benefit to clinical practice derived from an explosion of interest in merging clinical and social persuasion perspectives. He suggests that this increase of interest in viewing clinical phenomena as examples of social influence forces reflects convergence among the interests and methods of social and clinical psychologists, increasing national concern with practical rather than abstract problems in mental health, and the attention given to cognitive variables like attitudes and beliefs in neuroscientific investigations of psychopathology and illness.

A review of writings in the area of social persuasion will reveal that not all agree with the assertion that psychotherapy is a process of interpersonal persuasion. Certainly, we do not mean to imply that it is a process of "interpersonal persuasion" if that term is taken to mean that the therapist is either manipulative or coercive. To the degree that the therapist intends the process to create some change in a patient's feelings, insights, attitudes, viewpoints, or behaviors, however, the process is one of interpersonal influence. And to the degree that the therapist's ideas about what behaviors and attitudes constitute emotional health influence treatment aims, she or he must rely upon the powers of persuasion to accomplish the treatment goals. Identifying this process as "persuasion" simply recognizes that therapists *intend* to be agents for the changes which occur in perspectives, awarenesses, behaviors, and relationships and that they share, with their patients, some responsibility for defining what constitutes "improvement."

In the service of these ends, therapists attempt to establish an influential relationship. This relationship assumes a level of persuasive potency by directing patients to concentrate on certain experiences and to exclude others; by synchronizing patient and therapist verbal content, sensory experiences and feelings; by allowing patient and therapist to merge boundaries briefly; and from this merging to acknowledge unspoken patient feelings (Larson, 1987). To the degree that this relationship emerges as an alliance or mutual resonance, the atmosphere exists in which patients can be persuaded to change.

For example, only when J.I.'s therapist can convince her that he is trustworthy, that he resonates to her private experiences, and that he understands her unspoken beliefs will she be willing to have him direct her movement toward the sources of her anxiety (fears of losing control) and accept his support through the process of adaptation and change. The therapeutic bond is designed to foster persuasive power from which to initiate change.

If the processes of psychotherapy involve persuasion and interpersonal influence as we have defined it, then additional assumptions are invoked: (1) that persuasion is best accomplished within the context of a collaborative, supportive, caring, and respectful relationship; and (2) such a relationship is not accidental—it evolves from a complex interaction of the inherent dispositions contributed by the parties involved and the activities of the therapist that establish an environment that this patient will find conducive to change. In other words, persuasion is a process that derives its power from the felt compatibility, respect, and credibility that the participants share.

In turn, this compatibility derives both from extratherapy dispositions of both participants and from their specific interactions. These disposi-tional compatibilities and relationship-enhancing interactions are manifest in what has been called the "therapeutic" or "working alliance" (Bordin, 1976; Luborsky, McLellan, Woody, O'Brien & Auerbach, 1985).

In Chapter 2, we observed that patient-therapist similarities among inherent, extratherapy characteristics were central to developing a benefi-cial therapeutic alliance. On close examination, however, this assertion is far too simplistic. A good therapeutic alliance must also be built upon the presence of different but relevant perspectives and evolves out of what transpires within the treatment to enhance or inhibit the growth of the relationship.

This latter point is captured well in the writings of Kohut (1977, 1984) who proposes a tripolar concept of self, each aspect of which is associated with a certain environmental response. These tripolar needs to receive selective responses from the environment and the history of early environ-mental supply of these responses result in expectations and behaviors which serve as templates on which three types of relationships can be built. The first two attributes of self, *ambition* and *ideals,* grow from an environment that supports and acknowledges the differences which exist between one's self and others. Though the relationship is not precisely linear, it is assumed that if one's need to have differences acknowledged but valued (i.e., "mirrored") is frustrated, a demanding and grandiose transference relationship is likely to be developed. By contrast, if one's need for a benign model of ideals is frustrated, one may attempt to con-struct an idealized relationship with others and consequently to relate through the medium of dependency and self depreciation.

Kohut believed that these relationships were reenacted in psychother-apy, setting the nature of the therapeutic alliance (i.e., the type of transfer-ence that is experienced) and focusing the patient on the interpersonal differences which exist between the patient and therapist. For example, both the *grandiose* and *idealized* transference relationships described in the foregoing were thought to derive from the differences which are present between patient and parental figures.

In contrast, needs for *twinship* were thought by Kohut also to exist. Twinship needs reflect the desire to see one's self as similar to significant others. Frustration of these needs for similarity when interacting with objects of identification was thought to result in a sense of alienation and conversely, the acknowledgement of relevant similarities in the psychother-apy dyad was expected to contribute to a healing sense of human identity.

The present chapter is devoted to considering that broad network from which therapeutic alliances such as those proposed by Kohut derive. Thus, this chapter will explore the match of stable traits and indwelling character-istics which exist independently of one's role as patient or therapist, which promote compatibility among receptive parties and facilitate positive change. The next chapter will extend this consideration to the within treatment activities and treatment-specific attitudes which can be drawn upon to promote and enhance the treatment relationship, once initiated.

DIMENSIONS OF COMPATIBILITY

The power of the persuasive relationship is dependent upon the permutations among therapist qualities of interpersonal attraction, perceived expertness, and trustworthiness. These attributed qualities of the persuasive source (i.e., "source characteristics") have been extracted from research on interpersonal influence and have been widely applied to psychotherapy (Goldstein, 1966; Strong, 1978; Beutler, 1979b; Corrigan et al., 1980; Weary & Mirels, 1982; Brehm & Smith, 1986; Weary, 1987). These three qualities, attributed to effective therapists, are also captured in other, and often more general, concepts of "therapist credibility" and "persuasiveness" (Truax, Fine, Moravec & Millis, 1968; Corrigan, 1978; Heppner & Dixon, 1981).

A summarization of research on these persuasive characteristics reveals that the qualities of perceived expertness and credibility are consistently related to clinically important therapy processes and outcomes, accounting for upwards of 35 percent of variations among outcome rates (Corrigan et al., 1980; LaCrosse, 1980; Heppner & Heesacker, 1982, 1983; Beutler et al., 1986). Even the well known "facilitative" therapist conditions described by Rogers (1957) are probably best understood as qualities of patient perception as much as they are inherent qualities of the therapist (Gurman, 1977) and are, thus, subsumed by the attributed qualities of credibility and trustworthiness (e.g., Orlinsky & Howard, 1986, 1987).

The characteristics of credibility, trust, and persuasiveness that are attributed to the therapist in most effective psychotherapy derive both from preexisting attitudes or generalized expectations about therapists and therapy which patients bring with them to treatment and from the interactions that patients have with their specific therapists. While initial global attributions usually are positive, after patients enter treatment they begin to read facial changes (e.g., Berry & McArthur, 1986), postural cues (e.g., Robbins & Haase, 1985), and language styles (e.g., Horn-George & Anchor, 1982; Rosenthal, Blanck & Vannicelli, 1984) in order to refine their attributions of therapists' credibility and caring (Fretz, 1966; Edinger & Patterson, 1983; Maurer & Tyndall, 1983).

As patients become familiar with a therapist, their liking for the therapist and their willingness to commit themselves to making the changes implicitly demanded by the relationship become increasingly reliant on how similar and dissimilar to themselves they perceive the therapist to be. They begin to make increasingly more selective judgments of the therapist's credibility than those initially represented by the generalized expectations governing their response at the beginning of treatment (Corrigan et al., 1980). If these dimensions of similarity and difference comprise an initially good match, they go far to determine the degree to which an effective therapeutic alliance can be established.

The interpersonal match from which the therapist's influence potential derives reflects two major dimensions: demographic similarity and counterbalancing (i.e., different) interpersonal response patterns. Minimally, interpersonal response patterns include complex, interpersonal needs or strivings, belief systems, and attributional styles.

It is our contention that ideally one should consider both demographic and interpersonal response compatibility when assigning a psychotherapist. However, individual settings and circumstances will not always allow such specificity. The unavailability of the requisite types of therapists within a given setting, unbalanced treatment loads, and the clinic demands, which may make the ideal therapist unavailable, all require that adjustments be made, with the assurance that mismatches on any of the dimensions can probably be overcome by attention to other aspects of the patient's management.

Demographic Similarity

One's gender, ethnicity, and even features which identify one's age usually are easily observed (Shapiro & Penrod, 1986) and are used by patients to make relatively accurate judgments of therapists' status, even in short periods of time and with limited contact (Berry & McArthur, 1986). Because they are so readily observed, the effect of patient-therapist demographic similarities on treatment commitment and outcome have been extensively researched. While the results are far from consistent, they do allow for some tentative conclusions that demographic similarity between patient and therapist (1) facilitates positive perceptions of the relationship in the beginning stages of treatment; (2) enhances commitment to remaining in treatment, especially among disenfranchised groups; and (3) modestly accelerates the amount of improvement experienced by those who complete treatment.

More specifically, age (Luborsky, Crits-Christoph, Alexander, Margolis & Cohen, 1983), ethnic (Jones, 1978), gender (Blase, 1979; Jones, Krupnick & Kerig, 1987) and socioeconomic background (Carkhuff & Pierce, 1967) similarity have been associated with positive patient perceptions of the treatment relationship. These studies reveal that demographic similarity enhances patients' perceptions of their therapists' understanding and empathy, increases patients' liking for their therapists, and results in the relationship being judged to be more helpful than when such similarity is lacking. Patients apparently use relatively obvious similarities early in treatment to establish a basis for trust and for assessing how likely they are to be understood.

Demographic similarity also has been associated with the likelihood of returning for a second and additional treatment sessions, especially among ethnic minority patients (Abramowitz & Murray, 1983; Terrell & Terrell, 1984). Ethnic similarity between patient and therapist is preferred by many minority patients and is associated with an enhanced commitment to remain in treatment, thus frequently being associated with reduced early drop-out rates (Turner & Armstrong, 1981; Neimeyer & Gonzales, 1983).

The foregoing findings lend testimony to the role of background similarity in enhancing the early therapeutic alliance. However, only age (Morgan, Luborsky, Crits-Cristoph, Curtis & Solomon, 1982) and gender similarity (Kirshner, Genack & Hauser, 1978; Blase, 1979) have a predictable effect on outcome. On the other hand, even in these latter cases, the relationship between similarity and treatment outcome is not direct. In spite of persuasive evidence that female therapists are more likely than their male counterparts to facilitate therapeutic change, this gender effect is quite modest compared to other contributors to outcome (e.g., Jones et al., 1987). Moreover, flexibility and similarity of role attitudes rather than actual similarity *per se* account for even the modest outcome effects attributable to demographic similarities (Beutler, Crago & Arizmendi, 1986; Blier, Atkinson & Geer, 1987). Similarity of attitudes appears to contribute to the persuasive power of the therapist, enhances patient involvement, and facilitates treatment outcome, particularly in the form of attenuated drop-out rates (Luborsky, Mintz, Auerbach, Crits-Christoph, Bachrach, Todd, Johnson, Cohen & O'Brien, 1980; Beutler et al., 1986). Similar conclusions were reached by von Essen (1987), who observes that background similarities assist in recruiting involvement early in treatment but have a decreasing effect on final treatment outcome as treatment becomes longer term.

Similarity by itself may be of less importance to therapeutic processes than the level of interpersonal trust which such similarity often portends (Brody, 1987). Other dimensions besides background similarity can activate the trust and respect that characterize a helping alliance. Some of these general guidelines are outlined in Table 9.1.

Table 9.1
Compatibility: Demographic Background

Compatibility	Prescription for Noncompatibility
Similarity Ethnic Age Gender SES	Empathic listening and emphasis on similarity of viewpoints. Increased role of active listening and decreased role of directive interventions or instructional activities.

While initial similarity tends to foster the therapeutic alliance early on, it ultimately is the differences in interpersonal attitudes that seem to move the patient forward (e.g., Beutler, 1983; von Essen, 1987). Hence, we must look to interpersonal response patterns as another set of matching variables in order to ascertain how the therapeutic alliance might exert an effect on outcome over time.

Interpersonal Response Patterns

In their simplest form, interpersonal response patterns are enduring dispositions to action. Like the term "personality," they are associated with observable behaviors, but include attitudes (including conflicting attitudes), beliefs, and habits, all of which have accrued through each individual's unique history. In turn, these interpersonal patterns affect the therapeutic process.

Among therapists, such interpersonal characteristics as resistance to change (i.e., inflexibility) and rigidity of interpersonal boundaries may affect the therapist's tolerance of stressors (e.g., Hellman, Morrison & Abramowitz, 1987) and determine the selection of therapeutic styles (McConnaughy, 1987). No less among patients, interpersonal response patterns interact with background characteristics and therapeutic responses in very intimate ways and are distinguishable from these other constructs only by the convention of considering them to reflect inferred experiences.

Several authors (e.g., Strupp & Binder, 1984; Luborsky, 1984) have described the interpersonal nature of the conflicts from which recurrent interpersonal patterns of behavior arise. These authors have succeeded in reaching a meaningful balance between inference and description that is conducive to establishing realistic goals for psychotherapy. Following their lead, we consider *interpersonal response patterns* to be manifest as recurrent themes, expressing a core conflict. These interpersonal themes are distinguishable from personality both because they are restricted to the realm of interpersonal behavior and because they involve less indirect inferences than that which ordinarily is prescribed by personality theories.

The elements attributed to *conflictual themes* vary somewhat from author to author, but have certain common characteristics: (1) a recurrent need, impulse, or striving, (2) a stable set of expectations about the likely result of efforts to meet that need, and (3) a consistent introject or causal attribution which is activated when the striving is frustrated. The importance of the core conflictual themes to setting psychotherapy goals will be illustrated in Chapter 11, showing that excessive similarity on any of these dimensions calls for compensatory action on the part of the therapist (see Table 9.2).

Table 9.2
Compatibility: Interpersonal Patterns

Compatibility	*Prescriptions for Noncompatibility*
Strivings/Need Dissimilarity	Therapist identifies the conflictual element in the patient's patterns and highlights the discrepancies.
Belief Similarity & Dissimilarity	Therapist might emphasize the similarities of knowledge/social values, but stress and confront discrepancies in treatment goals and the degree of patient exclusive reliance on dependent or independent patterns, fears of environmental (world) instability, and excessive valuing or devaluing of social closeness and intellectual pursuits.
Attribution/Introjects General Dissimilarity	Accept patient's view of causal or punishment attributions; confront patient's attribution of control (external or internal). If patient is highly internal in expectations of and resistant to control, therapist should beware of potential countertransference struggles over control.

Interpersonal Strivings.   While all people develop their own private inferences or theories to explain behavior, the "truth" of these theories can be assessed only in terms of their functional value within a given circumstance. A theory of interpersonal behavior, for example, held by patients may be built principally around their own dominant needs and conflicts in a social world. Their theory is designed to help them predict and control the social environment, and their distress is an indication that the theory has less than optimal function for achieving those things for which they strive. Therapeutic intervention, therefore, is designed to alter these private meanings and theories so that they might be more functional (e.g., Frank, 1987).

The therapist's theory of behavior usually is more explicit and formalized than that of the patient. This formality allows communication among colleagues and also assists in defining the goals of treatment. Nonetheless, it is likely that private need systems affect how the therapist modifies and adjusts the formal theory which he or she uses. By maintaining this perspective, a therapist will consider the role of his or her own interpersonal needs when assessing the nature of the therapeutic relationship.

A considerable amount of research has been directed at the question of how differences between patient and therapist personality traits contribute to patient change. Early research suggested that initial similarity of global personality profiles was associated with improvement in psychotherapy (e.g., Carson & Heine, 1962; Mendelsohn & Geller, 1963). This general conclusion proved to be premature, however (e.g., Carson & Llewellyn, 1966; Mendelsohn & Geller, 1967). Nonetheless, as research on the topic has adopted a more specific and interpersonal definition of "personality," increasing numbers of studies have suggested that patient-therapist differences on certain dimensions of interpersonal striving or need may be associated with improved outcomes.

Most statistical descriptions of interpersonal traits suggest that there are relatively few dimensions on which most enduring behaviors can be arranged. For example, Widiger, Trull, Hurt, Clarkin, and Frances (1987) suggest three such dimensions: desires for social involvement, investment in power and dominance, and style of defense against anxiety. The latter two dimensions correspond closely with those of reactance and coping style that we have described in previous chapters. In the current context, we will focus on desires for social involvement, as a dimension of interpersonal functioning on which compatible patient-therapist matches may be developed.

Desire for social involvement, as defined by Widiger et al., has a counterpart in most descriptions of personality type. Millon (1981), for example, defines personality disturbance as reflecting various permutations of interpersonal attachment and levels of activity. Likewise, one of the most successful efforts to match patient and therapist descriptive personality traits has found interpersonal attachment to be useful in predicting treatment effectiveness (Berzins, 1977).

This study revealed that therapists who were most effective with dependent, attachment-oriented clients in a student mental health clinic were those who valued personal autonomy. The opposite relationship was also observed: Autonomy-oriented and self-sufficient patients did best when their therapists' needs were more attachment-oriented and affiliative. A pattern of dissimilarity in the dimension of social/interpersonal dependency-autonomy needs among good prognosis partners in marital therapy has also been noted (Jacobson, Follette & Pagel, 1986).

Observations such as the foregoing have led us to believe that patients and therapists work most productively with one another when they represent contrasting viewpoints around those patterns of interpersonal behavior that define the element of "striving" or "need" within the core conflictual theme (Beutler, 1979b; 1983). This point of view is compatible with the theories of Kohut (1977, 1984) referred to earlier.

It is probably a characteristic of the human organism to have both autonomy and affiliation strivings. Millon (1981) emphasizes that relative balances between autonomy and attachment strivings distinguish among the various personality styles represented on Axis II of DSM-III. He describes variations among four personality patterns: Dependent personalities, Independent/narcissistic personalities, Detached personalities, and

Ambivalent personalities. *Dependent* patterns, for example, represent relatively high dependent, attachment, and affiliation strivings compared to strivings for separation, individuation, and autonomy while *Independent* patterns reflect relatively high separation and individuation strivings. *Detachment* patterns are assumed to reflect comparatively low levels both of separation and attachment need systems and *Ambivalent* patterns portend relatively high but counterbalanced needs for both separation and attachment.

While Millon's conceptual framework is helpful for formulating the strivings from which interpersonal conflict patterns are derived, more systematic and specific information than that obtainable from interviewing the patient often is required in order accurately to place the level of contrast which exists between patient and therapist. Fortunately, dimensions of attachment/dependency and autonomy/independence also can be objectively assessed on a normative basis, separate from simple patient and therapist verbal report. Both Strupp and Binder (1984) and Luborsky (1984) have developed formal methods for assessing the nature of these strivings from a review of patients' histories. These methods emphasize the importance of staying close to observational descriptions, first drawing from the patient descriptions of how past relationships have begun, been maintained, and ended. Themes are then extracted from this information in order to capture the dominant strivings, attitudes, and attributions which have characterized the patient in these relationships. These themes are then used as focal targets for psychotherapeutic interventions. We will discuss this process in greater detail in Chapters 11 and 12.

The foregoing points can be illustrated in reference to J.I., the anxious and traumatized patient with whom we introduced this book. J.I. exhibited an Independent personality style in which the driving want was a degree of autonomy, which represented protection from being taken over, abused, or absorbed by others who might be stronger than she. This need formed the basis for her high reactance level, but stood in contrast to the ambivalent personality style of her therapist. His interpersonal wants reflected a stable but agonistic balance between needs for closeness and needs for independence and distance. Together, these two individuals represented a moderate amount of discrepancy on these need systems. Had the therapist had a level of autonomy drive that rivaled the patient's, they may have become too competitive, while a very attachment-oriented therapist may have threatened J.I.'s boundaries.

Personal Beliefs. Clearly, from a conceptual viewpoint, demographic qualities are related in complex ways to one's personal beliefs and values. Personal beliefs represent the cognitive elements that both comprise one's personal strivings and derive from one's demographic background. As one might expect, therefore, therapeutic compatibility among patient and therapist beliefs is defined by a complex pattern of similarity and dissimilarity.

This complexity can be illustrated by observing in juxtaposition the evidence that suggests that treatment outcome is related linearly to the degree to which patients acquire the global beliefs and values of their particular therapist, and the inconsistent relationship between initial patient-therapist similarity and belief system changes (Beutler, 1981; Beutler, Crago & Arizmendi, 1986; Hamblin, Beutler, Scogin & Corbishley, 1988; Tjelveit, 1986).

The most consistent evidence available suggests that treatment outcome is enhanced when patient and therapist similarities in the relative value placed upon such attributes as wisdom, honesty, intellectual pursuits, and knowledge are combined with differences in a variety of interpersonal beliefs and values. The dimensions on which patient-therapist differences have been found to facilitate improvement include: (1) a sense of personal safety in a social world (Beutler, Pollack & Jobe, 1978), (2) the value placed upon interpersonal treatment goals (Charone, 1981), and (3) such interpersonal attachment values as friendships and social recognition (Beutler, Jobe & Elkins, 1974; Beutler, Arizmendi, Crago, Shanfield & Hagaman, 1983; Arizmendi, Beutler, Shanfield, Crago & Hagaman, 1985).

The reader might reflect again on the case of J.I., whose history of remote as well as recent trauma induced strong feelings of depression and anxiety. Clearly, similarity of intellectual values may help develop the merging of identities that facilitate the therapeutic bond (Larson, 1987). At the same time, a therapist who is less fearful than she of personal safety, and who places greater value than she on personal attachment, might challenge her to grow and to accept the support available to her in the relationships she has with husband and friends.

These observations confirm the value of patient-therapist dissimilarity around those interpersonal values which comprise one's needs for attachment and individuation. However, they also place ethical issues in high relief. From the standpoint of a pragmatic ethic, the mere observation that persuasion of beliefs and values is associated with improvement may be enough to justify efforts directly to persuade patients to adopt therapists' value stances.

However, most of us who are trained in the tradition of free will and self selection have difficulty justifying such a position. Some comfort on this issue may be forthcoming in the observation that therapists' values ordinarily are more similar to those of their patients than they are different (Beutler, Pollack & Jobe, 1978). This finding may reflect some degree of self selection among patients and therapists when they decide who will be treated by whom.

Additionally, there is no indication that religious attitudes, those on which patients and therapists are most likely to differ (Bergin, 1980), are among those that either change during treatment or facilitate improvement (Hill, Howard & Orlinsky, 1970; Lewis, 1983). Finally, evidence suggests that it is the *acceptability* to the therapist of the patient's viewpoint (Beutler, Jobe & Elkins, 1974) and the therapist's ability to communicate within the patient's value framework (Probst, 1980; Probst, Ostrom & Watkins, 1984) more than either the particular values held by the therapist or the patient's persuadability which contribute to patient improvement. Even nonreligious therapists, if they are sufficiently accepting of the religious patient's values, can communicate within the patient's value system and effect improvement without threatening favored value stances (Beutler et al., 1986). J.I.'s therapist need not share her antagonism for fundamentalistic religious beliefs, for example, as long as he can accept her expressions of disbelief.

We conclude from reviewing available research on patient and therapist belief compatibility that therapists who share similar humanitarian and intellectual values with their patients and who have discrepant views of personal safety and the value of interpersonal intimacy and attachment comprise optimally compatible pairings. When differences occur in other belief and value dimensions, therapists who are sufficiently tolerant of and able to communicate from within the patient's framework may be as effective as those whose views are similar to those of their patients. Such therapists do not appear to exert undue influence over socially sensitive but nonpathological social and religious values.

Attributions.   Interpersonal patterns include dynamic processes of defense and control by which patients attempt to gratify their wants and control their anxiety. Among the dimensions of interpersonal behavior defined by these processes of defense and expectation, those of attribution may be especially important for psychotherapy (Beutler, 1983; Harvey & Weary, 1985). Concepts of attribution have been discussed widely under a variety of labels, generally reflecting variants of the construct of internal-external locus of perceived control of reinforcement originally formulated by Rotter (1966). This original concept has been expanded broadly since its inception (Lefcourt, 1980), and these expansions have included the introduction of a variety of measurement devices for capturing various aspects of the internal to external attributional dimension (Harvey & Weary, 1985). Indeed, the concepts of interpersonal defense which we discussed as therapy-relevant patient predisposing characteristics in Chapter 4 represent aspects of control attributions.

While there is some danger in equating attributional styles with broader personality types (Rotter, 1966; Lefcourt, 1980, Krause, 1986), there is evidence that these styles are relatively stable correlates of developmental stages (Deci, 1980; Lachman, 1986) and correspond both with coping adequacy and interpersonal styles (Lefcourt, 1980; Brehm & Brehm, 1981; Krause, 1986). Not only do attributions of control, reinforcement, punishment, and causation translate to corresponding, albeit limited, dimensions of personality and psychopathology, they also have relevance to the matter of establishing a compatible match between patient and therapist. For example, patient attributions of control seem to be conceptually similar to the Brehms' (Brehm & Brehm, 1981) concept of interpersonal *reactance.*

High-reactant individuals descriptively are similar to those who strongly adhere to internal attributions of control. That is, both the highly reactant individual and the person who is bound by an internal locus of perceived control resist persuasive influences (Biondo & MacDonald, 1971; Brehm & Brehm, 1981); perceptions and attributions of internal control are associated with patient resistance (Houston, 1972; Beutler, 1983) and correspond with poor treatment prognosis (Miller & Norman 1981).

Less highly reactant individuals and those with expectations of external control, on the other hand, are susceptible to external influence efforts. Indeed, the patient who is externally controlled is likely to manifest this susceptibility to influence by becoming more internally controlled in response to the therapist's efforts (Gillis & Jessor, 1970).

Because of the relative similarity of reactance potential, on the one hand, and attributions of control and punishment, on the other, it is logical to assume that certain types of introjects predispose one to high reactance and that patterns of patient-therapist similarity and dissimilarity on these dimensions facilitate and inhibit progress. Indeed, Tennen, Rohrbaugh, Press, and White (1981) maintain that a high status and authoritarian therapist is contraindicated when a patient is highly invested in attributing or maintaining internal control.

On the other hand, similarity of attributed locus of control (and punishment) between patient and therapist may facilitate a bond of commonality. Research on the dimensions of causal attribution suggests that patient-therapist similarity, as applied to self-vs-other blame and expected control, bodes positively for commitment to treatment and, to a lesser degree, for positive outcomes (Foon, 1986; Tracey, 1986).

While such findings as the foregoing are intriguing, they are not yet definitive. At this point, information is sufficient only to argue that a moderate amount of similarity between patient and therapist may facilitate treatment response. What is more important, however, is the conclusion that therapists should be well informed of the combative potential existing within a treatment relationship that is composed of individuals who are prone to resist each other's causal, reinforcement, or punishment attributions. We will address the implications of this point in greater detail in later chapters.

Again, the case of J.I. is illustrative. If the therapist were to be as protective of his own freedom from influence as J.I., a competitive relationship would be expected. The therapist, in fact, must be able to let the patient be "right." An interpretation should be withdrawn rather than forced, a homework assignment must be modified or discontinued, a therapy experiment must be allowed to fail, no matter how much the therapist believes in the value of any of these things, in order to avoid contributing to a patient's defeat. If there are instances in which a therapist must force an issue (e.g., involuntary hospitalization), it cannot emanate from his/her need to protect personal investments for freedom.

SUMMARY AND COMMENT

In this chapter we have proposed that a complex pattern of initial and background similarities and differences presents a solid footing for the establishment of stable working relationships. Theoretical concepts both from persuasion theory and from dynamic psychotherapy theories lend some support for this point of view. Available empirical evidence suggests that background and attributional similarities and perceptual or value dissimilarities combine to enhance the treatment relationship and further therapy outcomes. Patient-therapist differences in social attachment needs appear to facilitate therapeutic movement, perhaps by providing a counterbalancing viewpoint to the patient's style of interpersonal relationships.

These patterns of similarity and difference have implications for patient selection, but they also have implications for referral patterns. In the usual practice, a clinician defines what types of individuals he or she will work well with and what individuals will be referred. These decisions should include consideration of the patient's demographic and interpersonal similarities to the therapist. While neither dissimilarity in gender, ethnic background, SES, and age nor similarity of needs, beliefs, and attributions constitute insurmountable barriers to treatment when each is considered alone, therapists may especially want to consider referral for patients whose demographic characteristics are cumulatively incompatible with those of the therapist on several dimensions.

These matching dimensions also have implications for assigning the context of treatment. For example, patients whose personal characteristics (i.e., low SES, older adults from disenfranchised minorities) are associated with premature termination may be usefully considered for time-limited and highly-focused treatments. This decision may be especially advantageous in those cases where therapist-patient demographic dissimilarity inflates the probability of early or premature termination.

The initial compatibility of therapist and patient is only part of the story of the therapeutic alliance, however. While such initial compatibility may set the stage for treatment and facilitates a sense of being understood, the power of the relationship is not solely determined by those factors over which the therapist has little if any control. Though perhaps more difficult, a therapeutic relationship is very possible between patients and therapists who have unaccommodating differences and disparities in personal backgrounds.

It is the therapist's task to assess where the potential problems may occur because of incompatible backgrounds and learn to respond in anticipation of these difficulties in order to allay and prevent the interference. Learning to respond sensitively and wholly to problem areas can frequently overcome the disadvantages of problematic initial relationships. Therapist skill becomes all the more important in these circumstances, however (Foreman & Marmar, 1984). On this note, we will now turn to a consideration of what the therapist can do to enhance the initial level of compatibility and prevent incompatibility from becoming an insurmountable threat to the treatment relationship.

SUGGESTED READINGS

Beutler, L. E. (1979b). Values, beliefs, religion and the persuasive influence of psychotherapy. *Psychotherapy: Theory, Research and Practice, 16,* 432–440.

Beutler, L.E., Crago, M. & Arizmendi, T. G. (1986). Therapist variables in psychotherapy process and outcome. In S. L. Garfield & A. E. Bergin (Eds.), *Handbook of psychotherapy and behavior change,* 3rd ed. (pp. 257–310), New York: John Wiley and Sons.

Corrigan, J. D., Dell, D. M., Lewis, K. N. & Schmidt, L. D. (1980). Counseling as a social influence process: A review. *Journal of Counseling Psychology Monograph, 27,* 395–441.

Frank, J. D. (1973). *Persuasion and healing: A comparative study of psychotherapy* (rev. ed.). Baltimore: Johns Hopkins University Press.

Goldstein, A. P. (1966). Psychotherapy research by extrapolation from social psychology. *Journal of Counseling Psychology, 13,* 38–45.

Tjelveit, A. C. (1986). The ethics of value conversion in psychotherapy: Appropriate and inappropriate therapist influence on client values. *Clinical Psychology Review, 6,* 515–537.

10

Enhancing and Maintaining the Therapeutic Alliance

The nucleus of psychotherapy is the treatment alliance. This unique and healing aspect of human relationships depends upon reciprocal resonance and affirmation (Saunders, Howard & Orlinsky, in press). The power of the treatment alliance should not be equated with simple liking or attraction, however. Credibility and trust, as we have observed in previous chapters, are more substantial bases for therapeutic influence than the more fickle attribute of interpersonal attraction (e.g., Beutler, Crago & Arizmendi, 1986). This is true because attraction is largely influenced by such factors as physical appeal or beauty (Corrigan et al., 1980). Credibility and trust reflect patterns of interaction and collaboration which change within treatment and which can be altered by either patient or therapist.

At several points in earlier chapters, we have maintained that it is necessary to adjust treatment methods to fit the expectations and needs of patients who vary in diagnosis, background, personality patterns, symptoms, problem severity, and coping styles. This adjustment is no less a necessity among the methods for enhancing the treatment relationship itself. Throughout this volume we have emphasized the healing role of the collaborative treatment relationship. We now must emphasize the dynamic nature of this relationship. The therapist's task in this process is to maintain constant sensitivity both to problems which emerge in the collaborative alliance and to the current quality of that alliance, adjusting the approach applied accordingly.

Throughout Section III we discussed ways that patient predisposing characteristics might play a role in establishing a beneficial context in which treatment may be conducted. We turned in Chapter 9 to an exploration of patient and therapist compatibility and suggested that the effectiveness of psychotherapy can be enhanced by certain similarities and differences between patients' and therapists' backgrounds, beliefs, personalities, and interpersonal needs. In the current chapter, our attention shifts from that of patient and therapist inherent "fit," to methods that the therapist might use to enhance the compatibility between the patient and the treatment.

This chapter is designed to present methods for enhancing the fit between patient predisposing characteristics, on the one hand, and the demands of treatment settings and modalities, on the other. This task is an ongoing one, requiring moment-to-moment decisions about therapeutic implementation. These decisions constitute an ongoing "process diagnosis" of both the patient and the treatment context.

Procedures for enhancing the psychotherapy relationship generally fall into two classes. The first class of procedures aims to alter the status, expectations, and behaviors of patients to fit the treatment, while the second is designed to alter the treatment environment and procedures to fit the patient. We will refer to this first approach to enhancing the treatment process as *Role Induction* to distinguish it from the second class of procedures, to which we will refer as *In-Therapy Environmental Management.*

ROLE INDUCTION

Role Induction is a general term that describes efforts to prepare patients for treatment by educating them about treatment roles and outcomes *before* psychotherapy actually begins. While either allowing patients to select a preferred therapist or assigning a personally compatible therapist to them enhances the positive sense that the patient comes to attach to the treatment process, the possibility of doing this consistently does not usually exist within the constraints of clinic demands and therapist availability. If we could rely on compatibility matching and assignment to establish the therapeutic alliance, it is likely that some therapists would be extremely busy and others would have little to do.

Role Induction allows some opportunity to compensate for the limitations of natural selection and is a relatively powerful method for facilitating a positive treatment response. Most investigations of Role Induction, though varying in method, objectives, and patient sample, have supported the relative value of such preparatory activity (cf. Parloff, Waskow & Wolfe, 1978; Mayerson, 1984; Beutler, Crago & Arizmendi, 1986; Orlinsky & Howard, 1986). These studies suggest that Role Induction improves treatment retention rates (LaTorre, 1977; Wilson, 1985), facilitates positive perceptions and attractions to the treatment process (Yalom et al.,

1967; Jacobs, Trick & Withersty, 1976; Zwick & Attkisson, 1985), pro-
motes treatment compliance (Meichenbaum & Turk, 1987), and enhances
psychotherapy outcomes (Strupp & Bloxom, 1973; Childress & Gillis,
1977; Zwick & Attkisson, 1985). The procedures of Role Induction can
be subclassified under three headings: (1) instructional methods, (2) observational and participatory learning, and (3) treatment contracting.

Instructional Methods.   Instructional methods of inducing role behaviors
among patients consist of providing direct written or verbal information
about the nature of therapy and of the roles expected of patient and
therapist. In their simplest form, role instruction methods simply explain
what to expect and how to respond to the treatment. Most role induction
interviews are somewhat more elaborate than this, however.

In one of the best known studies of instructional methods for inducing
therapeutic roles, Hoehn-Saric, Frank, Imber, Nash, Stone, and Battle
(1964) constructed a pretherapy interview which outlined what behaviors
were expected of patient and therapist, described the nature of such therapeutic phenomena as resistance, provided suggestions for recognizing and
dealing with these issues when they arose, and specified the length of
time to be expected before improvement should be anticipated. When
systematically compared to the treatment of patients who did not receive
this method of retraining, the role induction interview was found to significantly enhance the process and outcome of psychotherapy.

While role induction interviews have occasionally failed to yield major
benefits (e.g., Yalom, Houts, Newell & Rand, 1967), most of the current
evidence indicates that instructional methods facilitate symptomatic
change, encourage the adoption of role appropriate attitudes, and promote
the development of positive feelings about treatment (cf. Mayerson, 1984;
Zwick & Attkisson, 1985). Other research suggests that direct instruction
reduces nonproductive advice-seeking and enhances involvement in short-
term treatment (Turkat, 1979). Moreover, the procedures translate across
patient groups, impacting many who present special problems or who
usually are considered to be poor risks for conventional psychotherapies.
For example, role induction interviews have been found to enhance the
relationship and process of conventional treatments provided to low socioeconomic class patients who have little treatment sophistication, when
compared to similar patients who were not instructed in roles and expectations (Heitler, 1976; Holliday, 1979).

Observational and Participatory Learning Methods.   A second role induction
method of enhancing treatment relationships consists of pretherapy modeling and/or practice, designed to develop the skills which facilitate treatment
response. Truax and colleagues were among the first to report positive

results with this procedure (Truax & Carkhuff, 1967; Truax & Wargo, 1969). Their induction procedure consisted of a 30-minute audio tape of representative therapy segments. The procedure was specifically aimed at facilitating group therapy process and modeled "good" and productive interchanges among group members.

In an effort to extend this procedure, Strupp and Bloxom (1973) employed a role induction film to prepare low socioeconomic class patients for conventional treatments. At the end of 12 treatment sessions, those patients who had been presented with film demonstrations reported more facilitative treatment relationships, exhibited more productive in-treatment behaviors, and experienced better treatment outcomes when contrasted with similar patients receiving a control film. A third group receiving a role induction interview demonstrated effects similar to those of the group observing the film; no significant differences appeared between the two role induction methods. Role induction films also have demonstrated a positive impact on drop-out rates, even among patients with relatively severe psychopathology (Mayerson, 1984; Wilson, 1985).

Another observational method has employed even a more active and participatory form of role induction. Warren and Rice (1972) suggest the value of therapy practice sessions in order to establish treatment roles and to stabilize or reinforce effective treatment behaviors. In this procedure, patients meet with someone other than their own therapist for approximately one-half hour following every third or fourth session during the course of time-limited psychotherapy. During these meetings, patients are encouraged to talk about problems which may arise with therapy or with the therapist, and then instruction, information, and suggestions are provided in order to enhance the effectiveness of the patient's response to these problems. The authors have demonstrated that this procedure reduces drop-out rates among poor prognosis clients.

Therapeutic Contracting. The third role induction method, therapeutic contracting, has a diverse history in psychotherapy. While it has been discussed widely in family systems theory (Madanes, 1981), Gestalt/Transactional Analysis (Goulding & Goulding, 1979), and cognitive therapy (Beck, Rush, Shaw & Emery, 1979), behavior therapists have been most active and explicit in defining its use. The specific techniques have ranged from signed agreements (Alexander, Barton, Schiavo & Parsons, 1976) to requiring the patient to deposit money which can be returned if the contract is kept and the predetermined goals are achieved (e.g., Pomerleau, 1979; Pomerleau & Pomerleau, 1984). These various behavioral contracting procedures can be viewed as components of several lockstepped but supraordinate phases. One view of these phases begins with (1) initial decision making and proceeds through (2) the generation or modification of expectancies, (3) the identification of target objectives of change, (4) monitoring progress, (5) delivering consequences, and (6) programming generalizations (Kirschenbaum & Flanery, 1984).

The role of contingency contracting is currently receiving wide usage in marital therapy where it is employed to facilitate communication and the provision of mutual support (Azrin, Naster & Jones, 1973; Emmelkamp, 1986; Weiss, Hops & Patterson, 1973).While the effectiveness of behavioral contracting, as used in this way, has been demonstrated (Emmelkamp, 1986), its usual use is to instigate therapeutic change rather than to prepare patients for therapy. For example, much of the activity in treatment programs which use behavioral contracting has centered around negotiation of the contract itself and, concomitantly, on the acts of assessing and reinforcing compliance. While important, this is a task that is different from preparing patients for the demands of treatment and enhancing their involvement in the process.

The role of contracting as a procedure for enhancing patient involvement in therapy is best seen in studies of time-limited psychotherapy. One of the most surprising conclusions to come from this literature is the serendipitous finding that an explicit, preset time limit results in patients remaining in treatment longer than when no such explicit contract is present. While the usual treatment duration in outpatient clinics is approximately five sessions and the usual duration of outpatient psychotherapy in private practice is approximately eight sessions (Butcher & Koss, 1978; Koss & Butcher, 1986), judging from a sampling of literature (e.g., Sloane, Staples, Cristol, Yorkston & Whipple, 1975; Elkin, 1986; Beutler, Scoggin et al., 1987), time-limited therapies may have a mean treatment duration closer to twice this amount.

Reasonably good evidence exists to suggest that patients treated under time-limited contracts tend to express satisfaction with the time limits, although the latter conclusion may be somewhat less warranted with certain, dynamically focused treatments than it is for behaviorally oriented methods (Koss & Butcher, 1986). Clearly, what we have traditionally thought of as "short-term" treatments, by this standard, are not short-term at all, on a relative scale. Perhaps, if therapists were to make explicit the long-term nature of the treatment contract, the high drop-out rates in the early stages of long-term treatment might be allayed.

One can conclude that contracting procedures can be used within individual treatment sessions themselves (e.g., Stuart, 1975) to facilitate treatment gains and to focus treatment activities. While the ingredients of the contract will vary with these several goals, one might extract certain ingredients that can be expected to enhance treatment involvement and prolong therapy commitment. Our conclusions and readings emphasize the following points:

(1) The time limits of the treatment should be explicit. This can be accomplished either by using a time-limited therapy or by specifying a renewable trial period of a designated length, during which time the effectiveness and usefulness of the treatment are to be assessed.

(2) The contract should also specify treatment goals even though these frequently will change in the course of treatment. To the degree that the treatment goals can be specified in terms of current behaviors and anticipated changes, they can serve as reference points for helping patients accurately assess the treatment. Specificity allows goals also to be used therapeutically both to assess gain and to explore changes in values and beliefs about self and others.

(3) The contract should be two-sided, specifying the roles of the therapist as well as those of the patient in order to facilitate the adoption of therapeutic behaviors.

(4) The contract may well emanate from other role induction procedures in order to capitalize on and reinforce the behaviors that are considered to be valuable and conducive to beneficial treatment outcome.

(5) It is helpful if the contract also specifies consequences of failing to comply with the agreement. These consequences may be monetary or symbolic but, in either case, should be specific and relevant to the treatment goals.

(6) The treatment contract can be written out in detail. While such explicitness may be difficult for some patients, and hence undesirable, it does facilitate keeping a focus on treatment aims. In any case, a method should be provided for referring back to the conditions of the contract as the need arises.

Summary of Role Induction Methods

The methods of Role Induction have several characteristics in common, whether constructed as direct instruction, through contracts, or through modeling and observation. Wilson (1985) has provided a helpful compilation of the recommended ingredients into a procedure which combines both instructional and observational methods. As he notes, a central tenet of most procedures is that pretherapy training will help establish treatment as a collaborative adventure, shared by both patient and therapist. The various other aspects of role induction simply reinforce and operationalize this concept of collaboration.

Prescription of Role Induction Methods

Once one decides that certain patient roles should be induced rather than adopting procedures which accommodate to patient expectations, the method to be used for role induction becomes a critical variable. A careful distinction between the induction and the treatment cannot always be maintained. Hence, the role induction should be selected to fit patients' needs for personal contact, structure, and reassurance, as well as their preferential defensive styles.

Overall, it seems that combining procedures is more advantageous than using single role induction procedures (Mayerson, 1984), but this is seldom feasible in view of time demands and convenience. For most cases, we are left to rely on clinical experience and common sense to tell us how to prepare a given patient for treatment.

Table 10.1 summarizes some of the major conclusions from the prior pages. We urge the reader to be cautious in accepting our recommendations on this topic. As is often the case with prescriptive treatment assignment, clinical intuition has preceded empirical data. Although we must urge respect for research findings when they occur, we cannot wait for their advent. Like all clinicians, we must assume the value and validity of clinical wisdom until scientific investigations provide more information.

Table 10.1
Indicators and Enabling Factors for Role Induction Procedures

---

Instructional Methods
   Enabling factors include verbal and/or written fluency.
      Indicated for patients with little prior experience with psychotherapy; has a positive impact with low SES adults and difficult to treat children; may reduce drop out rates in group therapy.
Observational and Participatory Methods
      Indicated with low SES clients and those with few written or spoken language skills; role modeling/participatory procedures may be especially useful for low prognosis groups who find talking to their therapist difficult.
Therapeutic Contracting
      Indicated use of preplanned time limits for patients who have a difficult time delaying gratification and making long-term commitments; especially helpful in marital and family therapies; valuable whenever early termination represents a risk; helps direct treatment goals and serves as a focus for active intervention and communication skills training.

Heretofore, we have considered two major classes of variables which bear upon fine tuning the prescriptive assignment of relationship enhancement methods—predetermining patient characteristics and characteristics of the treatment context. Building upon and extending the material summarized in Table 10.1, we can now provide some tentative suggestions for adjusting Role Induction procedures as a function of these two dimensions.

Predetermining Patient Variables. Many if not most patient predetermining variables can be applied prescriptively to decisions about role induction methods. That is, predetermining variables can be differentially used to select and modify the content and methods of implementing or delivering role induction programs. However, of the predetermining variables discussed in prior chapters, Axis I and Axis II diagnostic labels enter into decisions about methods of role induction the least reliably, doing so only insofar as they suggest the presence of deficits in the patient's ability to process information and comprehend social meanings. Among the predetermining variables which may augur for the selection of one or another role induction method, demographic and coping style variables offer the clearest decisional criteria.

Among patients with intellectual deficits or cognitive impairments, or for those with limited educational and social resources, observational and practice methods of preparation may be preferred to instructional ones. For obvious reasons, such deficits in predisposing characteristics argue against the use of preparation methods which require reading recognition and comprehension skills. Research has consistently emphasized the value of contracting methods and of methods which engage the patient's participation through practice or direct observation. To this conclusion, we add the need to develop preparation materials which are consistent with patients' verbal level and which use examples and language which are consistent with their usual experience.

Such strategies as informing the patient in advance of the therapist's gender, ethnicity, and perhaps even age will go far to align therapist-patient similarity, especially if an effort has been made to respond to the patient's expressed preferences when making therapist assignments. When the patient has expressed a more specific preference that certain attitudes and characteristics be present in the treatment, as when a religious patient specifically requests that the therapist share certain religious values and beliefs, some reassurance of being responsive to this request may also be provided during role induction interviews in order to facilitate the initial engagement process.

Personality and coping patterns also can effectively be considered prescriptively when selecting a method of role induction. For example, knowledge of the adequacy and stability of the patient's coping abilities and of the problem-solving phase which characterizes the patient's current dilemma may be of assistance in selecting the specific role induction method used. The poorer the patient's coping ability, for example, the greater the value of employing very careful and intensive therapy preparation. Individuals with poor coping skills can be expected to be intolerant of group-based preparations and those which provide little support, such as is often true of verbal or written instructional methods. Individual attention in a quiet and unstressful environment is likely to be productive with these patients. Observational methods that require little participation may also be more helpful than direct role playing interviews, under these circumstances.

When selecting a method of role induction, it may also be helpful to attend to the patient's phase of problem resolution. Because of the different methods typically used at different stages of problem resolution, the patient who is in the contemplation phase of problem resolution, for example, may be better able to benefit from instructional methods than the person in the active phase of problem resolution. The latter individual, on the other hand, may benefit from observational or contractual methods of preparation.

Some of the recommendations implied by these suggestions will be found to contradict one another when applied to the unique combination of characteristics presented by a given patient in a given setting. One might expect, for example, that among the patients described throughout this volume, the relative ego integrity of J.I., in spite of her traumatically induced phobias and recurrent depression, may make her a candidate for a larger number of role induction options than would be true of J.C., whose rather fragile belief in his own deity (recall that he believed that he was Jesus Christ), may lend itself better to participatory methods than to observational or instructional ones.

We wish principally to emphasize, by the foregoing considerations, that a single preparation procedure for all patients probably is inappropriate and the more one can tailor the preparation method to fit the given patient, the better the likely effect. We suggest that the therapist have available a set of basic instructional materials that can be delivered both in writing and via verbal instruction, along with examples of effective individual and group (including marital therapy) interactions. We further suggest that the presentation of these prepared materials be preceded and followed by an individually tailored interview which is sensitive to the desires and wishes of the particular patient. This unstructured clinical interview can be responsive to patient questions and sensitive to those nuances of patient behavior that may suggest the need for special considerations in selecting treatments.

Treatment Context.   It should go without saying that the environment or context in which the patient is to be treated should also play a role in selecting and constructing role induction methods. Certainly it would seem to be sensitive, if not directly facilitative of treatment process and outcome, if the patient were provided in advance with information about the treatment setting and conditions of payment and service. With those whose social skills and achievements allow, a written description of the treatment setting and conditions may suffice, if appropriately followed by an expressed opportunity for discussion.

In discussions with our own patients, many of whom present with confusion and disorientation associated with aging and disease, we find it useful to provide an instructional tour of the facilities and some personalized instruction on how to find the office, the billing clerk, the lavatories, the pharmacy, etc. Those in smaller offices should nonetheless take equal care in orienting patients, with particular attention given to those whose condition and major symptoms may interfere with their comfort in the treatment surroundings.

Treatment length and frequency are particular aspects of preparation which should be routinely provided to all patients. Even those who are to be seen in long-term treatment may benefit from some discussion about what is to be gained in such an extended treatment regimen. Especially in this latter case, one must be careful to provide a rationale for the program which does not make the patient's anxiety worse. A recommendation of frequent or long-term treatment may be presented by emphasizing that the patient has ego resources to tolerate and move quickly in treatment of the assigned intensity, rather than as suggesting the lack of coping skills and the seriousness of the patient's problem. Great care should be given to making these explanations acceptable, positive, and supportive.

Medical, group, and family treatments require special preparation, once again with due consideration given to tuning the explanation to the common experiences and expectations of the patient. For example, when we reach a point in treatment that we want to include J.I.'s husband, a special preparatory interview with the couple together may be advantageous for setting the roles and limits of this format of treatment. This introductory session would explore the husband's objectives and fears of treatment, as well as confirming the confidentiality of prior work with J.I.

We particularly recommend observational methods for preparing patients for group therapy (Daldrup, Beutler, Engle & Greenberg, 1988). Patients whose defensive style is one of inhibition and constraint especially need to be provided with time in the group setting during which they may be assured of not being required to take undue risks. These protected periods may be less necessary for the emotionally expressive and socially extraverted (externalizing) patient than for the inhibited one.

Finally, the patient should be provided with an overview of the treatment philosophy of the therapist. Especially with the highly reactant patient, care must be taken in this presentation to avoid the impression that these beliefs and philosophies are to be adopted or believed by the patient. Indeed, if there is an exception to the rule that such philosophies should be shared, it may be for the patient whose investment in personal freedom is very strong (i.e., those with high levels of reactance). Symptomatically, this description roughly can be applied to severely compulsive individuals and to those with paranoid or antisocial patterns of interpersonal defense.

IN-THERAPY ENVIRONMENTAL MANAGEMENT

While role induction methods are useful and relatively easy to implement, they also have certain limitations. Not only is it unlikely that all people will be able to adapt to the demands of conventional treatment, but there are, in the methods of role induction, certain philosophical underpinnings which may be counterproductive for some purposes. For example, the implication that patients must change to fit the treaters' methods and environments is a potentially dangerous assumption because it may lull one into blaming the patient if treatment is not successful. It is this very attitude which may hamper the effective treatment of patients whose ethnic and socioeconomic backgrounds are very different from their therapists' (Goldstein, 1971; Garfield, 1978; Lorion & Felner, 1986).

When we speak of environmental management in this chapter, we do not refer to manipulating or changing the formal aspects of treatment— those procedures that are associated with and advocated in the context of different theories. The distinctiveness of environmental management, in comparison to these other aspects of technical eclecticism, is partially paralleled in the differences that have been drawn between therapist *styles* and *interventions* (Lambert & Bergin, 1983; Beutler, Crago & Arizmendi, 1986). Therapist interventions are those operations and procedures whose applications are guided by the therapist's theory of psychotherapeutic change and will be discussed at length in Part V of this volume. Communication styles are usually employed with little conscious awareness. Moreover, when they are employed intentionally, these styles seldom derive specifically from theories of psychotherapy and generally arise from more general notions of social influence and communication.

In this chapter, we will use the term "Environmental Management" to refer to methods of initiating and systematically using styles of communication and interaction which cut across theories and formal procedures. Procedures of in-therapy management are designed to maintain and further the relationship rather than treatment outcome directly and characterize the in-treatment environment. The focus is upon bringing into the therapist's conscious control those verbal and nonverbal mannerisms and cues by which information is transmitted. These styles convey information about the communicator, separate and apart from the content of the communication; hence, their role in enhancing the quality of the relationship.

Therapeutic Styles

It should be recognized that the distinction between therapeutic styles and therapeutic interventions is becoming more difficult to maintain, especially as writers increasingly advocate the intentional use of stylistic patterns of communication and incorporate theoretical formulations about these styles into formal theories of psychotherapy. While somewhat arbitrary, environmental management methods of enhancing the relationship will be discussed for the current purposes under three headings: (1) Nonverbal Styles, (2) Situational Stimuli, and (3) Verbal Behavioral Styles.

Nonverbal Styles. While a good deal of research has accumulated in the past three decades on the communication value of nonverbal behaviors, this research seldom has been conducted in actual psychotherapy. Nonetheless, analogue research has addressed such therapy-relevant issues as the recognition of arousal and attachment (Burgoon, Buller, Hale & de Turck, 1984), the establishment of trust and intimacy (Mintz, 1969; Haas & Tepper, 1972; Burgoon et al., 1984), conveying the communicator's attitudes about the listener (Ekman, 1964), and the establishment of interpersonal control (Ellsworth, 1975).

Depending on the aspect of attitudes being influenced, this research suggests that nonverbal communication cues exert from five to 20 times more influence on listener attitudes than does the verbal content of the message, even though listeners frequently are not aware of this influence. While even subtle cues can influence attitudes, their effect is frequently less predictable than if these nonverbal cues are both clear and prominent (cf. Robbins & Haase, 1985). Thus, nonverbal cues are most likely to convey the message intended by the therapist if they are different from the usual behavior of the therapist and carry a message that is consistent with those that precede and follow them. This conclusion implies that some intention in their use may be helpful in transmitting therapeutic understanding.

In a review of current literature on the social roles of one important nonverbal dimension, that of gaze and eye contact, Kleinke (1986) emphasizes that *mutual gaze* is a correlate of liking and attraction, *continuous gaze* reflects interpersonal dominance, *infrequent gaze* is perceived as a lack of involvement, *frequent gaze* is judged by respondents to reflect a high intensity of feelings, and *selective changing of gaze* regulates the flow of communication among people.

The effects and correlates of gaze are not always positive or consistent, however. For example, gaze may be a poor indicator of whether the communicator's feelings are positive or negative (Kimble, Forte & Yoshikawa, 1981), may be utilized to deceive as well as to convey accurate information (Riggio & Friedman, 1983), and can be used to threaten others as well as to assert oneself (Hughes & Goldman, 1978). It is because of this ambiguity that message vividness—clarity and prominence—is so important (Robbins & Haase, 1984). Collectively, the multiple roles of gaze and eye contact suggest that these behaviors can be used therapeutically to enhance and facilitate the development of a treatment alliance.

The experimental research done on gaze and other nonverbal styles to date, while clearly limited, has been quite positive. The most realistic conclusions to be drawn from this research are the suggestions that forward posture, mutual gaze, and responsive facial expressions and movements enhance the quality of therapeutic contact (Ekman, 1964; Haase & Tepper, 1972; Maurer & Tyndall, 1983), encourage patient's openness to treatment influence (Patterson, 1982), facilitate client satisfaction levels (Fretz, 1966), and reduce premature termination rates (Howard et al., 1970). It also seems justified to conclude that the systematic use of silence, gaze, posture, and nonsexual touch can facilitate the development of trust and liking (Forer, 1969) and can increase the therapist's level of perceived credibility and expertness (Hubble, Noble & Robinson, 1981). However, it is also clear that the use of nonverbal cues should coincide with therapist intent and be presented as part of the general communication effort rather than being arbitrarily applied independently of other verbal and nonverbal messages (Hermansson, Webster & McFarland, 1988).

In spite of these positive and promising findings, the effective therapist must be aware of our current ignorance in how nonverbal variables operate when applied to actual therapy, the selective impact of these communication styles on different patients, and their potential danger. We do not know for certain if the observed correlations between eye contact and posture, on the one hand, and openness and liking, on the other, are causally related, nor if they function in actual treatment in the same way they do in laboratory settings. Similarly, we cannot be certain if one can really increase the quality of a treatment relationship by planfully altering posture and gaze or if qualities of these experiences simply follow from and reflect the level of intimacy established (Beutler, Crago & Arizmendi, 1986). Such gaps in our knowledge should not constrain our efforts to use nonverbal communication styles in a selective and explicit fashion, but they should argue for the use of sense and judgment in the process.

The selective nature of the impact of nonverbal cues should also be considered. For example, males and females appear to respond differently to gaze and touch (e.g., Buchanan, Goldman & Juhnke, 1977; Hughes & Goldman, 1978), with women being more tolerant and favorable in their reactions than men. A persistent gaze may indicate either sexual or nonsexual intimacy between a man and a woman, and may signal competitiveness between two men (Kleinke, 1986; Valentine & Ehrlichman, 1979). Women may be disposed to help other women who manifest closeness in nonverbal ways, while the same nonverbal behavior between two men is likely to result in avoidance (Kleinke, 1986).

Personality variables may also determine both the use of nonverbal cues and one's response to them. Characteristic and distinguishing nonverbal patterns of communication appear to develop early in life (Coates, 1978) and to bear a relationship to established personality characteristics among both psychotherapists (Smith, 1972) and other groups (e.g., Exline, 1963; Mischel, 1968). For example, the intensity and frequency of interpersonal eye contact reflect affiliation needs, and women who have high needs for affiliation gravitate to and utilize nonverbal approach behaviors in conducive situations. However, at the same time, women may avoid and retreat from nonverbal approach behaviors in competitive situations. The reverse pattern has been observed among women with low affiliation needs (Exline, 1963).

It may also be that individuals who are especially sensitive and resistant to persuasive efforts by therapists may respond negatively to attributes of liking and empathy that may be conveyed through nonverbal and verbal means (Kolb, Beutler, Davis, Crago & Shanfield, 1985). Patterson (1982) proposes that changing one's nonverbal approach behaviors can induce either a positive or negative effect in another person, depending upon the recipient's predisposition to interpret the experience in given ways. He suggests that these approach or "intimacy-arousal" behaviors induce physiological changes in the recipient, roughly corresponding to the intensity of the communication.

Preestablished dispositions toward interpersonal distance or attachment may set the interpretations given to these changes and correspondingly may induce either avoidance or increased intimacy. While those whose thematic needs reflect attitudes of trust and affiliation interpret such cues positively and reciprocate by intimacy seeking, those whose thematic needs suggest distrust and competitiveness may respond negatively to their own arousal and withdraw from or avoid those who emit approach behaviors. These findings may serve to remind us that nonverbal cues, by their nature, are ambiguous, are subject to diverse interpretations, and are capable of eliciting diverse effects (Kleinke, 1986). The need for selective application of the nonverbal cues becomes clear when one has this awareness.

While an intentional forward lean and eye contact may have been quite helpful in conveying therapist interest and support to M.S., the anatomy student whose fears of contamination forced her withdrawal from school, these same verbal cues could be expected to be threatening to J.I. The relatively low reactance level of M.S. as well as her tendency to seek attachment may have allowed her to perceive the intended meaning of these cues. In early treatment, these strategies may foster the development of the relationship, but at a later time withdrawing these nonverbal signs may better serve the therapeutic objectives by highlighting her reliance on others for direction and support.

In contrast, the relatively high reactance level of J.I., as manifest in her intense needs to maintain autonomy and to resist external influence, may have contaminated the intended nonverbal message of support. Early in treatment, such nonverbal messages may have resulted in her sensing a threat to her safety. Later in treatment, such cues may direct her attention to the sources of her conflicts by selectively raising her anxiety. In each case, the decision to employ or not to employ nonverbal cues must be based upon what is desired at a given phase of treatment—relationship building or exposure to unfounded fears.

Situational Stimuli. Stimuli that are not transmitted directly by the therapist's behavior may also serve as nonverbal messages of support. Characteristics of the setting, the arrangement of the room, the availability of support staff, and the procedures used for registering and billing patients all comprise situational cues that reveal therapist attitudes.

Relatively little research has accumulated on the role of situational cues in altering specific aspects of the psychotherapy relationship, although an increasing amount of research has accumulated on how aspects of the inpatient psychiatric environment may hamper or facilitate emotional healing. This research has suggested that such architectural design features as the number of beds on a ward, their juxtaposition with respect to one another, and the number and size of rooms for social gatherings may either promote or reduce social withdrawal (Ittelson et al., 1970, 1972; Bell, Fisher & Loomis, 1978).

When building design allows institutionalized patients to maintain freedom of movement, privacy, and control over their social contacts, social interaction is facilitated (Snyder & Ostrander, 1972). Large, abundantly furnished day rooms are used less efficiently and with less social interaction than small, more sparsely furnished, and relatively private rooms. Moreover, hospital environments in which rooms are designed for easy access and viewing by staff may retard patient freedom, disregard patients' needs for privacy, and hamper social contact. Patients who feel violated by the unhampered intrusion of ward staff may attempt to reestablish control over their worlds by avoiding social contact and by developing other symptoms of institutionalization (Ittelson, Proshansky & Rivlin, 1972).

Many of the negative responses to environmental order and constraint observed in the foregoing paragraphs reflect on human needs for personal space. Overcrowding, seating arrangements which violate one's need for distance, and lack of control over one's environment all negatively impact emotional healing. Clearly, these observations carry major implications for hospital and partial care environments. There are also less obvious implications for psychotherapy. Individual needs and sensitivities to change and encroachment are characteristics of those with high *reactance* (Brehm & Brehm, 1981) and tendencies to withdraw or act out may reflect more general coping styles (see Chapter 4). The implications of these variables for the use of various types of therapeutic procedures will be discussed in Part V of this volume (Chapters 11–13). There are additional implications for office practice, however, as suggested in our previous example of J.C., whose tenuous identity may be threatened if offices are too confined and crowded. Similarly, some phobic patients may be especially needy of space and vistas to enhance a feeling of safety, while others avoid such openness and seek enclosed offices.

As a general rule, the location in which therapy takes place and its surrounding environment should be one of relaxation, safety, and peace. Many things can be done to enhance patient comfort and subjective safety. A formal office environment may facilitate beliefs in the therapist's credibility (Kerr & Dell, 1976; Childress & Gillis, 1977). Allowing a patient freedom in seat selection, maintaining an interactional space free of physical barriers between patient and therapist, and providing relatively small waiting areas that allow either privacy or interaction may facilitate positive attitudes toward treatment (Bell, Fisher & Loomis, 1978). Office practices which minimize patient frustration, such as clearly specified billing procedures and sensitive support staff, are at least as important as other aspects of the environment to enhancing patient safety and comfort.

Aside from providing safety and privacy, psychotherapy is also designed selectively to arouse, confront, explore, and extinguish patients' fears. In the service of these objectives, there are aspects of the treatment environment over which the therapist may exert control in order to intensify or reduce patient arousal levels as needed. Patients who lack clear boundary and personal definitions (Greene, 1976) and those who are relatively high in authoritarian attitudes but low in self esteem (Frankel & Barrett, 1971) especially may avoid proximity to the therapist. This pattern may represent indirectly either a patient's conflicts with attachment and intimacy or the presence of high levels of reactance.

As a microcosm of the patient's interpersonal world, the psychotherapy relationship is designed to confront and expunge patient fears of closeness and separation, but doing so requires the ability progressively to change patient-therapist proximity. The availability of different seating arrangements and the use of a rolling chair may provide this flexibility. By moving his or her position in order to alter proximity to the patient, selectively changing seating patterns in group therapy environments, and by selectively altering room lighting, the therapist may be able effectively to increase or reduce patient arousal levels as needed.

In the case of J.I., for example, early treatment may be enhanced by proxemic distance until the anxiety symptoms associated with her automobile accident subside. In these early phases of treatment, alterations of therapist posture and of patient-therapist distance within sessions may be too threatening to provide the sense of safety required to allow her to become desensitized to automobiles and travel. Because she relies on repressive coping styles, however, increasing therapist proximity may assist in later efforts to arouse repressed memories and to undermine unproductive denial regarding the events surrounding the rape and death of her girlfriend and her own traumatic loss of the ability to walk.

Verbal Behavioral Styles.   Most of psychotherapy consists of verbal activity. Interpretations are made, directives are given, homework is assigned, feelings are discussed, interactions are observed. Deciding which of these activities to employ and how to do so constitute the technical aspects of treatment. Often more important than the actual procedures, however, is the method of their implementation. The quality of the therapist's voice, rather than its content, the perceived emotion behind the words, rather than the words themselves—these subtle aspects of treatment are only partially understood and are seldom addressed by the therapist's theory.

Such speech patterns are used to convey therapist attitudes toward patients and attitudes about life more generally (Rosenthal, Blanck & Vannicelli, 1984; Beutler, Crago & Arizmendi, 1986). Direct self disclosures of such information may be weighed in contrast to that which is communicated by voice quality before it is allowed to exert any influence on patient disclosure. If consistently conveyed, disclosure of personal beliefs through verbal content and lexical style may facilitate perceived helpfulness of the therapist's intervention (e.g., Davis & Skinner, 1974; Mann & Murphy, 1975; Remer, Roffey & Buckholtz, 1983).

Research on patient and therapist verbal patterns suggests that the frequency and type of speech patterns of participating members converge with time in effective therapy. Effective outcomes may be enhanced when both patient and therapist maintain relatively high verbal activity levels (Pope, 1979; Tracey & Ray, 1984) and adopt similar patterns of word usage (Horn-George & Anchor, 1982). However, when patients are very distressed and agitated, adopting relatively low levels of activity seems to exert a calming and healing effect (Staples & Sloane, 1976).

Patterning of verbal activity within sessions and across treatment phases may also facilitate patient involvement, attention to focal themes and symptoms, and achievement of treatment goals (Beutler, 1983; Tracey, 1987). Maintaining relatively high levels of therapist activity focused on the mediating and final objectives of treatment, both throughout early treatment sessions and in the final minutes of each treatment session, while at the same time encouraging high levels of patient activity in late phases of treatment and early in each session may be an ideal pattern. This general goal must be adjusted by observing the verbal activity level of the patient, however, since the treatment relationship is probably not enhanced when therapists' levels of activity are highly discrepant, in either direction, from those of their patients (Grigg & Goodstein, 1957; Tracey & Ray, 1984).

Prescriptive Decisions

In the foregoing pages, we have supplied a number of recommendations for the implementation of environment management methods for enhancing the treatment relationship. The enabling and indicating factors for these procedures are summarized in Table 10.2.

Table 10.2
Indicators and Enabling Factors for Environmental Methods

Nonverbal Styles

Enabling factors for the use of touch and frequent or intense eye contact include tolerance for closeness and emotional arousal, a sense of interpersonal boundaries and low levels of interpersonal reactance; prolonged gaze and touch may be *contraindicated* between two male members of the dyad, especially if patient reactance level and competitiveness are high; may induce further distrust among individuals who are highly suspicious.

Indicated for those with high affiliation needs, especially if both members of the treatment dyad are female.

Situational Cues

Indicated use of open spaces and private spaces among psychiatric inpatients and institutionalized elderly; self selection of seating arrangements indicated for those with interpersonal distrust and/or high interpersonal reactance; physical distance and seating arrangement may be used to increase arousal levels among overcontrolled and emotionally insulated patients; proximity may also be indicated to control the undercontrolled and externalizing patient; proximity and distance may be helpful in individuals who are avoidant of social intimacy.

Contraindications of open spaces include risk of suicide and danger to others; close proximity is contraindicated when attempting to establish a treatment relationship.

Enabling factors for selective distance include a positive therapeutic bond.

Verbal Styles

Indicators of therapist verbal activity level are patient disturbance level and verbal facility; therapist activity level should match or be slightly discrepant from that of the patient; high therapist activity is *contraindicated* when patients have few verbal skills or are extremely distraught and agitated.

Several points bear emphasizing from the foregoing table, especially as applied to predisposing and treatment context variables. These can be summarized in reference to patient predisposing and treatment context variables.

Predisposing Patient Variables.   Patients seeking psychotherapy are typically in need of comfort, a sense of safety, and reassurance of personal control in the treatment environment. A place that is conducive to relaxing, a competent staff, and clear procedures for intake and billing enhance attachment and comfort.

Unlike the stable environmental cues required for patient comfort, however, therapist-controlled environmental cues are often used to increase arousal and focus treatment efforts rather than to decrease patient discomfort. It seems apparent that certain diagnostic, demographic, and personality variables may serve as indicators for use of these latter environmental management methods. For example, disorganized patients—those with major thought disorders, dementia and tenuous ego boundaries—may respond poorly to therapists who intrude on personal space with the use of touch and proximity. While some aspects of proximity and movement-oriented therapies may enhance boundary definitions among those with severe psychopathology (e.g., Muzekari & Kreiger, 1975), frequent changes of posture and distance by the therapist may be upsetting.

Likewise, the use of touch between members of different sexes and ethnic groups always runs the risk of being interpreted as being sexual or dominating in nature and, thus, may interfere with treatment progress. Holroyd and Brodsky (1980), for example, suggest that therapists who routinely touch their patients are at greater risk for engaging in potentially damaging sexual encounters with patients than those who don't. Even when such behavior is not carried to this extreme, physical touch can be interpreted negatively by some people and can disrupt the process of treatment (Tyson, 1979). Touch by a majority therapist of a minority member patient may be intrusive and insensitive to cultural differences in personal boundaries (Frankel & Barrett, 1971).

The foregoing concerns suggest that patient sensitivity to interpersonal control (reactance), external defensive strategies, demographic differences, and disorganized pathologies all serve as indicators for the cautious implementation of distance and touch either to enhance patient arousal or to provide comfort in times of stress. The examples of J.C. and M.D. again come to mind. Both of these individuals presented with high problem severity and poor ego integrity, J.C. by his detachment and belief in his own deity and M.D. by her Borderline cyclic patterns of making and ending intense relationships with suicidal gestures. J.C.'s lack of self identity and M.D.'s high reactance, tendency to sexualize relationships, and explosive externalization all prove to be indicators for considerable caution in the use of closeness and touch.

Context of Treatment.   In the previous section, we briefly discussed some of the ways in which the context of treatment will affect the use of environmental control to enhance the treatment relationship. Providing safety through environmental constancy and comfort is a uniform requirement for effective treatment relationships to develop regardless of other aspects of the treatment context such as duration, frequency, setting, and format.

Some aspects of the environment are especially critical in different settings, however. For example, constancy and low levels of stimulation are critical for acute care treatment settings. Similarly, in an inpatient treatment program, respect for privacy and opportunity for self control of social contacts may be especially critical in preventing symptoms of institutionalization and should be provided even at the increased inconvenience that such flexibility may portend for ward staff. Translated to the outpatient environment, waiting areas which allow the choice of privacy or socialization may encourage patient comfort and security. Only when issues of patient physical safety and the safety of others arise should the rule of privacy and comfort be sacrificed.

In group and family therapies, it may be especially advantageous periodically to reconstitute seating patterns, thereby clarifying and altering the issues of safety and distance which are reflected in these self-selected and routinized patterns (e.g., Greene, 1976). Freedom in the therapist's movement may also be used to approach, provide comfort, and confront different patients in these multiple person treatment formats, as the need arises. Conversely, freely allowing patient movement in group treatments may encourage a feeling of personal involvement and drawing attention to the patterns of these movements may clarify personality and conflictual issues of intimacy and control which the patterns may belie.

We can see how seating arrangement may be used differentially in the clinical examples previously discussed in this chapter. Specifically, we would want to allow both J.C. and M.D. considerable initial seating and movement latitude in group treatments because of the lack of clarity that characterizes both of these patients' interpersonal boundaries. As treatment progresses, however, our use of seating patterns would begin to differ for these two patients. We may want to confront M.D. with her inability to maintain interpersonal distances. In contrast, we may want to introduce some constancy of seating arrangements for J.C. in order to increase his sense of safety.

SUMMARY AND COMMENT

This chapter has attended to matters of enhancing the quality of the therapeutic relationship. It is intended to supplement the advantages obtained by selecting compatible therapeutic matches between patient and therapist and at the same time to provide guidelines for overcoming the barriers which occur when good matches are foiled or impossible to find. Our discussion has taken us through a review of a variety of procedures, both in the realm of therapy preparatory procedures and in therapy enhancement procedures. By and large, we recommend the use of role induction methods for preparing patients for the activities assigned to them by the nature of the treatment provided. Beyond this, however, managing and controlling the treatment environment and flexibly selecting appropriate technical procedures work both to provide safety and comfort and to allow maximal power by which to confront and expose patient fears.

To accept the value of role induction without accepting either the role of in-therapy environmental management or the role of selecting technical procedures to fit patient needs conveys the belief that patients have the responsibility to mold their lives to fit the often foreign demands of treatment. On the other hand, to argue for modifying treatment without also accepting the value of role induction procedures runs the nearly equal risk of ascribing too much importance to treatment and therapist variables. By accepting the value of role induction procedures and the potential benefit of both in-therapy management and selective technical application, one acknowledges the mutuality of the endeavor. It is our belief that a preeminent acceptance of the value of the collaborative relationship and, concomitantly, a respect for the patient's needs, fears, views, and strengths are the core of the treatment process. All other decisions flow from these. These evaluative beliefs, in turn, cannot be lost to view as one debates theories, selects discrete procedures, and evaluates the dynamics of change.

SUGGESTED READINGS

Goldstein, A. P. (1971). *Psychotherapeutic attraction.* New York: Pergamon.

Harper, R. G., Wiens, A. N. & Matararazzo, J. D. (1978). *Nonverbal communications: The state of the art.* New York: John Wiley & Sons.

Ittelson, W. H., Proshansky, H. M. & Rivlin, L. G. (1972). Bedroom size and social interaction of the psychiatric ward. In J. Wohlwill & D. Carson (Eds.), *Environment and the social sciences* (pp. 95–104). Washington, DC: American Psychological Association.

Meichenbaum, D. J. & Turk, D. C. (1987). *Facilitating treatment adherence: A practitioner's guidebook.* New York: Plenum Press.

Rosenthal, R., Blanck, P. D. & Vannicelli, M. (1984). Speaking to and about patients: Predicting therapists' tone of voice. *Journal of Consulting and Clinical Psychology, 52,* 679–686.

PART V

Tailoring Strategies
and Techniques

We are aware that some would have had us address the principles of psychotherapeutic strategy earlier in our presentation. However, the delay represents our belief in the relative importance of carefully assessing patient predisposing characteristics, considering the contextual elements of treatment, and developing a caring therapeutic relationship. Consistent with current empirical research, we consider the role of specific interventions to be of lesser importance to ultimate treatment outcome than any of these latter variables.

The first two objectives of this section will be to explore the differences that exist among the methods deriving from different theories and then to present a system for classifying psychotherapeutic procedures.

A third objective of this section is to develop and apply a model of psychotherapy selection. Hence, in the following three chapters, we will delineate how the various differences among psychotherapies can be translated into a four-step system for matching the procedures of psychotherapy to the characteristics of patients described in Section II. Each step invokes a set of treatment decisions. Collectively, these decisions narrow the treatment menu provided to the patient to those that are likely to be maximally successful.

Figure V.1 illustrates the concepts to be discussed in the three chapters comprising Section V. We will address specific aspects of the matching process, beginning at the most general level of abstraction and proceeding with progressive specificity to address the implementation of specific interventions within the ever-changing, moment-to-moment interactions that occur between patient and therapist.

Chapter 11, after presenting an overview of the treatment selection scheme, is devoted to a special aspect of the treatment process, that of selecting the focal issues that will guide treatment. We propose that the breadth of the selected outcome (Step #1 in our decisional hierarchy) derives from a thorough understanding of the complexity of the patient's difficulty. These goals serve both as a beginning point in the development of a focal theme to guide treatment and a global measure of treatment effectiveness.

Chapter 12 considers both the levels of experience addressed by various treatment models and the tasks associated with each stage of the treatment cycle (Steps #2 and #3 in selective psychotherapy assignment). Decisions about the selection of what experience levels and tasks to address complement the selected therapeutic foci and help the therapist maintain therapeutic consistency and progress.

Chapter 13 is the most specific to the issue of moment-to-moment deci-

sions and will address the methods for selecting the procedures that constitute the internal structure of psychotherapy (Step 4). The reader will note
that in Figure V.1 relationships are especially interactive (i.e., arrows go
both up and down among the dimensions). This degree of interaction
emphasizes the importance of constant monitoring, analysis, and correction. At the conclusion of Section V, the reader should have a general
understanding of the complexity and beauty of the differential treatment
process.

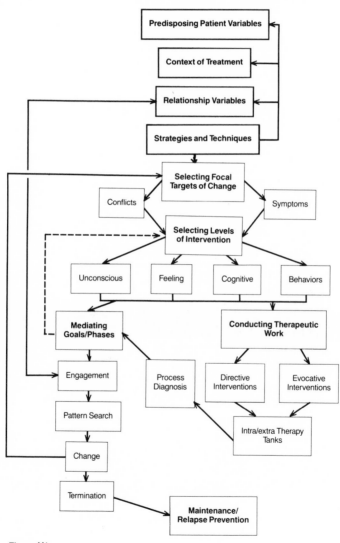

Figure V.1

11

Selecting Focal Targets of Change

Pain
As I put away
The glossy idealism of childhood
The faintly held notion
That a blissful dance through life
Has brought me here
To this stage of uncertainty
And Loss

Struggle
I must
To sort through the past
Separating out what I need to keep
For future wear
And giving up the chaps of childhood
That no longer fit
Or apply

Hope
I will
even as I always have
That the pain and the struggle
Will combine to give birth
To an embryo of insight
And that I will feel and understand
Its birth

(S.B., four months into therapy)

Psychotherapy involves a struggle against demoralization and pain. The overall therapeutic task is to keep the patient in the struggle and to encourage movement toward resolution. But, resolution of what? Should we attempt merely to reduce the level of J.I.'s anxiety about driving a car or should we try to improve her marriage as well? Should we go even further and offer her the opportunity to grieve the loss of her friend and of her own mobility that occurred 21 years earlier? With so many issues before us (her car accident, her marriage, her stabbing and attempted rape, the murder of her girlfriend when J.I. was 13), how will we know when psychotherapy is finished? Will it ever be finished?

Psychotherapists have few guidelines by which to select goals and apply specific treatment interventions. Usually such guidelines are thought to arise from the therapist's theories of behavior, psychopathology, and psychotherapy. However, therapists are typically schooled in the procedures of only one or two systems of treatment and, thus, may be ignorant of some important treatment options that arise from unfamiliar models of change. Even if therapists were more broadly schooled in the theories of their trade, theoretical concepts are frequently too general to meet the needs of selecting the specific interventions that will prove fruitful for specific patients at specific moments.

In this chapter, we will begin the discussion of matching patients to therapeutic procedures by exploring some of the many ways in which psychotherapies differ and the dimensions that define their similarities. From this brief analysis, we will develop the basic structure of a four step model that both differentiates among therapeutic procedures and guides their differential application. Different aspects of this model will be selected for expansion and explication over the next three chapters. At the beginning of each of these chapters we will explore the similar and distinctive elements of various psychotherapies as pertains to the dimensions of our differential decision model. From the vantage point of these similarities and differences, we will describe the dimensions whereby the various psychotherapeutic practices can be matched to relevant predisposing patient characteristics.

After presenting the basic structure of the differential psychotherapy decision model, the second half of this chapter will concentrate attention on the nature and indicators for the first set of decisions. Specifically, we will observe that psychotherapies differ in the relative value placed upon one of two broad classes of treatment goals, conflict resolution and symptom change. We will explore what implications these different outcome goals have on the assignment of treatments and will develop guidelines for selecting between these broad classes of objectives.

DIFFERENCES AMONG PSYCHOTHERAPY METHODS

Before we can address the problem of matching treatment technique to patient needs, we must define the nature of the interventions currently available. In a linear world, every theory of psychotherapy would be somehow distinct from every other theory and each would result in discriminatively different treatment decisions, intervention packages, and outcomes. However, there are striking similarities in the practices of experienced clinicians who represent different theoretical frameworks (Sloane et al., 1975; Beitman, 1987) and only some of the areas of actual difference are captured in theoretical distinctions (e.g., Parloff, 1986; Strupp, 1986).

To the degree that there are systematic differences among practitioners from different orientations, these differences generally are consistent with the theoretical frameworks to which therapists adhere (Sloane et al., 1975; Sundland, 1977; Brunink & Schroeder, 1979; Larson, 1980). Yet, there are nearly 400 different theoretical systems, and it is unlikely that all of these embody unique aspects of either theory or practice. The probability that there are a relatively few clusters of representative approaches and theories has sponsored several efforts to find dimensions of basic commonality and distinction.

The principal method used for reducing the number of theoretical systems into clinically meaningful groupings has been that of rational reductionism—seeking common philosophical positions and/or developmental roots. As one views the many rational approaches to collapsing the number of theoretical systems, two points become clear: (1) there currently is no consensually accepted set of dimensions that allows one to make rational distinctions among theoretical systems, and (2) the effort to find commonalities is hampered by the tendency to equate theories with therapeutic procedures and formats.

In reference to the first of these conclusions, for example, opinions vary widely about the number of useful categories that can be formed by collapsing theories. Corsini (1981) lists over 140 theories, with little effort to combine similarities; Smith, Glass, and Miller (1980), utilizing a combination of rational and empirical methods, collapsed 19 theoretical systems into nine basic categories; and Rachman and Wilson (1980) maintain that a clear distinction is possible only among four general systems.

In counterpoint to those who consider all theories to be transposable to distinct methodologies, "common factors" theorists take the view that all psychotherapies can be condensed to a common set of effective principles (e.g., Frank, 1973; Garfield, 1980; Beitman, 1987). This argument effectively considers all distinctive elements of various theories to be of limited importance. Clearly, a systematic method for viewing similarities among *procedures* rather than among broad theories may circumvent some of the disparities in these approaches.

In viewing this confusing picture, we agree with Beitman (1987) who urges that the mental health disciplines turn their attention from the perennial search for new theories to understanding what is actually done in practice. In pursuit of this understanding, research has revealed few specific procedures that are unique to any given theoretical system. Without going so far as to suggest that all therapies are the same, it may be possible to define a finite number of categories, both of therapies and outcomes, which represent dimensions on which differential treatment assignment may be based.

While most writers would agree that the many different theoretical approaches cluster into some finite number of procedural similarities, many will urge us not to disengage from theoretical systems too quickly or too completely. There is at least one major advantage that accrues from keeping in mind the theoretical understructures of different procedures. Theories go beyond immediate data and are creative in nature; they hold potential for providing guidelines by which old procedures may be applied in new ways or entirely new procedures may be developed (Arkowitz & Messer, 1984). If we restrict ourselves to a search for commonalities based solely on what procedures now exist, the field is unlikely to circumvent the tendency merely to repeat the past.

On the other hand, we are impressed that theoretical terminology can mask both similarities and differences among approaches. Classifying therapeutic approaches on the basis of the technical similarities that are observed in the process of application, rather than on the basis of theoretical constructs, may result in dimensions that are more easily subjected to empirical verification. Ultimately, we must seek some balance between adopting a very abstract classification system that has little reference to the actual procedures used, on the one hand, and a catalogue of concrete therapeutic procedures with no underlying order, on the other.

A classification of theoretically derived procedures, when coupled with empirical demonstrations of their distinctiveness, may represent such a balance, and may overcome the problems that arise when different theories use different terms for the same phenomenon or the same term for different phenomena.

A Comparison of Manualized Therapies

A review of the many brief therapy treatment manuals that have been recently constructed is instructive. These manuals allow a ready comparison of the actual goals and methods of therapy that distinguish approaches. The manuals we will review in this section were selected to represent a wide range of procedures and treatment philosophies, but are neither exhaustive nor mutually exclusive. They include: (1) The Behavioral Treatment of Agoraphobia described by Barlow and Waddell (1985); (2) Cognitive Therapy (CT) of Depression described by Beck, Rush, Shaw, and Emery (1979); (3) Focused Expressive Psychotherapy (FEP) described by Daldrup, Beutler, Engle, and Greenberg (1988); (4) Interpersonal Psychotherapy (IPT) described by Klerman et al. (1984); (5) Time-Limited Dynamic Psychotherapy (TLDP) described by Strupp and Binder (1984); and

(6) Structural Family Therapy as described by Minuchin and Fishman (1981).

From these manuals, we will consider the variations that exist in defining the objectives, tasks, and selection criteria that characterize these different treatments. Over the next three chapters, the descriptions of these manuals will be revisited and their distinctions will be extended to a variety of therapy decisions in order to illustrate the systematic selection and application of interventions.

Behavioral Treatment. The behavioral couples group treatment of agoraphobia (Barlow & Waddell, 1985) was developed for application among adults with agoraphobia with and without panic attacks. Patients with psychotic disorders, bipolar disorders, and organic disorders are considered to be relatively inappropriate for this treatment.

The objective of behavioral treatment is modifying phobic behaviors, the motoric behaviors that occur in the presence of the phobic situation, and the cognitions and feelings directly associated with the phobic response. Ancillary aspects of treatment are addressed to the role of the patient's spouse and activities that are antiphobic (e.g., using coping statements, *in vivo* exposure). Collectively, the treatment addresses change in the symptom manifestation and the constellation of cognitions, environmental supports, and reinforcing behaviors supporting that symptom complex.

Therapy Process and Procedures. In the first session, the therapist emphasizes that the treatment goal is symptomatic and devotes no attention to why the problem began. Descriptive information is given about the nature of agoraphobia and a reinforcement rationale is provided for the treatment. In subsequent sessions, the therapist reviews the treatment rationale regularly and tracks patient change through records of daily activities. The patient is instructed to pay particular attention to thoughts that occur while in anxiety-provoking situations, coping self-statements are introduced, the patient is instructed in the use of a fear hierarchy, and education is used to ensure the patient's understanding.

Role playing and homework are used to develop coping skills, especially as applied to meeting and talking with others. Homework assignments include recording and using coping self-statements. These assignments are reviewed weekly and new assignments are developed to address areas of avoidance. Periodically, the patient is assured that heightened anxiety is a sign that the treatment is working.

Comment. Exposure is probably a sine qua non of the successful symptomatic treatment of agoraphobia. However, Barlow and Waddell acknowledge that there are a number of patients who do not respond successfully to this treatment. A broader focus on interpersonal or intrapsychic conflicts may be helpful in such cases. This point at least is partially supported by evidence that treatment of target phobias generalizes to non-targeted phobias at different rates and in different patterns than would be predicted by situational similarity (Williams, Kinney & Falbo, in press). Such idiosyncracies suggest that for some patients, processes of generalization may follow rules set by the nature of an underlying conflict rather than the nature of the environment.

Cognitive Therapy. The cognitive treatment of depression (Beck et al., 1979) is applicable to adult outpatients who complain of a range of unipolar, depressive symptoms. Patients with hallucinations and delusions, those with a diagnosis of schizoaffective disorder and/or organic brain syndrome, severe endogenous depression, and borderline personality disorders are considered to be relatively inappropriate for cognitive therapy without adjunctive somatic treatment (Beck et al., 1979; Beck & Emery, 1985). Patients who are considered to be most amenable to cognitive therapy are those who are introspective, can reason abstractly, are well organized, are good planners, can responsibly carry out tasks, and are not excessively angry.

Like behavior therapy, the objectives of cognitive therapy are at the symptomatic level—depression. However, more attention is given to the cognitive patterns that mediate between the environment and the patient's depression than is true in behavior therapy. Correspondingly, less attention is given to the overt manifestations of depression, except in the case of the socially inactive and/or motorically retarded patient for whom behavioral interventions are implemented as precursors to cognitive interventions.

Therapy Process and Procedures. Beck and colleagues (Beck et al., 1979; Beck & Emery, 1985) have emphasized that the good cognitive therapist must reason logically, plan strategies, spot subtle flaws in another person's reasoning, and skillfully elicit a more convincing interpretation of the same event. The therapeutic techniques that the cognitive therapist uses to identify and change depressogenic cognitions include: behavioral experiments, questions, logical discourse, examination of evidence, problem solving, role playing, and imagery restructuring.

The therapist plays an active role in assessing and then keeping the therapeutic activity focused on the patient's cognitions. At the beginning of each session, an agenda for that session is agreed upon. Particular emphasis is placed upon collaboration and feedback. Feedback is designed to occur at three points in the session: while preparing an agenda for the session, at the midpoint of the session, and at the end of the session when the therapist recapitulates the main points of the session.

Major therapeutic goals, from the first interview, are to provide symptomatic relief and to identify the problems that serve as a treatment focus. The therapist works to clarify the goals of treatment, reinforces the patient's hope for change, and explains the value of focusing on targeted problems. Concomitantly, the therapist interrupts patient efforts to speculate about the origins and dynamics of their problems.

Early in each session, the therapist reviews homework assignments and sets an agenda for the day's work. The therapist establishes priorities by focusing on the relationships between the patient's thoughts, life situations, and depressive moods (the A-B-C relationship). These A-B-C relationships represent the guiding themes and are illustrated by using the patient's experience to emphasize the correspondence between thoughts and depressive emotions. After the focal problem has been selected, the therapist chooses and applies procedures from a repertoire of cognitive and behavioral techniques. At the end of each session, homework is assigned to help the patient identify or change cognitive patterns.

The middle and late sessions focus on problems that are more deeply embedded in the patient's experience and that are less accessible to direct awareness. This task involves the examination of *schemas*, which are generalized cognitive assumptions about self and life.

Comment.   Recent evidence suggests that the cognitive distortions hypothesized by Beck et al. are not characteristic of all depressed patients (Hamilton & Abramson, 1983). Moreover, when they do occur, they appear to be additional symptoms of the depression rather than etiological or maintaining variables (Lewinsohn, Steinmetz, Larson & Franklin, 1981). Hence, they can be changed indirectly or not at all when treating depression symptomatically. For example, pharmacotherapy reduces maladaptive cognitions as effectively as does cognitive therapy (Bellack, 1985), while the techniques of cognitive therapy may alter depression without inducing the expected changes in cognition (Beutler, Scoggin, Kirkish et al., 1987). These observations introduce concerns about the validity (or at least the uniqueness) of the focal patterns identified as the targets of cognitive therapy.

Experiential Psychotherapy.   Focused Expressive Psychotherapy (FEP) (Daldrup, Beutler, Greenberg & Engle, 1988) is a gestalt therapy applied in a group format. The treatment was designed especially for overcontrolled, covertly angry individuals who present with a constricted range of affect. FEP is considered to be less valuable for individuals who repetitively and inappropriately undercontrol anger through tantrums and tirades or for those with inadequate social and personal resources.

In contrast to cognitive and behavior therapies, overt symptoms are not considered to be either the direct objectives of the interventions or good indicators of the treatment's effectiveness. Symptoms are a side effect of inadequately resolved (i.e., "unfinished") interpersonal conflicts arising during development. Ordinarily, problems are assumed to arise when unwanted feelings are managed and redirected by the use of such defenses as deflection (i.e., redirecting the anger), projection (i.e., reattributing the source of anger), introjection (i.e., adopting a parental injunction which explains or excuses anger), retroflexion (i.e., inhibiting and self-directing the anger), and confluence (i.e., superficially accommodating to others) (Polster & Polster, 1973). Improvement is indexed by alterations in these defensive patterns and by the "completion" of unfinished relationships.

Therapy Process and Procedures. The therapist plays a central role in developing the formulation of the patient's defense against feelings, and this formulation serves as the focus of treatment. The therapeutic task is to identify the unfinished experience and the defensive pattern that prevents completion. Then the therapist guides each patient through a series of "experiments" designed to bring to life, in the here-and-now, a painful interpersonal event in the memory of the patient. The therapist attempts to intensify blocked emotions and sensory experiences by forcing the patient into contact with the feelings that were suppressed or denied during past events.

The experiment is the reliving of an interpersonal event, with the therapist serving as choreographer and guide, mediating the transmission of the past event into the present moment. The goal of the experiment is to vitalize the "dead" memory so that it can be resolved in a new way. In the service of this end, the therapist uses active and directive techniques such as the empty chair, directed and free fantasy, role playing, exploration, and exaggeration of verbal and nonverbal behavior patterns.

After the enactment of the painful event of the past through such procedures as the foregoing, group feedback is used to help the patient integrate the experience. Homework is assigned in order to transfer the in-session experiment into the daily life of the patient and into his/her relationships with significant others.

Comment. Experiential and existential therapies are probably among the least researched and understood of the available treatment models. While they have been described at some length, only recently has an effort been made to assess the reliability of their application and the effectiveness of their methods (e.g., Johnson & Greenberg, 1985; Beutler et al., 1987, 1988). To date, the focus of the interventions remains somewhat confusing, and they continue to be very reliant on the creative processes of the therapist for determining the nature of the treatment procedures used.

In view of the very directive and therapist-controlled interventions of FEP, it is important to question what patient enabling factors are required for a person to benefit from the treatment. For example, to engage in many of these directed procedures, the patient must be motivated and interested in exploring his/her difficulties in this way. Some patients may be less willing or able to do this and more likely to resist or reject the formulation presented by the therapist. Considerable work is needed to validate the procedures advocated and to assess their similarity to those deriving from other models.

Interpersonal Psychotherapy. Klerman et al. (1984) have manualized an individual format of Interpersonal Psychotherapy (IPT) for outpatients who experience mild to moderate depression. The treatment is based on the assumption that depression is related to the disruption of interpersonal relationships. Largely, these disruptions evolve from four types of experience or problems: (1) loss experiences leading to grief reactions, (2) interpersonal disputes leading to internalized anger, (3) role transitions leading to helplessness, and (4) interpersonal skill deficits leading to loneliness and social isolation. Each of these areas constitutes a potential focus of therapy.

Overall, the objectives of IPT are to develop effective interpersonal relationships. Symptomatic focus is not lost, however, and changes in depression are considered to be good but indirect indices of specific treatment effects. The more important goals are interpersonal events and patterns that make one vulnerable to recurrent depression.

Therapy Process and Procedures. The procedures of IPT include clarification, directed confrontation, interpretation, and analysis of transference. There is a significant commitment to education, moreover, which departs from the psychodynamic roots of the treatment. The patient is instructed in the cyclical nature of depression, in the four basic interpersonal situations that evoke depression and in the importance of social support in coping with the symptoms of depression. Specific skills are not taught, although these may be reinforced as the patient experiments with the ideas developed from the discussions.

The treatment is occasionally supplemented both with homework assignments and with the inclusion of significant others in the treatment setting. However, neither of these procedures is considered to be central to the treatment. More central is the patient's understanding of the problem and willingness to accept the natural course of the depression experience.

Comment. IPT provides one of the clearest descriptions of nonbehavioral treatments currently available. The model is specific in its description of depression, flexible in observing that depression represents a number of different problems, and explicit in its technology. IPT has been widely researched in a variety of settings and this research has demonstrated both the efficacy of the treatment and the reliability of its procedures (Rounsaville et al., 1987).

In spite of its explicitness, there probably is more skill required for implementation of IPT than for applying *in vivo* exposure among patients with specific phobias. Required therapist skills are very broad and great sensitivity is necessary to identify and formulate the problem, and then to articulate this formulation in an understandable way to the patient.

Psychodynamic Psychotherapy. There are a number of writers who have written manuals for short-term psychodynamic psychotherapy. Moreover, there is considerable overlap of perspective among most of these manuals, especially in defining the objectives of change. Indeed, three of the major manuals (Horowitz, Marmar, Krupnick, Wilner, Kaltreider & Wallerstein, 1984; Luborsky, 1984; Strupp & Binder, 1984) derive directly from psychotherapy research programs and two of these (Strupp & Binder; Luborsky) emphasize very similar, conflict-oriented goals. Formulations about the nature of internal and interpersonal conflicts serve as the therapeutic foci. These manuals draw heavily from the writings of David Malan (1976). It was Malan who first attempted systematically and reliably to define a dynamic focus of treatment in the form of a persistent or repetitively expressed conflict. The authors of these manuals assume that the therapeutic relationship is a reenactment of interpersonal needs and conflicts, thus extending Malan's methods to encompass interpersonal, transferential patterns.

The patients described as appropriate for treatment in Strupp and Binder's studies of Time-Limited Dynamic Psychotherapy (TLDP) are diagnostically heterogeneous. Most present with mild to moderate depression and/or anxiety. They are all assessed to be capable of insight and to have the ability to establish meaningful relationships, and they are considered to be capable of being treated safely on an outpatient basis.

Therapy Process and Procedures. The therapeutic procedures of TLDP rely heavily upon those that enhance the therapeutic bond. The therapist provides support, interprets transference relationships, and confronts resistance, but most of all attempts to be a credible and empathic resource person. The therapist initially develops the therapeutic focus, or core theme. Priority is given to pointing out the way this dynamic interpersonal theme is reenacted in the therapy session.

The Strupp and Binder manual does not address the issue of how to focus differentially at various stages of the treatment. Hatcher, Huebner, and Zakin (1986), however, observe that the focal theme is likely to undergo change over the course of treatment, particularly in long-term treatment. As new patterns emerge, they are explored as a patient-therapist response, and improvement is indexed by changes in the thematic enactments themselves rather than by symptomatic change.

Comment. TLDP is an elegant procedure with well articulated goals and focal objectives. As in IPT, the specific procedures are clearly reliant on the therapist's ability to create a warm and caring environment. Using this environment to develop a focus on the patient-therapist interaction also requires great self awareness and insight on the part of the therapist. What is still missing in TLDP is an understanding of the limits of its effects.

TLDP is most directly applicable to individuals who exhibit repetitive interpersonal difficulties. Although it is assumed that symptoms will be alleviated by a sustained focus on interpersonal problems, this assumption appears most relevant to generalized and subjective discomforts rather than to well defined, external symptoms like agoraphobia. This observation raises the theoretical issue of the relationship between symptoms and interpersonal behavior.

Family Therapy. Family therapy manuals have been much less specific and detailed than manuals on group and individual psychotherapies. While behavioral marital therapy has been described and manualized (Jacobson & Margolin, 1979), there are broad differences between these approaches and traditional family-based therapies. Though it is less systematically described than other manuals, it is clear that in the structural family treatment described by Minuchin and Fishman (1981; Minuchin, 1974), the patient is the family, not the individual. Little attention is given to individual cognitive patterns, symptoms, or extrafamily interactions.

Minuchin and Fishman have presented many clinical vignettes that illustrate their method of identifying the repetitive family interactions that are believed to be related to the manifest problems. These vignettes illustrate how various foci serve to direct treatment, but each is selected without benefit of consistent attention to a common set of principles. At times the focal objective is symptomatic (e.g., the absence of social skills in a family) and at other times it represents an interpersonal conflict pattern (e.g., a son whose drug use diverts focus from his parent's marriage).

Therapy Process and Procedures. In structural family therapy, the therapist is extremely active in observing, eliciting the enactment of problematic behaviors, and focusing on what are considered to be recurrent interpersonal sequences of behavior that are the foci of intervention. There are few general principles by which to define the nature of the treatment procedures or the explicit outcome objectives. The preponderance of treatment is evocative in nature, but includes some direct guidance and instruction as well.

Comment. Controlled research on the effectiveness of structural family therapy is lacking. While the general focus on the repetitive family behaviors around the problem area is clear, Minuchin makes no attempt to define the indications and contraindications for selecting interventions, or, for that matter, for electing a family format of treatment over the more usual individual format.

One of the recurring difficulties in this as well as in some other manualized therapies is the tendency to define a therapeutic focus on a model of the problem/disorder that is inadequately researched. This point is most clearly seen in the intense disagreement among the proponents of different therapies about the specific role that cognitions play in the arousal, generation, and maintenance of depressive moods and affects (e.g., Arkowitz & Hannah, in press; Beutler & Guest, in press; Coyne, in press).

A MODEL FOR MATCHING THERAPY TO PATIENT

The preceding review of manualized treatments illustrates wide diversity both in procedures and in therapeutic goals. Some therapies emphasize conflictual change, while others focus solely upon symptomatic changes. Some therapies are reliant on evocative procedures, while others direct the patient's activities. Some focus on the therapy relationship while others focus on interpersonal relationships outside of therapy. Some therapies concentrate on experiences within the session itself, while others advocate the importance of extratherapy activities. In the diversity of these approaches, the question remains unanswered as to how to select among and within these various dimensions of procedure to fit the therapy goals to the tasks and procedures.

Several eclectic systems have been developed to guide the selection of treatment strategies across theoretical systems. We explored several of these systems in Chapter 2. From among these, we have extracted a set of principles that we believe to represent a practical balance between those who favor theoretical integration and those who favor technical applications across theories. This balance is achieved by the development of a decisional model that is directed by the sequential processes that enter into psychotherapy decisions. Our resolution has been to differentiate among interventions in terms of their distinctive goals, tasks, and procedural requirements.

A preview of the dimensions we will discuss is presented in Table 11.1. As this Table illustrates, the levels of analysis through which similarities and differences among psychotherapies will be described are not independent of one another. The Table reflects our belief that the various distinctions among psychotherapies are best understood as representing hierarchies of preferred strategies based upon progressively refined levels of analysis.

We propose that any therapeutic procedure can be understood in terms of four layered dimensions, proceeding from relatively grossly defined distinctions among theoretical systems to specific listings of procedures. These four levels of therapeutic selection include: (1) the breadth of the focal objectives of treatment, (2) the depth of experience level targeted for change, (3) the mediating phases and goals required by the intervention, and (4) the intratherapy structure required for initiating and maintaining productive work.

Each of these levels contains two or more subcategories, representing choices that, collectively, narrow the selection range of potential and meaningful techniques. The categories of choice alternatives within each layer of this model are portrayed in Table 11.1.

Table 11.1
The Dimensions of Technique: Decisional Alternatives

Breadth of Focal Goals	Depth of Experience	Levels of Analysis Mediating Tasks	In-Treatment Structure
(1) Conflict Focused	(1) Unconscious Motives		
	(2) Misidentified Feelings		
(2) Symptom Focused	(3) Dysfunctional Thoughts		
	(4) Excessive/ Insufficient Behavior	(1) Engagement (2) Pattern Search (3) Change (4) Termination Planning	(1) Evocative-Directive (2) In session-Extra session activity

The hierarchical organization of decision points, we believe, effectively bridges the gap between the advantages of abstract theoretical formulations and those of procedural catalogues. Each level of analysis yields a different type of data, which when integrated with patient characteristics provide the basis for constructing a menu of high probability and appropriate psychotherapeutic procedures.

Four general steps for "fitting" the treatment to the patient coincide with the four levels of therapeutic procedure (Table 11.2). These steps include: (1) fitting the *focal goals and objectives* of the treatment to the complexity of patient problems; (2) selecting the level of intervention to fit patients' methods of coping (i.e., screening, assimilating, and accommodating experience); (3) altering treatment menus to fit the mediating tasks and goals that define the *phases* through which treatment progresses; and (4) adapting specific in-therapy procedures to the moment-by-moment *treatment states* that occur between a patient and a therapist.

Table 11.2
Matching Patient and Therapy

Steps in Selection	Patient Dimensions	Therapy Decisions
(1)	Problem Complexity	Breadth of Focal Goals
(2)	Coping Styles	Depth of Experience Addressed
(3)	Problem Solving Stage	Mediating Tasks to Fit Treatment Phase
(4)	Therapy Structure Coping Adequacy Reactance Level	Treatment States Maintaining Arousal Amount of Directiveness,
	Mediating Task Changes	Intrasession to Extratherapy Activity

In this and the following chapters, we will illustrate this model of therapeutic decision making by exploring each of the four proposed steps of
differential psychotherapy selection, in turn. This chapter will address the
first step in therapy assignment, that pertaining to the selection of outcome
goals, while the next two chapters will address the increasingly specific
decisions involved in the remaining steps of our model.

FORMULATING FOCAL TREATMENT GOALS

It is clinical truism that different forms of treatment are designed to
induce different types of outcomes. As a general rule, these outcomes are
of two general types—altered symptoms or resolution of internal conflicts.
The difference between these two categories is most obvious when the
effects of broadly focused psychological therapies are compared to more
narrowly focused somatic therapies (Klerman, DiMascio, Weissman,
Prusoff & Paykel, 1974; DiMascio, Weissman, Prusoff, Neu, Zwilling &
Klerman, 1979; Christensen, Hadzi-Pavlovic, Andrews & Mattick, 1987).
Somatic therapies are designed to effect change in the symptoms that
constitute the patient's diagnosis. Behavioral and cognitive psychotherapies, in a similar fashion, are directed specifically at altering symptomatic
presentations over the course of treatment.

In contrast, therapies such as interpersonal, experiential, and psychodynamic therapies place higher priority on changing patterns of coping than
on changing symptoms per se. Though not ignoring the importance of
symptomatic change, these theories add to the definition of improvement
alterations of internal and nonobservable characteristics. Indeed, to most
clinicians of these latter persuasions, changing symptoms is the easy part

of treatment; it is not unthinkable that some improved patients will continue to have symptoms at treatment's end. These clinicians recognize that for someone like our schizophrenic student J.C., learning to cope with some symptoms may be a more realistic alternative than eliminating them.

An analysis of the differences in philosophies that lead one to select either symptomatic or conflictual targets of change suggests that these outcome goals reflect a dimension of "breadth" in the desired spread of effect. Symptomatic change assumes only a limited need for treatment effects to generalize beyond the symptoms themselves, while conflictual change efforts are based on the assumption that changes will be observed beyond those manifest in any single symptom or complaint.

Therapy models that emphasize symptomatic change do not ordinarily devote time and attention to the genesis of symptoms or the presence of unconscious motivations, while those that emphasize conflictual change do not devote a great deal of time and energy to discussing symptom intensity or consequence. In other words, the definition of outcome goals has a direct bearing on what will be addressed in and serve as the focus of the psychotherapy.

Because of the importance of the collaborative, helping relationship, it is critically important that the goals of therapy that are selected by the therapist can be accepted by the patient. Hence, irrespective of theoretical leanings, the patient's initial complaints must be incorporated into the criteria by which the success of treatment is judged. This observation underlies the critical importance of collaboration (e.g., Beck et al., 1979; Strupp & Binder, 1984), and it also emphasizes the value of a well-defined treatment focus by which to direct and integrate the goals and subgoals of treatment. Defining the general goals of treatment represents the first of our psychotherapeutic decision points.

Step #1—Selecting a Therapeutic Focus

The importance of defining a focus and following the plan that evolves from this focus is seen in the observation that the amount of focal concentration upon the problem constituting this formulation (Strupp, 1980a, 1980b, 1981), as well as the degree of adherence to the structure and processes defined by the therapeutic plan, is related to patient outcome (Luborsky et al., 1985; Rounsaville et al., 1988). In other words, consistent attention to the relationships and goals that constitute the focus of treatment may well be more important to treatment outcome than either the strength of the techniques employed or the accuracy of the theory from which these techniques are derived.

The therapeutic focus bridges the gap between the *breadth* of the treatment goals and the *complexity* of the patient's problem. In its simplest form, the development of therapeutic focus begins with the question, "Are these problems simple habits maintained by the environment or symbolized expressions of unresolved conflictual experiences?'' Historical data and careful observations are critical in answering this question. Recurrent symptom patterns that have long since departed from their original and adaptive form, that are evoked in environments that bear little relationship to the originally evoking situations, or which exist with little evidence of specific, external reinforcers, represent *complex symptom patterns* indicative of underlying conflict. On the other hand, isolated symptoms that are environment specific or that are supported by reinforcing environments, and that bear a clearly discernible relationship to their original adaptive form and etiology, represent *habitual or simple symptoms*.

Fundamentally, there are two types of therapeutic foci, symptomatic and conflictual, corresponding to the global objectives of psychotherapy. However, the focus extends beyond the outcome goals to include aspects of mediating goals, as well. *Mediating goals* represent the means-ends relationships required to accomplish the final goal, symptomatic or conflictual. For example, cognitive therapy, a symptom-focused treatment, incorporates in the focal pattern cognitive events and processes that mediate between the symptom and the environment. At times, various of these mediating goals form the targets of specific treatment procedures, even though the end goal is symptom relief. Focal themes represent the assumed relationships that exist between mediating goals and outcome objectives and thus define both the end point sought and some of the steps in the treatment process. This point is illustrated further for the cases of depression and agoraphobia in Table 11.3.

In a technically well-executed treatment, the treatment focus consists of a chain of hypothesized relationships between precipitating (i.e., evoking) events and the final objectives of change (i.e., specific symptoms or conflict

Table 11.3
Focal Chains in Treatment

Depression

Observed Symptoms (e.g., Depression)   social skills deficits associated with the presenting problem (e.g., lack of communication skills) ← cognitions directly related to symptoms (e.g. negative self attributions) ← feelings and affects masked by the symptom (e.g., primary emotions such as anger at a significant other)   unconscious conflicts (e.g., mourning for a lost mother-child relationship).

Agoraphobia

Observed Symptoms (e.g., inability to go in a crowded building) ← coping skill deficits (e.g., inability to control arousal level) ← cognitions associated with symptoms (e.g., anticipations of death) ← emotions associated with or covered by symptom (e.g., fear of losing a significant other) ← unconscious conflicts (e.g., conflicts over seeking dependency).

---

patterns). In conflict-oriented foci, the evoking events are often considered to be rooted in the inability to escape from one's history, while in symptom-focused treatments, the evoking events are more often considered to be in the immediate environment. In either case, each of the links in the chain of events comprising the focus represents a potential objective of change.

Assessing Symptom-Based Foci. Once the decision has been made about whether the manifest problem represents a transient response or a persistent and recurring pattern maintained by internal conflict, it is the task of the therapist and patient collaboratively to define the specific symptoms or conflicts that require work. In the event that the symptoms are seen as situational manifestations of habits and current reinforcements, one can begin to develop the therapeutic focus by specifying the variety of symptoms present and assigning each symptom a priority for intervention. Symptoms should be defined in as much detail as possible, including the frequency of their elicitation, their evoking environments, and their consequences.

Most diagnostic dimensions can be reduced to sets of common problems reported by patients as significantly interfering with their lives (Montgomery, Shadish, Orwin & Bootzin, 1987; Dubro, Wetzler & Kahn, 1987). If one looks at DSM-III-R not as a categorical diagnostic system but as a collection of symptoms and behaviors that reflect the kinds of difficulties that patients bring to mental health practitioners, the criteria can be conceptually grouped as follows: symptoms of mood (depression, anxiety), symptoms of thought (thought disorder), faulty interpersonal behaviors (e.g., shyness) and habitual motoric behaviors that are disruptive (e.g., drug abuse, anorexia, bulimia, specific fears, and phobias).

One helpful aspect of the general diagnostic categories, especially those that are close to problem descriptions, is the opportunity they afford for accumulating information about the range of treatment foci expected when one is dealing with a symptomatic complaint. With reference to substance abuse, for example, McCrady (1985) has noted that the treatment packages that are most successful in treating alcohol abuse utilize a treatment focus that includes both the substance abuse itself and social-support and network systems. It will be recalled that H.D., the 44-year-old alcohol abuser described in Chapter 3, for example, was being supported financially by his family, but that they rejected and criticized his destructive behavior. Following McCrady's suggestions, treatment would be concentrated first upon controlling drinking behavior and then upon bolstering family supports for appropriate behaviors.

In analogous fashion, let us consider the case of J.I., our 34-year-old patient with PTSD. If we elected to treat J.I. in symptomatic fashion, we would begin by defining a priority of treatment targets, beginning with her anxious mood. As we developed the symptomatic focus, we would include an assessment of the patient's disruptive cognitive patterns, these being dominated by flashbacks and negative expectations about riding in an automobile. We then would begin to gather data on how frequently the patient experienced anxiety attacks and in what circumstances these occurred. From this information, we would develop a formulation about the relationship between evoking events, mediating cognitions, and consequent anxiety responses. As we successfully intervened with the patient's anxiety responses, we might extend the analysis to a consideration of the patient's depressed feelings and proceed from there to other symptoms in our hierarchy of symptoms requiring attention (e.g., marital difficulties, etc.).

It is revealing to explore the symptom-oriented treatment manuals previously described to obtain information about how treatment foci are assessed and used. The focus of treatment in Barlow and Waddell's (1985) behavior therapy for agoraphobia is determined both by clinical interviews and structured assessment instruments. The Anxiety Disordered Interview Schedule (ADIS) is utilized in order to establish the presence of the symptoms outlined in DSM-III, differentially to diagnose subcategories of anxiety disorder, and to rule out mood disorders and other co-morbidity. The clinical interview also is used to assess the degree of reliance on safe places and persons and the patterns of avoidance behavior across time.

In addition, a number of paper-and-pencil self-report questionnaires are administered to assess levels of fear, depression, and dyadic adjustment. Using these instruments, a major differential is made between agoraphobia with panic, generalized anxiety disorder, and panic disorder. Then the clinician develops a formulation that defines the behavioral objectives and specifies the hypothesized relationship among avoidance behaviors, cognitive patterns, the experience of anxiety, and associated internal and/or external cues. These behaviors and the pattern among them constitute the therapeutic focus; changes in various components of this focus are used to evaluate treatment progress.

Beck et al.'s (1979) cognitive therapy of depression also employs clinical interviews, supplemented by self-report instruments (e.g., Beck Depression Inventory, Young Loneliness Inventory, Dysfunctional Attitude Scale) to define the symptomatic therapeutic focus. The therapist constructs a list and profile of the patient's distorting cognitions, along with an index of the patient's level of depression. From this profile, the therapist develops a hypothesis about the nature of patient cognitive distortions and the relationship of these cognitive patterns both to evoking environments and to symptoms of depression.

The specific focus of cognitive therapy is described in an A-B-C sequence, defining the mediation of thoughts and beliefs (B) between precipitating events (A) and depressed feelings (C). Thought patterns are believed to be relatively idiosyncratic but to fall into distinctive and identifiable classes, the collection of which serves as the initiator and maintainer of the symptoms.

Assessing Conflict-Based Foci. The choice between symptomatic and conflictual goals begins with the idiosyncratic descriptions of problems that are listed by patients upon their entry to therapy. In Chapter 3, we noted that these complaints constitute both the reasons for seeking treatment and the motivating forces to remaining in treatment. Yet, patient complaints cannot always be trusted to define the most beneficial objectives of treatment. In some cases, the symptoms are vague and changing across situations, bearing little relationship to current events. Yet, the clinician can observe in the symptoms certain common symbols, and within the recurrent events certain patterns of similarity. Unlike symptom-based foci, the focus of treatment in these latter instances is organized around a formulation that accounts for the common elements that exist across situations and which are not readily apparent in the concrete events that serve as the background for problem occurrence.

While both symptomatic and conflictual goals are manifest in symptom patterns (Mintz, 1981; Beutler & Hamblin, 1986), the goals expressed by patients with complex, neurotiform problems may be distorted by the patients' defenses. Hence, among these patients, the more obvious elements of initial complaints as well as expressed goals frequently undergo change over the course of treatment (Sorenson, Gorsuch & Mintz, 1985; Hatcher, Huebner & Zakin, 1986). Since patient-reported goals may change with treatment, the therapist must work to define relevant treatment goals at a level of experience which will remain stable in spite of variations in the overt manifestations of complaints. Once defined, the conflictual themes express direction of treatment and define the specific changes in those conflicts that are sought in the course of psychotherapy. If the clinician is careful and sensitive, the formulation of conflictual themes will specify a recognizable set of behaviors and activities that will signal the resolution of the conflict across situations (Malan, 1976; Horowitz et al., 1984; Luborsky, 1984; Strupp & Binder, 1984).

Manuals for conflict-focused psychotherapies provide more help than DSM-III or DSM-III-R in defining the therapeutic focus. Experiential (Daldrup et al., in press), interpersonal (Klerman et al., 1984), psychodynamic (Strupp & Binder, 1984), and family (Minuchin & Fishman, 1981) therapies all define therapeutic foci somewhat differently and utilize different procedures for arriving at a formulation. Some of the variations in conflictual themes can be illustrated best by an example.

A 42-year-old married, male college professor (P.O.) entered psychotherapy with depression and suicidal ideation. An only child, he presented a history of being abandoned by his mother at age four. He was left to a paternal aunt to raise until his father remarried some years later. His father and stepmother were conservative and religious, and held high standards for the patient's achievement. Always dogmatic, the patient's father was periodically abusive and the two never achieved a sense of closeness until shortly before the father's death when the patient was 38 years old.

After several weeks in therapy, P.O. admitted that he was unhappy in his marriage. He had been married on two prior occasions, each ending because he felt his wife did not support his career. His third wife was described as warm and caring, but the patient reported being unable to feel close to her, a feeling that was similar to that described in earlier relationships. Eighteen months into the treatment process, the patient expressed his conflict in a first poetic effort.

> *Why is it so hard to let go and at last*
> *step forward or back to the future or past?*
> *I think of my life and with struggle I know*
> *what piece is missing and how I must grow.*
> *I've spent my days in a search, to at last*
> *find someone to fill a hole from the past.*
> *I'm living with needs gone but not yet lost,*
> *the plain between child and man never fully crossed.*
> *Can any love settle that old score,*
> *to calm the child and the man restore?*
> *No! But I spend my life in desperate deed,*
> *to frustrate my child and deny my need.*
> *Nothing can quell a child's past cry,*
> *but I avoid today in order to try.*
> *I continue to try, my Mother to know,*
> *only to lose the things by which I grow.*

This poetic rendering can be viewed from a number of positions, depending upon one's particular orientation. For example, in experiential therapy (Daldrup et al., 1988), the conflictual focus selected for this patient will be the relationship with the patient's absent mother. Anger arising from abandonment will form one focal quality and the effort to deny and discard that anger will represent a second aspect of the focal experience. Still a third component to the focus will be the patient's avoidance of present commitment while mourning his mother's loss.

As one can see, experiential therapy as described by Daldrup et al. defines the theme through a variable set of symptom behaviors, constellations of which are taken to reflect the presence of emotional constraint. Objective scales are used to disclose the patient's intensity and methods of expressing anger (coping styles). Direct observation of in-therapy processes following the role play of anger also are used to fine tune the therapeutic focus.

From a different perspective, IPT (Klerman et al., 1984) defines four fundamental themes: (1) loss experiences, (2) interpersonal disputes, (3) role transitions, and (4) interpersonal skill deficits. While the themes are quite specific to the nature of treatment, the symptomatic presentations are not. The low correspondence between symptom and theme is revealed by the fact that all of the themes are manifest in a common set of symptoms—depression.

For our poetic patient, P.O., a focal IPT theme may be developed around the concept of "grief." The failure to complete the grief cycle subsequent to his mother's departure may move the therapist to explore a range of feelings, including anger, fear, and guilt. Depression and withdrawal may be interpreted as reflecting fear of being abandoned once again. Current relationships, it can be seen, may have more salience from this point of view than from the experiential viewpoint.

In developing the focus, during the first few sessions, the IPT therapist explores the symptomatology of depression and then asks the patient to review the potential interpersonal problem areas listed above. After the range and intensity of depressive symptoms have been scored, the patient is asked to review his or her current and past interpersonal relationships. It is from this interview that the problem areas are defined.

A still different method of defining the focal theme is found in Minuchin and Fishman's (1981) family therapy model. In this model, the therapist develops a formulation of the problem by defining the allegiances that exist among family members. This formulation includes hypotheses about the way these allegiances are protected.

It is hard to see this family theme in P.O.'s poetry. Instead of focusing on the patient, family therapy would concentrate upon the depressed marriage. While family patterns may reflect individual struggles, it would also be argued that they have a life of their own. Hence, an analysis would be made of how the depression is supported and even encouraged by family interactions and this process of encouragement and maintenance would become the focus of treatment.

The therapist's technique of choosing a focus in a family session is based on the clinical interview with the whole family present. In this interview, the verbal as well as the nonverbal enactments of patterns are observed and from these observations hypotheses are developed about family interactions, bonds, and allegiances.

Among the conflict-oriented methods, psychodynamic theorists have been most explicit in the development of methods for defining the therapeutic focus. There are actually several methods for assessing themes in psychodynamic psychotherapy. These range from efforts to define relationships between patient goals, pathogenic beliefs, and self-defeating behaviors (e.g., Rosenberg, Silberschatz, Curtis, Sampson & Weiss, 1986) to elaborate descriptions of patient character styles (Horowitz et al., 1984). Horowitz and colleagues (1988) have begun successfully to identify the common principles among these various approaches, emphasizing that all reflect a relatively finite set of interpersonal conflicts relating to power and dependency.

Strupp and Binder (1984) define the dynamic focus of treatment as a individualized theory which the therapist uses to integrate behavioral and experiential aspects of the patient into a coherent whole. Two principles are annunciated for the TLDP focus. First, it is assumed that the kinds of problems treated by TLDP are intimately related to how the patient characteristically construes his/her interpersonal life experience. Second, it is assumed that the primary mode of construing life experience is the "narration."

The narration is the patient's story about how he/she relates to others. The focal narrative is composed of four elements: (1) human actions—thoughts, feelings, images, verbalizations, and other behaviors of the patient and others; (2) the interpersonal transactions and relationships in which these actions are embedded; (3) the repetitive, persistent, and inflexible patterns that these actions take; and (4) the problems in the daily life of the patient caused by these actions.

Strupp (1981) defines the reliable therapeutic theme by the recurrent interplay of four sequential elements: (1) the wishes, feelings, impulses, and wants that motivate the patient; (2) the expectations the patient has about how the expression of his wishes will influence others; (3) the acts of others perceived to occur as a function of the patient's efforts to express the wishes; and (4) the respondent acts of the patient toward themselves, particularly those that define the participants' opinions of themselves.

For the patient in our example, the first element in the thematic focus would be the striving or need for attachment. The second element might be identified by the patient's belief that expressing this need may result in abandonment. The third element in the conflictual theme, in turn, may consist both of the patient's withdrawal and the perceived withdrawal of others, confirming his initial expectation. Finally, the fourth element in the chain may be described as the feeling of inadequacy emanating from another failed relationship or rejection.

Comment. At this point, it may be important to remind the reader that psychotherapy is a process of altering the patient's view of the world. The benefits of treatment are significantly and positively related to the way patients view and discuss their problems, to whether these views come to correspond with those of the therapist (Beutler, 1981), and the degree to which these views incorporate a belief in one's own responsibility for problems and solutions (Orlinsky & Howard, 1986).

Since the formulation of a problem depends so heavily on the therapist's philosophy, therapists always will differ in their views of patients' problems. Indeed, we encourage this diversity and believe that it need not interfere with the discriminating selection of treatments. We encourage only that the focal theme or pattern be explicitly related to the complexity of the problem, be reliable, and be used consistently throughout treatment.

Beyond this principle, in order maximally to be useful within our framework of differential treatment selection, the focal conflict-oriented theme should include benchmarks by which to judge progress and be acceptable to the patient.

We want to emphasize that a clear distinction should be maintained between symptom-oriented and conflict-oriented themes. Because it is so persuasive for those of us trained in viewing the world complexly to conclude that all symptoms are symbolic of persisting conflicts, the laws of parsimony must be applied to our formulations of the problem complexity. We believe that the initial assumption should be that any problem is a simple habit or transient adjustment problem. Only when it can be demonstrated with reasonable reliability and confidence that the symptoms represent a link in a recurrent and debilitating pattern of interpersonal relationships should the focus of treatment be upon the symbolically represented conflict rather than upon the symptom alone. If such evidence is not forthcoming—if the symptom cannot be consensually demonstrated to be other than an isolated reaction to a specific environmental change, either current or past—a narrow range of goals can be defined based upon the specific symptoms and areas of distress observed or expressed.

Returning to the now familiar example of J.I., the reader can observe that the patient's history of early trauma is seductive and could easily lead to the development of any of several dynamic formulations of conflict to serve as the basis for planning intervention. For example, we might propose that J.I.'s anxiety symptoms are exaggerated because the recent automobile accident has reactivated long denied rage, and that this rage threatens her protective defenses by penetrating her awareness. However, while J.I.'s marital problems might be found to arise from a recurrent inability to trust men sufficiently to allow intimacy, there is little to suggest that her PTSD symptoms represent a *recurrent* pattern. Even if the extent of anxiety symptoms are overdetermined by her early trauma, there is a reasonable correspondence between the evoking events and the protective function of the symptoms themselves. The nature and form of the symptoms are a natural reaction to threatened loss of life. There is no evidence of symbolic transformation and, hence, we believe, there is little justification for treating these symptoms with a conflict-focused treatment. However, as symptoms of acute anxiety dissipate and *if* there emerges evidence that marital conflicts reflect recurring thematic patterns that supersede situational expectations, a conflict-based theme may be considered for continued work.

Support for beginning with symptomatic-focused treatments unless there is clear evidence for the conflictual basis of the problems is found in the observation that while the use of a conflict-focused treatment (i.e., broad band) to treat a simple problem may be inefficient, the reverse is not true. There is no indication that the application of a symptom-focused treatment (i.e., narrow band) to a complex problem invokes negative results. While symptom patterns may recur when narrowly focused treatments are applied alone to complex problems (Beutler et al., 1987; Coyne, in press), mixing treatments of varying breadths actually may allay this recurrence.

On the other hand, it stands to reason that as the number of treatment foci increase and as the assets of the patient decrease, the treatment will be of correspondingly longer duration (see Chapter 8). The field has begun to be precise about the foci of brief treatments, but the definition and sequencing of treatments that are long-term is still somewhat beyond the state of the art in clinical research. There are some data suggesting that target complaints (Beutler & Hamblin, 1986) and focal themes (Hatcher et al., 1986) both change over time. To date there are but a few examples of efforts to manualize long-term treatments and address these changes (Linehan, 1987; Kernberg, Selzer, Koenigsberg, Carr, & Applebaum, 1989), however.

Since transient changes in the significance of various symptoms may require the use of focused interventions to reduce the symptomatology before conflicts can be addressed, we will return to the foregoing issues in subsequent chapters as we address increasingly specific aspects of applying psychotherapy procedures.

SUMMARY AND COMMENT

This chapter has explored some of the efforts to reduce the many theories of psychotherapy to meaningful dimensions. From these efforts to describe the nature of psychotherapy, we have presented a general model for developing psychotherapy treatment plans. In doing so, we have attempted to reconcile some of the arguments in favor of seeking theoretical similarities among various systems with those of seeking procedural similarities. This has been accomplished by considering the process of differential treatment selection to be one of progressively filtering the decisional field through a series of increasingly refined steps. The initial decisions in this process rely upon making distinctions among global goals, while later decisions and interventions become more specific and discrete.

A major portion of this chapter has been devoted to describing the relationship between global outcome objectives and the nature of therapeutic foci. We have suggested that treatment outcomes vary in breadth, ranging from symptomatic (narrow band) change to conflict resolution (broad band). The more specific and behavioral the focus of treatment, the more narrow the impact of the intervention (Willis, Faitler & Snyder, 1987).

Concomitantly, patient problems range along a dimension of complexity. Some problems are quite situation- and symptom-specific while others represent neurotiform needs and repetitions of stable life themes. The focus of therapeutic work represents a conceptual marriage between the complexity of the problem being presented and the differential outcomes to which different treatments are targeted. Thus, the interface of these dimensions, one patient-based and one therapy-specific, suggests directions for defining a pattern of responses around which therapeutic procedures are integrated.

From our comparison of treatment manuals, it is possible to extract some generalizations about when and how different types of therapeutic foci should be developed. In doing so, however, it should be clear that we do not advocate the truth of any one particular manual or method of treatment. Rather, exploration of alternative procedures has allowed us to decipher some guiding principles for selecting a therapeutic focus.

(1) In the patient with a simple, unidimensional symptom or situationally specific problem, the treatment focus reasonably can be on those behaviors that define the symptom. Cognitive-behavioral and behavioral treatments that focus specifically on symptomatic complaints provide examples of how the focus of treatment is defined in these cases. The treatment focus, in both of these instances, consists of the symptoms themselves, precipitating environments, consequences, and mediational processes such as perceptions and dysfunctional beliefs.

(2) In working with patients who present with complex problems that are not easily understood in terms of environmental demands or stresses, the treatment foci are likely to be more complicated than in the case of simple problems. This complexity is noted both in the identification of the focus and the sequence of mediating objectives. It is here that the therapist's theory of psychopathology and change is relevant because it is from this theory that the focus is likely to derive. Several models have been presented for defining a reliable formulation of the patient's complex problem, around which the therapeutic methods may come to be organized. In the next chapter, however, we will see

that some aspects of the focus selected may be adapted to the patient's type of psychological defense or coping style.

(3) Fundamentally, the focus of treatment represents a rationale for understanding the patient's difficulty. It is this rationale that is the philosophy that implicitly and explicitly is taught in the course of treatment. There are no data to indicate that one formulation of focus is better than another. It is important, however, that both participants believe the formulation offered. Only when both agree and accept the rationale can the formulation really serve as the focal point of the interventions. The foci of treatment, therefore, whether symptomatic or thematic, must be negotiated with the patient in some direct or indirect manner.

(4) When the objectives of treatment are symptomatic and correspond to the patient's chief complaints, the treatment focus will include relatively objective intervening variables to serve as mediating goals between the symptom and the treatment. In contrast, complex problems call for treatment foci that consist of abstract and often complex formulations of the causes of the problems. The explanatory variables that are incorporated into the treatment foci in these cases are hard to validate and are often very dependent upon one's particular theory of behavior.

We encourage the general principle of parsimony and emphasize that simple formulations should be tested first. This simple focus should not be discarded simply out of preference, but evidence for and against it should be considered before beginning to develop a more complex treatment focus.

(5) In those clinical situations in which the problem is multidimensional, the therapist must incorporate symptomatic considerations into the conflictual theme and associated treatment. The therapist must define the hierarchy of problem areas that are implicated in the treatment foci, and proceed in a sequential fashion, from symptom to conflict. This sequencing of interventions necessitates a theoretical rationale for describing how the various layers of problem difficulty and presentation are interrelated and how they will respond sequentially to intervention.

Once the complexity of the problem is defined and both the breadth and the nature of the desired treatment outcomes are specified, the therapist is ready to become more specific in the selection of treatment menus. As the next few chapters unfold, it is our hope that the reader will see the complex interaction of the several types of experience and goals that compose psychotherapy. The nature and breadth of the mediating goals of treatment as well as the means-ends goals will enter into our discussion as we define both the use of treatment menus and the selection of specific interventions.

SUGGESTED READINGS

Barlow, D. H. & Waddell, M. T. (1985). Agoraphobia. In D. H. Barlow (Ed.), *Clinical handbook of psychological disorders: A step-by-step treatment manual* (pp. 1–68). New York: Guilford.

Beck, A. T., Rush, A. J., Shaw, B. F. & Emery, G. (1979). *Cognitive therapy of depression*. New York: Guilford Press.

Daldrup, R. J., Beutler, L. E., Greenberg, L. S. & Engle, D. (1988). *Focused expressive psychotherapy: Freeing the overcontrolled patient*. New York: Guilford Press.

Minuchin, S. & Fishman, H. C. (1981). *Family therapy techniques*. Cambridge, MA: Harvard University Press.

Strupp, H. H. & Binder, J. L. (1984). *Psychotherapy in a new key*. New York: Basic Books, Inc.

12

Selecting the Level of Intervention and the Mediating Goals of Psychotherapy

I promised you honesty and diligence;
You promised to listen and accept.

But somewhere along the way we added more.
I wanted you to understand as well as listen,
to care as well as accept.

You wanted me to question my feelings
as well as be honest
and evaluate as well as work hard.

I had to function on two levels—
experience my world
and then observe that process.

I have often struggled with the effort to do both—
extending the process of self-discovery
from the walls of your office
to every facet of my life.

Our time together was filled with experiencing,
my time away filled with observations
of the many parallels that now seem everywhere.

That dual process forced me to grow out of the old automatic
patterns
into more thoughtful, purposeful ones.

I have learned from you and learned from me
and I think that when I look back at my life
this will be one of the parts
I wouldn't have wanted to miss.

(S.B., sixteen months into treatment)

At some point in the treatment process, it becomes apparent that caring and support are not enough; that learning and experiencing are not restricted to the treatment hour; and that the passage to feeling better is through struggle and pain, a process that is shared by both the patient and therapist. As this awareness unfolds, the skill by which the therapist can select and apply appropriate methods from her or his technical armamentarium assumes increasing importance. It is this technological expertise which the trained therapist brings to the treatment that allows the relationship to provide more than the comforting support of a good friendship. Yet, this technical skill must be applied selectively and thoughtfully, always within the context of a supportive relationship and caring alliance.

In the foregoing chapter, we suggested a rather simple connection between the complexity of the problem presented by the patient and the breadth of the outcomes to which the therapeutic procedures should be addressed. It is explicitly assumed that the objectives of different treatment models have led to procedures that differentially are effective at addressing different degrees of problem complexity. Procedures that focus on narrow goals (i.e., symptomatic behaviors) may be best used when symptom removal is the desired aim but may have correspondingly less effect for overcoming complex problems based upon forgotten and denied wishes and interpersonal experiences. Conversely, procedures that are designed to focus on conflictual themes and recurrent interpersonal patterns may not be particularly effective for changing focal symptomatic complaints.

Our example of J.I. is a case in point. It is unlikely that the patient's anxiety symptoms that arose in response to her automobile accident efficiently would be alleviated by a treatment that focused on the conflictual themes of anger expression and control arising from her early history of attempted rape, stabbing, and parental neglect. On the other hand, the use of relaxation training, desensitization, and cognitive control strategies are not likely to alleviate her conflicts over control and anger.

In this chapter, we will address the second and third steps in differential psychotherapy assignment, both of which are designed to expand upon the objectives of treatment. These two steps include: (1) determining the level of experience to which the therapy should be addressed (i.e., unconscious, emotional awareness, cognitive habits, behavior change), and (2) identifying and prioritizing the mediating tasks and goals of treatment.

TYPES OF PSYCHOTHERAPY EXPERIENCES

In addition to the breadth of goals targeted by different procedures, theoretical systems also differ in the *types of experience* valued. These valued experiences range along a dimension of "depth" to complement the dimension of "breadth" addressed in the previous chapter. Addressing psychotherapy differences at this level of analysis allows us to take theoretical constructs and conceptual differences a step closer to the selection of particular procedures.

Variations in Types of Experience

We can define the "depth" of a therapeutic experience by the degree to which the procedures employed emphasize unconscious experience, historical determinants, and involuntary behavior, as opposed to emphasizing conscious experience, contemporary determinants, and voluntary behavior. This definition parallels various distinctions between "action" and "insight" (London, 1986) or "reality-oriented" and "insight-oriented" (Thorpe, 1987) therapies.

An understanding of the different "depths" of experience addressed by different procedures requires translating theoretical formulations into their implicit value systems. The analysis of differences and similarities among theoretical systems can then proceed by noting the realms of patient experiences to which the mechanism of change is attributed. For example, all theories value change at numerous levels, but some theories consider the means by which change occurs to be through the recovery of unconscious experience (i.e., "insight"), others attribute change to increasing awareness of feelings or sensations, and still others attribute change to alterations in either cognitive habits or overt behaviors.

Most analyses of therapeutic depths or levels define three or four groupings of theories, based upon which combination of these levels of experience they most consistently attend. Unfortunately, the underlying dimensions characterizing many of these classification systems are occluded. One of the most traditional classification systems (e.g., Kolb, 1968) succeeded in ordering interventions along a continuum of depth, ranging from behavioral interventions, the least deep of the approaches, through supportive and crisis management approaches, to psychoanalysis, the deepest approach. Unfortunately, the discrete categories in this conceptual ordering fail to capture the uniqueness of the experiential and cognitive therapies that have recently come into their own and which may be applied to a variety of levels of depth.

To avoid this problem, the first author (Beutler, 1983) derived a fivefold theoretical classification of therapy systems based upon their empirical distinctiveness (Psychoanalytic, Interpersonal, Experiential, Cognitive, and Behavioral). These five therapeutic systems were found to be distinguished by several dimensions, including the relative value given to the use of evocative and directive interventions, the degree of intratherapy versus extratherapy focus, their emphasis upon structural or symptomatic change, and the formality or informality of the therapeutic atmosphere desired.

The fivefold classification system proposed by Beutler is relatively unconfounded by issues of format, duration, and involvement when compared to other approaches. Indeed, within each of the five categories there exist representative models for time-limited and long-term treatments and for group, individual, and family interventions. However, because of their varying points of entry within the history of psychotherapy, the descriptive differences may be somewhat time-locked. For example, traditional psychoanalytic theory is probably not reflective of that practiced by current psychoanalytic practitioners. Psychoanalytic theory and early interpersonal theories have largely fused with the advent of a unifying object relations theory.

Another approach has been proposed by Prochaska (1984; Prochaska & DiClemente, 1982, 1986). He and his colleagues differentiated among therapeutic schools on the basis of the levels of change addressed or valued by the various theories. These levels included: symptom/situational, cognitive, interpersonal, family, and intrapersonal.

While the system proposed by Prochaska and colleagues represents an improvement over many others, both by its adherence to a relatively consistent underlying dimension and by its specificity, it still embodies some conceptual limitations. On the one hand, the distinctions offered by Prochaska et al. fail to acknowledge the different levels of experience represented by experiential and psychodynamic therapies (both are grouped under "interpersonal" levels). On the other hand, the system treats interpersonal and family conflict as if they existed as places along the dimension of depth or levels, thus confounding the format of treatment with the level of experienced change.

From the foregoing considerations, we propose an integration of the model suggested by Prochaska and his colleagues with those proposed by Beutler et al. (Beutler, 1983; Daldrup, Beutler, Engle & Greenberg, 1988) and by Frances, Clarkin, and Perry (1984). We propose that the levels of experience to which change mechanisms are addressed can be ordered, thusly: (1) unconscious motivation, wishes, and conflicts; (2) unidentified feelings and sensory experiences; (3) dysfunctional cognitive patterns; and (4) behaviors of excess and insufficiency.

While all theoretical systems implicitly or explicitly address each of the foregoing levels of experience, each theoretical system attempts to implement change in its preferred level by defining the therapeutic focus and associated mediating tasks in a theory-compatible way. It is only when we inspect how these levels of patient experience serve the therapeutic focus that we begin to see the differences in implementation that actually characterize therapeutic systems. These differences are reflected in the refinement of the therapeutic focus as we move toward the development of increasingly specific treatment *menus*. This refinement, in turn, derives from matching the depth of intended intervention both with the coping styles that uniquely characterize patients and with the variations in outcome goals associated with problem complexity.

Step #2—Selecting the Depth of Intervention

As we begin to turn our attention to the development of specific treatment menus, we must keep in mind that different menus must address problems that differ in degree of complexity. In the case of relatively situational, transient, or simple (i.e., noncomplex) problems, there is a wide latitude in the variety of procedures selected. Thus, for such problems as simple phobias, situational anxiety, and other mildly impairing disorders, virtually any symptom-focused procedure applied within the context of a supportive therapeutic environment will achieve the desired ends of symptom relief (cf. Berman, Miller & Massman, 1985).

As problem complexity increases, technical procedures become more important. These technical procedures vary in terms of the level of patient experience addressed, the phase objectives of the treatment process, and the characteristic modes of patient defense to which they are best applied (Rounsaville, Chevron, Prusoff, Elkin, Imber, Sotsky & Watkins, 1987; Jones, Cumming & Horowitz, 1988).

While reducing the complexity of decisions to a set of precise and unvarying matching relationships is not possible, there is reason to believe that relatively consistent benefits derive from matching the depth of experience addressed by the treatment procedures and the dominant coping styles presented by patients.

The treatment menus that result from matching the intended depth of the intervention and the patient coping styles are based more upon principles of intervention than they are on specific procedures. As we continue to move from gross to refined distinctions among the psychotherapies in the next chapter, however, the specific procedures will become clearer.

At least one reason that an unvarying fit cannot be found between any specific patient coping style and a corresponding level of experience addressed by a menu of interventions is because of the dimensional nature of both experience level and patient coping patterns. In both cases, a categorical system is imposed (for convenience and clarity) on a quality that is distributed in a continuous fashion.

Beyond the matters of convenience and convention, there is evidence for the efficacy of matching the level of experience addressed by the therapy intervention with a categorical index of patient coping style among patients with complex problems. For example, Beck (1982) has defined two personality styles, which he called "sociotropic" and "autonomous" types, that he found responded to different therapeutic methods. The sociotropic patient was described as socially active and responsive, similar to our description of "externalizers," and was thought to need reassurance, direction, and assistance in taking risks. In contrast, the autonomous style, like our description of the "internalizing" patient, was considered to be self-directed, self-controlled, and insensitive to feeling or sensory states. Beck proposed that such patients require less behavioral direction than their counterparts and may benefit from attending to internal experiences. Likewise, interactions between similarly defined patient coping styles and the levels of intervention have been shown to affect the nature of the therapeutic alliance among depressed and anxious patients (Gaston, Marmar, Thompson & Gallagher, 1988), as well as to enhance treatment outcome among alcoholic patients (McLachan, 1972).

Specifically, behaviorally targeted therapies appear to induce better results than those that focus on unconscious processes among patients who are prone to externalize their distress (e.g., Sloane et al., 1975; Beutler, 1979a). Conversely, therapies which address the level of unconscious motives and feelings are more effective than those that address the level of behavior change among patients who internalize sources of stress (Calvert, Beutler & Crago, 1988). Other research suggests that therapies that implement change by arousing awareness of sensations and feelings are somewhat more effective than therapies that address the level of unconscious motives when applied either to patients with externalizing or those with cyclic (i.e., mixed and unstable) defenses (Beutler & Mitchell, 1981). Such research allows us to begin to narrow our list of symptom-oriented and conflict-oriented procedures sufficiently to construct general menus of procedures for use within the categories of coping styles.

Procedural Menus for Treating Symptoms.   As we have indicated, there is considerable flexibility in the selection of procedures among patients whose problems are of relatively low complexity (i.e., situationally induced or monosymptomatic). The guiding rule is only that the procedures are appropriately symptom-focused and occur in the context of a supportive and caring relationship. Therefore, it will be useful to consider symptom-oriented and conflict-oriented treatments separately when assigning treatment levels.

Ordinarily, simple (i.e., unisymptomatic and situational) symptoms will reflect either behavioral deficits, impulsive and extrapunitive behaviors, or reactive (usually intropunitive) responses in the form of acute anxiety or depression. Corresponding to these patient manifestations, treatments that have symptomatic goals will be focused at the levels of experience required to change cognitive patterns and/or to control socially excessive and/or insufficient behaviors.

These interventions will largely include methods for identifying contingent events, antecedent stimuli, mediating cognitions, and sustaining reinforcements (both positive and negative). The specific therapeutic foci, therefore, will be consistent either with the behavioral (Barlow & Waddell, 1985) or the cognitive therapy (Beck et al., 1979) foci described in the previous chapter. Selection between these two procedures will depend upon the degree to which the behavioral manifestations of the symptoms are overt. The more overt or external the symptomatic display, the more convenient a behavioral therapeutic focus, while the less overt (i.e., subjective) the symptom, the more convenient the selection of a cognitive focus on automatic thoughts and deficient cognitive skills.

The example of J.I. again comes to mind. Efforts to ameliorate the PTSD symptoms associated with her car accident would address cognitive distortions (negative anticipations and overgeneralization) and behaviors (phobic avoidance). A behavioral treatment focus would be developed by means of an analysis of contingent events and evoking environments. The objective of treatment would be upon overt behavior, but the focus of treatment would also extend to include a systematic description of the evoking environment, mediating events, and reinforcing consequences, much as described by Barlow and Waddell (1985) with respect to agoraphobia and by Meichenbaum (1977) for impulse control problems and disorders of concentration.

In a more general way, the treatment menu associated with a symptom-based behavioral focus consists of such procedures as:

(1) Social skills training (assertiveness or communication),

(2) *In vivo* or *in vitro* exposure to avoided events,

(3) Graded practice,

(4) Reinforcement.

If the symptom is more subjective than overt, the development of a treatment focus around the A-B-Cs described by Beck et al. (1979) is used to guide treatment. The therapeutic focus, in this case, highlights subjective distress as the symptomatic target and includes an identification of evoking situations and a specification of the types of cognitive distortions characterizing patient responses to these situations. The cognitive components of this focus are automatic thoughts, but the guiding formulation extends to cognitive schemas, the latter of which represent a "deeper" (i.e., involving less easily accessible material) level of experience.

(1) Identification of cognitive errors,

(2) Evaluation of risk or degree of distortion,

(3) Questioning dysfunctional assumptions and beliefs,

(4) Self monitoring,

(5) Self instruction,

(6) Practicing alternative thinking,

(7) Testing new assumptions.

All of these behavioral and cognitive procedures may be applied within a group, family, or individual environment, depending upon the indicators for treatment context. Throughout, the tasks of the therapist are to focus these interventions on the symptoms identified, present the hypothesized interrelationship of events and symptoms proposed by the therapeutic focus, test and address these associated variables in the order of their priority, instruct the patient in the procedures of cognitive or behavioral change, and provide practice in applying these methods of problem resolution. In this process, one may utilize a variety of extratherapy supports and contingencies, as the case permits, to facilitate and activate direct instruction and guidance. The specific nature and indicators of these external supports will become clearer as we proceed to look at moment-to-moment treatment decisions in the next chapter.

Procedural Menus for Treating Complex Problems. While therapeutic foci usually are constrained to the levels of dysfunctional cognitive and behavioral patterns among patients with uncomplicated, transient, and habit problems, the range of foci for patients with complex, conflictually-based patterns of disturbance is much broader. The general rules that apply to matching patient coping styles to the levels of experience addressed by the therapy procedures are presented in Table 12.1.

The level of experience selected for attention when one is developing a differential therapeutic focus depends upon the nature of the patient's coping style. Here we find currently available treatment manuals of little help. Manuals like those described in earlier chapters limit the variety and type of interventions to those that are consistent with the theory from which the manual is derived. Hence, we find treatment manuals to be useful for describing how procedures might be employed once they are

Table 12.1
Match of Coping Style to Level of Experience

Dominant Coping Style	Matched Level of Therapy Intervention
(1) Internalization	Unidentified/Misidentified Sensory and Feeling States
(2) Repressive	Intrapsychic Conflicts and Unconscious Motives
(3) Cyclic	Dysfunctional Cognitive Patterns and Behavioral Variation
(4) Externalization	Excessive and Insufficient Behavior

selected in a particular case, but we must look beyond current manuals for the actual selection of specific therapeutic procedures.

In making treatment selection specific, we seek to develop crosscutting treatment menus by observing concomitantly, the nature of the patient's predominant coping methods and the types of experience addressed by given procedures, independently of the specific theories on which these procedures are based. These menus can then be refined further to fit the phase and state of treatment, as well.

As a general rule, we believe that the more reliant the patient is on internalizing defenses, the more valuable experiential and expressive procedures will be found to be, and the more reliant the patient is on externalizing defenses, the more valuable will be found cognitive and behavioral procedures. As illustrated in the case of J.I., however, it is important to note that symptom-based foci often are targeted first and treated directly even when the overall guiding focus is conflictual. This is done by using procedures that address behavioral and cognitive levels of experience as entry points to the levels of sensory/affective experience and intrapsychic processes.

(1) Internalized Coping Styles are defined by a preferential use of the specific defenses of undoing, self punishment, intellectualization, isolation of affect, and emotional overcontrol or constriction (see Chapter 4). These patterns of response are designed specifically to contain the expression of unwanted feelings. Therefore, patients who use internalized coping styles have both little tolerance for and high resistance to feelings and sensations. They tend to split off the affective elements of experience from the content of those experiences, focusing upon the latter and avoiding sensory/affective stimulation (Gleser & Ihlevich, 1969). Hence, they ordinarily present with blunted or constrained affect and with very constrained interpersonal relationships.

We propose that, as a general rule, patients with complex conflictual patterns, who adopt predominantly internalizing defenses against feelings such as anger or guilt, will benefit from treatments designed to magnify and expose the affective and sensory levels of awareness. Such procedures are also designed to produce dramatic relief through expression of these feelings and to enhance tolerance for such experiences. These things, in turn, may smooth the course of interpersonal relationships in which negative feelings are ordinarily evoked (Rice & Greenberg, 1984; Beutler, Engle, Oro'-Beutler, Daldrup & Meredith, 1986; Beutler, Daldrup, Engle, Oro'-Beutler, Meredith & Boyer 1987; Daldrup et al., 1988).

One method for developing a therapeutic focus at the level of sensory/emotional experience has been described by Daldrup et al. (1988). The objective of this therapeutic focus is identified principally in terms of arousing feeling states that have been avoided. The denied and disowned emotional states usually are thought to center on anger or rage, and the original targets of those feelings are typically parental figures.

Suppose, for example, that J.I. had responded to her automobile accident with increased constraint and overcontrol rather than with phobic anxiety. If she had presented in this fashion, the therapeutic focus would have targeted anger inhibition as a central aspect, and the mediating goals of treatment would be to magnify and clarify the nature of the inhibited feelings. Therapeutic procedures for initiating affective and sensory arousal and abreaction would have been given prominence in the treatment plan. These experiences would allow her to revisit the loss of power represented first in her automobile accident and secondarily in her original trauma.

In identifying the problematic feelings that are to be brought to awareness with such interventions, it is important to differentiate among primary, secondary, and instrumental emotions (Greenberg & Safran, 1986). Primary emotions are defined as those that are uniform and unlearned responses, usually including anger, sadness, joy, fear, disgust, and surprise (Burgoon & Ruffner, 1978; Ekman, 1982; Siegman & Feldstein, 1985). Secondary emotions arise from these primary or spontaneous affective states; they are reactive and protective in nature. As a special case of secondary emotion, instrumental anger is the manifestation of angry behavior supported by secondary gain. While primary anger serves to protect one against threat, instrumental anger has the additional quality of being manipulative, often even characterological, in nature. Uncovering emotions is most likely to lead to a therapeutic response if the affective target of therapy is a primary rather than an instrumental or secondary emotion.

To put the affective level of therapeutic depth into context, there are additional elements of the focal theme that can be described when one targets emotional recognition and expression as the mediators of change. These elements include the nature of the particular relationships in which emotional constriction is displayed, the instigating parental relationships associated with learning this pattern, and the processes of redirection (i.e., retroflexion, introjection, confluence, deflection, and projection) employed during the process of transforming these unwanted emotions into symptoms.

The therapist's task with internalizing patients is to observe, exaggerate, reiterate, and challenge the patient's thematic pattern. The therapist intensifies unwanted emotional experiences, most notably anger, in order to promote awareness of these feelings and their associated thematic pattern of expression. Once identified, the patient is encouraged to explore and practice emotional expression through both cathartic release and role-playing dialogues with an imagined other. The procedures for addressing this level of experience have been applied to individual therapy (Gendlin, 1969; Rice & Greenberg, 1984), to group therapy (Daldrup et al., 1988),

and to family therapy (Johnson & Greenberg, 1985). Some of the procedures that various authors have identified for enhancing emotional and
sensory awareness are:

(1) Focusing on sensory states,

(2) Reflection of feelings,

(3) Two-chair work on emotional "splits,"

(4) One- and two-chair work related to unfinished business,

(5) Structured imagery,

(6) Gestalt dream work,

(7) Reflective mirroring of the hidden self,

(8) Enacting emotional opposites,

(9) Free association to sensory cues, and

(10) Physical expression and release exercises.

A specific description of these therapeutic techniques and their applications has been provided by a number of authors (Gendlin, 1969; Perls,
1969; Polster & Polster, 1973; Goulding & Goulding, 1979; Mahrer,
1986; Daldrup, Beutler, Greenberg & Engle, 1988).

(2) Repressive Coping Styles are characterized by the preferential reliance
on denial and reversal. These patterns are observed as overt responses that
are in direct counterpoint to internal states, unconscious motives, or the
social demands embodied in the circumstances. The specific defenses involved in repressive patterns include denial of negative feelings, reaction
formation, repression of the content that arouses uncomfortable experiences, minimization of the significance of events, negation of the meaning
of negative social stimuli, insensitivity to one's impact on others, and the
introduction of either a positive or, at best, a neutral response by which
to react to these negative events.

Theoretically, repressive coping patterns are associated with unrecognized wishes and desires that evoke strong injunctions against direct expression. Coming to recognize the nature of these wishes, impulses, and
injunctions is assumed to reduce conflict and to allow one's behaviors to
become more consistent with the demands of the environment.

In treating the patient who presents with complex problems and a repressive coping style, we believe that the approach of highest yield will be
one that addresses the level of unconscious experience. Hence, the therapeutic focus for patients of this type may incorporate the principles outlined by writers such as Strupp and Binder (1984), Luborsky (1984), and
Bond, Hansell and Shevrin (1987). The focus includes recurrent interpersonal patterns, with emphasis upon uncovering the needs and wants driv-

ing these transactions. The focal theme also includes the expectations the patient has for others' responses, the experiences encountered when needs are expressed, and the introject or conclusion that typifies the patient's efforts. The patient's behavior in the face of both unrecognized needs and more apparent expectations is likely to solicit or invite the very responses that are feared from others, however unwanted and disliked these responses are.

For example, J.I.'s presentation consisted of exaggerated positive affect, even in the midst of decided symptoms of PTSD following her accident. Given this style of defense, the therapeutic focus might logically be directed at uncovering the nature of denied experiences. After initially addressing J.I.'s symptomatic complaints, treatment would begin to explore the recurrent pattern of denial and control that characterizes her relationships with intimates, most recently her husband. Efforts to define this theme and to relate it to her early experience of having been stabbed and left for dead may work to break her tendency to deny the memory and impact of this traumatic experience.

Therapeutic procedures for addressing patients who rely on repressive coping styles seek to uncover hidden motives, such as J.I.'s hidden fear of dependency; bring to awareness unexpressed wishes and impulses; and evoke changes in the schematic systems that maintain response rigidity beyond their due. All of these tasks rely on the mechanisms of confrontation and interpretation. Indeed, the accuracy of interpretations designed to evoke insight (Crits-Christoph, Cooper & Luborsky, 1988), as well as the acceptability to the patient of interpretations offered (Silberschatz, Fretter & Curtis, 1986), has been found to be related to therapeutic response. Among the procedures comprising interventions whose mediating task is the development of insight are:

(1) Free association,
(2) Dream interpretation,
(3) Encouragement of transferential projections,
(4) Interpretation of resistance and defense,
(5) Analysis of hidden motives through assessment of common mistakes or slips,
(6) Free fantasy explorations,
(7) Discussion of early memories,
(8) The construction and analysis of genograms, and
(9) Two-chair work on intrapersonal "splits."

Like the other procedures to be discussed in this chapter, the foregoing ones can be implemented with considerable variability of method. For example, problem severity modulates the use of various of these interventions and tempers the relative emphasis that the therapist might give to interpretation versus support (Jones, Cumming & Horowitz, 1988). These considerations will be refined and addressed more completely as our discussion proceeds.

(3) Cyclic Coping Styles call for variability in the nature of therapeutic interventions to match the variations observed in patient behavior. By their nature, cyclic coping patterns are ones of change and instability. Patients with such coping styles exhibit ambivalence (Millon, 1969) and, alternately, may act out, somatosize, become blaming and vengeful, or withdraw and become guilt-ridden and self-blaming. They have very low tolerance for frustration and do not have the verbal labels and cognitive constructs to help differentiate among emotions. Thus, they respond in an overdetermined but similar fashion to a variety of social experiences. Quite minor stressors may provoke very primitive behaviors, and these behaviors seem to bear little relationship to realistic demands of the environment.

Pursuing our example of J.I. further, imagine how treatment might have been different if she had responded to her early trauma with the type of cyclic instability described here. She might have presented with a history of dependency relationships interspersed with periods of aggressive demands. Her behavior would show a general correspondence with her mood, being up at early points in relationships and depressed when those relationships could no longer support her demands for attention.

If J.I. had presented a cyclic coping style to her original trauma, we might expect that her reaction to the more recent automobile accident would have been overwhelming. Rather than presenting with anxiety and phobic symptoms alone, she may have regressed significantly, perhaps requiring hospitalization to prevent suicidal behavior. Histrionic symptoms would be expected, including exacerbated paralysis and other physical complaints.

Even under the best of circumstances, an abreactive treatment may be expected to exacerbate these intense behavioral and mood swings. On the other hand, an insight-oriented treatment may be expected either to produce little response if J.I. is well defended or decompensation if the treatment relationship becomes too intense for her defenses to withstand.

Because of the variation and inconsistency that exist between overcontrol and undercontrol among patients with intense cyclic defenses, the therapist's treatment menu must include both procedures that focus on internal experience and those which focus on external behavior. The level of depth tends to remain relatively close to the symptom, however, until stability is achieved, in spite of the conflictual basis of the problem. Hence, the experiences addressed by the procedural menu are at the behavioral and cognitive habit levels. This is not to say that the therapist discontinues her/his emphasis on the underlying conflict during this time; formulations of the conflictual pattern continue to be the binding elements of treatment. However, direct attention to the conflictual underpinnings of cyclic instability is reserved until behaviors are modulated.

A distinguishing feature of the cognitive procedures used among those with simple or noncomplex problems and those addressed to these complex problems is the inclusion of schematic themes in the latter case. As defenses become external and behaviorally disruptive, controls are placed on behavior through the construction of environmental contingencies. As the patient becomes more introspective, sullen, or withdrawn, attention is given to dysfunctional thought processes and schematic patterns. Treatment menus designed for impacting patients who have cyclic coping styles include:

(1) Identification of cognitive distortions,

(2) Labeling of emotions and their relation to thoughts and situations,

(3) Questioning assumptions,

(4) Exploring alternatives to automatic thoughts and associated assumptions,

(5) Self monitoring of behavior and thoughts,

(6) Analyzing the validity of assumptions,

(7) Behavioral contracting for change,

(8) Instruction in reinforcement principles,

(9) Thought stopping,

(10) Hypnosis and pleasant imagery to lower arousal,

(11) Counterconditioning,

(12) Stimulus control of thoughts and behaviors, and

(13) Self instruction.

Examples of how these procedures may be implemented can be found in a variety of source books and manuals (Goldfried & Davison, 1976; Bandura, 1977; Meichenbaum, 1977; Paul & Lentz, 1977; Beck et al., 1979; Yost et al., 1986). The procedures are collectively devoted to controlling the intensity of both internal arousal and disruptive behaviors. Hence, they characteristically fall within the two domains of experience here referred to as "cognitive dysfunction" and "behavioral."

Cognitive and behavioral procedures represent an unusually robust and adaptable set of interventions and are applicable to a wide variety of conditions (Shapiro & Shapiro, 1982; Miller & Berman, 1983; Berman,

Miller & Massman, 1985); hence, their suitability to the unstable and inconsistent patterns typified by the cyclical patient.

(4) Externalizing Coping Styles characterize and identify a fourth group of patients for whom procedures are addressed to the most symptomatic and behavioral level. Externalizing patients represent the contrasting extreme of our coping style dimension, when compared to those patients defined as "internalizers." Externalizing patients share many of the undercontrolled, acting-out and projective patterns of behavior observed in the patient who manifests a cyclic pattern of defense, but they do not present with the degree of ambivalence, vacillation, and instability of that latter group.

Externalization is defined as the process of limiting anxiety by transferring responsibility for one's own behavior to external sources of influence, and/or discharging this anxiety directly through overt behavior. In the interpersonal domain, it consists of moving against others and acting against the environment. Those with well developed externalizing defenses are successful at keeping intense feelings at a distance. Their symptoms are quite ego syntonic and include such patterns as true conversion symptoms, projection and paranoid reactions, unsocialized aggression, and manipulative or impulsive suicidal behaviors, as well as other forms of controlling others.

Here we should also distinguish between acting out as a hedonistic response and acting out as a neurotic defense. Behaviors in the former domain may be treated symptomatically as simple habits, while behavior in the latter domain is usually more complex.

As an example, consider H.D., who you will recall from Chapter 3 exemplified a chronic externalizing coping style. This 44-year-old man had obtained several graduate degrees in spite of overt rebellion against scholastic authority, and remained unemployed, usually drunk, relying on his parents for financial support. While these symptoms might represent a relatively uncomplex pattern that is maintained by secondary gain (financial support from parents), they might also constitute an effort to self medicate his anxiety about losing a parental bond. In this latter case, H. D.'s drinking would be judged to be a complex problem because it represents an indirect but repeated symbol of an unexpressed need, embodying the neurotic paradox—i.e., it either results in increased anxiety or exhibits behavior that actually diminishes the likelihood of gratifying the need that it is designed to serve.

The treatment of externalizing patients is constructed to parallel their patterns of social acting out and avoidance. The therapist develops a formulation of the repetitive nature of the symptom and the interpersonal contingencies that account for the similarity of behaviors across those situations that are not overtly similar to the original evoking events. The level of these treatments is defined by their attention both to behaviors to be eliminated or reduced in frequency (i.e., excessive behaviors) and to socially appropriate behaviors that need to be developed or increased (i.e., insufficient behaviors). Since behavioral excesses and insufficiencies are two sides of the same behavioral coin, the procedures addressed to these two aspects of experience are not mutually exclusive.

Frequently, behavioral excesses are treated by the training of patients to produce high frequencies of competing and more appropriate responses. In these cases, it is assumed that reinforcement of desirable behavioral responses will introduce and maintain these appropriate behaviors once trained. The specific strategies used for intervening with externalizing patients include:

(1) Behavioral contracting for change,
(2) Counterconditioning,
(3) Covert and overt practice,
(4) Graded exposure,
(5) Withdrawal of reinforcement,
(6) Direct instruction and advice,
(7) Role enactment,
(8) Self monitoring, and
(9) Contingency management/token economies.

As noted, the indicated procedures for externalizing patients are aimed at the level of behavior—i.e., the symptomatic level of experience. However, the relationship among symptoms cannot be ignored and for the patient with complex problems this relationship is assumed to be reflected in the conflictual theme. This theme is constructed to include the common sources of anxiety that stimulate the various avoidance responses and that provide the guiding thread for prioritizing the order of interventions. While this theme is subject to some change over the course of treatment for all patients (Hatcher, Huebner & Zakin, 1986), it may be most stable for externalizing patients, whose symptoms are such direct manifestations of their defensive styles.

MEDIATING GOALS AND PHASES OF PSYCHOTHERAPY

In contrast to outcome goals, mediating goals define the sequence of anticipated change. In a broad sense, therefore, the type of experience (unconscious motives, feelings, cognitive habits, overt behaviors) targeted for change represents a mediating goal in the process of achieving symptomatic or conflictual change. It is a means-end goal; by attending to the level of experience selected, we assume that we efficaciously will achieve our outcome objectives.

However, *mediating* goals, in the more narrow sense that we desire to use the term here, have the added quality of defining the order of events that we anticipate will lead to treatment success. Knowing the level of experience to be addressed does not provide the practitioner with this needed degree of specificity regarding the course of treatment.

Within the context of different theories of treatment, mediating goals are represented with various degrees of specificity. Hence, before we address the problem of selecting among these goals, we must develop a system within which the various mediating goals that characterize different treatments can be organized.

Defining Mediating Goals

Typically, the nature of mediating processes and objectives selected by a given therapist reflects his or her theoretical adherence. The level of flexibility required for differential treatment decisions necessitates a general procedure for classifying mediating goals that cuts across theoretical philosophies, however. A temporal system of classification promises this flexibility. For example, Blau (1988) presents an example of how mediating psychotherapy goals can be defined within the phases of psychodynamic psychotherapy. He defines three comprehensive phases of psychoanalytic treatment based upon patient tasks: exploration, experiencing, and integration.

Beitman (1987) proposes a more comprehensive and eclectic system than Blau, suggesting that all therapy models encompass four treatment phases, each of which embodies relatively specific goals and procedures. These goal-oriented phases include: (1) facilitating patient-therapist *engagement,* (2) *pattern search* to identify the objectives of change, (3) instigating *change,* and (4) preparing for *termination.* One will note that the mediating goals, when defined in this way, describe the tasks that must be accomplished in order to move to the next stage.

Beitman's model of psychotherapy phases is quite concise and offers the advantage of being independent of a specific theory. However, to fit the needs of differential treatment assignment, we must identify the potential treatment processes that will be addressed by different clinicians within each of these treatment phases. This level of description represents a second layer of mediational processes, the awareness of which will help narrow the range of therapy procedures that are appropriate at given points in time.

There are two promising systems that address this second layer of specificity. Each of these two systems was particularly developed to include the degree of flexibility required by eclectic treatment applications.

The first system derives from the first author's prior description of systematic eclectic psychotherapy. In this work, Beutler (1983) proposed that six types of mediating processes define the variations among different models of treatment. The system of Prochaska and DiClemente (1984, 1986) for classifying mediating processes is more extensive than that of Beutler, purporting to represent all the basic "change processes" embodied in psychotherapy procedures.

These two lists are not mutually exclusive. Moreover, various items on each list appear to be more characteristic of one phase of treatment than another. This is important since it suggests that by assigning these processes to specific treatment phases, we can achieve the degree of specificity needed to move treatment forward. Perhaps even more important, each mediating process can be associated with a variety of relatively specific procedures.

To illustrate these latter points, step three in our decisional model will describe methods of matching the intermediate treatment goals to patient needs.

Step #3—Matching Mediating Goals to Treatment Phase

Table 12.2 illustrates the expansion of treatment processes that results when we assign the various mediating goals defined by Beutler (1983) and Prochaska and DiClemente (1984) to a place of priority within the phases of treatment. With a little imagination, one also might be able to identify the level of intervention and the breadth of focus to which each of these processes might be best addressed. If one were to expand the list in this way while recognizing that mediating objectives may operate in more than one treatment phase, the intermixture of treatment phase objectives and level of experience addressed in the therapeutic focus will result in a large variety of therapy processes that potentially characterize treatment.

Table 12.2

Mediating Goals Characterizing the Phases of Treatment

| | Treatment Phase | | |
Engagement	Pattern Search	Change	Termination
Dramatic Relief	Insight	Self Liberation	Social Evaluation
Catharsis	Emotional Awareness	Social Liberation	Changing Environment
Helping Relationship	Contingency Awareness	Increased Arousal	Enhancing Social Liberation

(Continued)

Table 12.2 *(continued)*

| Engagement | Treatment Phase | | |
	Pattern Search	Change	Termination
	Raising Consciousness	Decreased Arousal	Establishing Stimulus Control
	Self Reevaluation	Behavior Change Perceptual Change Counterconditioning Establishing Stimulus Control Changing the Environment	

By identifying the procedures that are appropriate to each treatment phase, we can refine the menus outlined in earlier pages of this chapter by selecting the procedures that are most consistent with a given phase of treatment. As a prelude to the paragraphs to follow, these relationships partially are illustrated in Table 12.3, which suggests some tasks that may be appropriate at each level of experience and within each of the treatment phases that follow initial engagement.

Table 12.3
Level of Experience by Therapeutic Phase/Task

Level of Experience	Tasks Interpolated to the Phase

A. Misidentified and Unidentified Feelings
  (1) Pattern Search = Sensory and affective awareness.
  (2) Change = Dramatic relief or enhanced emotional arousal; enhanced expression of emotions.
  (3) Termination = Acknowledging and accepting one's emotional reactions; retaining focus on current emotional and sensory experience.
B. Unconscious Motives, Wishes and Conflicts
  (1) Pattern search = Insight into unconscious and schematic beliefs.
  (2) Change = Changing schematic beliefs; becoming free from parental injunctions/introjects.
  (3) Termination = Acknowledging those aspects of past relationships that cannot be changed and maintaining awareness of motives and defensive dispositions.

(Continued)

Table 12.3 *(continued)*

Level of Experience	Tasks Interpolated to the Phase

C. Dysfunctional Cognitive Patterns or Habits
  (1) Pattern search = Identification of automatic thoughts.
  (2) Change = Correct dysfunctional thoughts; alter social expectations.
  (3) Termination = Checking and monitoring unchanged assumptions and automatic thoughts.
D. Behavioral Excess or Insufficiency
  (1) Pattern search = Becoming aware of contingencies.
  (2) Change = Reinforcing and changing behavioral habits; altering social skills.
  (3) Termination = Acknowledging habitual behaviors; maintaining stable contingencies.

Engagement. It is at the beginning of treatment that the foundation of trust must be laid. No specific designation of psychotherapy procedures, medication regimen, or hospital treatment plan can be expected to be maximally successful without ensuring that the patient and therapist are working collaboratively. Even if the patient is forced to attend treatment by an act of family or legal authority, the first working goal is to establish a basis for engagement.

Among the specific processes of change listed by Prochaska and DiClemente (1986), two are of particular relevance to the goal of inducing engagement. These are the promotion of expression, including the induction of dramatic relief (i.e., catharsis) and facilitating a helping relationship. Beyond these general processes, we have addressed the specific procedures of therapeutic engagement in Section IV (Chapters 9 and 10), and do not need to reiterate those processes here.

The relationship enhancement methods discussed in Chapter 10 are designed to provide the atmosphere of safety and support that will allow these goals to be achieved. Indeed, for many patients whose problems are either transitory or mild, the successful application of procedures to enhance engagement may be sufficient for treatment to proceed through its various other stages. For most of those who seek treatment, however, the processes of engagement must be partially supplanted by other procedures in order to accomplish the mediating goals represented by the other treatment phases.

Pattern Search. Pattern search reflects the mediating objectives of acquiring knowledge, insight, and awareness. In noncomplex problems, accomplishing these goals may simply be a matter of defining the nature of contingencies and evoking events. In the case of complex problems, pattern search is more intimately involved with defining and then learning to recognize the recurrent theme that characterizes one's problematic adjustments. Beutler (1983) and Prochaska and DiClemente (1982, 1986) express the various goals of this phase as: (1) insight enhancement or understanding (Beutler), (2) emotional awareness or sensitivity to sensory experience (Beutler), (3) inducing self-reevaluation (Prochaska & DiClemente), and (4) provoking reevaluation of the environment or social condition (Prochaska & DiClemente) (refer to Table 12.2).

Among patients with dominantly *internalizing coping styles,* it will be recalled, the level of experience addressed is that of affective and sensory awareness. The specific procedures that characterize the pattern recognition phase of treatment at this level of experience include such activities as sensory focusing, one- and two-chair work on "unfinished business," dream work, free association, reflective mirroring, enacting opposites, and reflection of feelings.

Alternatively, procedures addressed to the level of uncovering unconscious motives and impulses are advantageous for patients who present with dominant *repressive coping styles.* Among the procedures we suggest as most relevant for use with patients with these coping styles, free association, interpretation, encouraging projections, free fantasy explorations, recalling early memories, and the use of genograms all seem suited to pattern search.

Among patients with *cyclic coping styles,* we wish to intervene at the level of dysfunctional cognitions. Procedures for identifying cognitive distortions, pinpointing characteristic A (situation)—B (intervening thought)—C (emotion or behavior) sequences, questioning assumptions, self monitoring thoughts and behaviors, and direct instruction are all ways that may be particularly appropriate to the phase of pattern search for these patients.

Finally, there also are pattern search procedures that address the behavioral level of experience that is targeted for focus among patients with dominantly *externalizing coping styles.* These procedures include direct observation, instruction, and self-monitoring.

For example, if J.I.'s symptomatic intensity has not responded to the supportive process of engagement, her phobic avoidance would be treated as an externalization; during the phase of pattern search, the therapist would encourage self-observation, record keeping, and self-monitoring of fears and avoided situations. If, on the other hand, symptomatic relief has been achieved during the first treatment phase, patterns associated with the conflictual pattern of intimacy avoidance would be sought, utilizing procedures that accommodate to the patient's repressive coping style.

These procedures may include exploration of early memories, free association, exploration of dreams, and use of free fantasy. Material obtained via these procedures would be used to construct a dynamic formulation of the patient's motives and fears, incorporating the essential nature of the patient's recurrent interpersonal theme (e.g., the pattern of wishes, expectations, compromises, and introjects; Strupp & Binder, 1984).

Change. Specific changes are sought based upon the information that comes to light during the phase of pattern search. Even then, change is accepted only as a mediating goal of treatment when the treatment relationship is sufficiently strong to provide a sense of safety as the patient begins to take risks. Within such an environment, the nature of the changes sought in various treatments can be subdivided into two major categories: personal (or intrapersonal) and interpersonal changes. By incorporating both of these types of change into this phase of treatment, the therapist ensures that all treatments attend to the social significance of treatment gains. As we pointed out when discussing variations in treatment formats, the patient's position in the problem-solving cycle defined by Prochaska and colleagues (1982; 1988) (precontemplative, contemplative, action, and maintenance) might help determine whether one focuses on personal or interpersonal changes.

As suggested in Table 12.4, one implication of matching treatment task to Problem Solving phase is that this match ensures that all therapies have an interpersonal component. In contrast to the distinction proposed by many authors between interpersonal or family therapies, on the one hand, and various other, assumedly noninterpersonal therapies, on the other, the current model holds that all effective treatment must attend to interpersonal processes.

The foregoing viewpoint does not necessarily mean that marital, family, or group therapy uniformly will be the format selected during this interpersonal phase. However, it does recognize the role of personal change in altering interpersonal systems. Whether patients are treated in multiple person settings and contexts will depend upon many factors, but the inclusion of interpersonal changes as an intermediate task of therapy recognizes that there are specific aspects of improvement which may be best imple-

Table 12.4
Matching To the Phase of Therapy

Patient Problem-Solving Phase	Matching Treatment Task
(1) Precontemplative (2) Contemplative (3) Action (4) Maintenance	Understanding/Awareness and Personal Change Interpersonal Change

mented by changing the context of treatment from individual to group or family settings at certain points in the treatment process. When patients are in the action and maintenance phases of the change process, they may be most susceptible to the influences and benefits of these multiple person interventions. If other indicators for such treatments are present as these treatment formats are initiated (see Chapter 7), entry to the interpersonal and the action stages of change may require a shift in treatment format in order to ensure maximal gains at these times.

Both Beutler and Prochaska and DiClemente recognize a variety of personal change objectives. These include increasing arousal level; reduction of emotional states; behavior change; and perceptual change promoting dramatic expression of feelings and cathartic relief, reducing constraint against feelings, counterconditioning, and reevaluation of the environment or social condition in which one lives.

Interpersonal changes potentially include altering the environment that elicits the symptom, introducing a new environmental stimulus, reevaluating the social environment associated with the problem, and practicing behavior change.

Among the procedures that promote the type of sensory awareness changes which we consider most appropriate for the patient with dominantly *internalizing coping styles,* sensory focus, two-chair work on emotional "splits," structured imagery and practice, physical expression, and cathartic release exercises may be quite helpful.

Alternatively, free association, dream interpretation, confrontation, interpretation of resistance and defense, two-chair work on interpersonal "splits," and rehearsal are likely to be helpful for uncovering unconscious motivations among patients who dominantly utilize *repressive coping styles.*

In similar fashion, patients with *cyclic coping styles* may be responsive to interventions that address the level of dysfunctional cognitive patterns. This may include such change-inducing methods as questioning assumptions, construction of perceptual and behavioral alternatives, analyzing the social validity of assumptions, thought-stopping procedures, hypnosis and pleasant imagery, counterconditioning, and self-instruction.

Finally, patients who tend to rely on *externalizing coping styles* require procedures that directly impact the behavioral level of experience. In the change phase of treatment, these patients may be well served by behavioral contracting, reinforcement, withdrawal of reinforcement, graded exposure, and contingency contracting.

To use J.I. as a continuing example, let us look at the difference between the symptomatic treatment of her phobia (excessive fear behavior) and the thematic treatment of her intimacy avoidance pattern. Considering her anxiety symptoms within a narrow band (i.e., symptomatic) set of treatment objectives, graded exposure and desensitization would be implemented in accordance both with the nature of her symptom and the nature of her repressive defenses. On the other hand, as we began treating the recurrent interpersonal pattern of avoiding intimacy, change would be sought by interpreting and confronting the patient with the avoidant pattern, especially as this pattern occurs in the therapeutic relationship.

The rationale for selecting confrontational and interpretative interventions invokes the assumption that the patient's repressive style will be best served by inducing awareness of repressed material. Hence, recovering early experiences may be assisted through two-chair work around unfinished relationships with parental figures and figures of abuse, with resulting coping styles interpreted and translated to current situations.

At a later point in treatment, as the patient moves to the stage of action in the problem-solving cycle, marital therapy may be implemented. The focus of this format would be to translate the patient's learning to more immediate situations and to gain control of the interpersonal pattern within the most pressing social environment available.

Termination Planning. The principal tasks of termination planning are to: (1) ensure that the patient has a supportive social system available after treatment, (2) anticipate potential problems, (3) prepare plans for handling future stress, and (4) plan for follow-up meetings with the therapist.

Preparing for termination calls for a shift from a past and present focus of treatment to a future-oriented one. In this treatment phase, interpersonal changes are of particular importance since lack of social support is such a strong determiner of symptom recurrence (see Chapter 5). Accordingly, this phase of treatment begins when the patient achieves what Prochaska (1984) has called the stage of maintenance. Interpersonal treatments and procedures designed to alter the patient's social environment are to be used at this point whenever feasible.

By asking patients to anticipate potential problems, the therapist provides an opportunity for the patient to test, in a safe way, how effective his or her new learning might be for coping with anticipated stressors. The skills and knowledge acquired during treatment may need to be supplemented by some specific translation to anticipated, extratherapy situations in order to help the patient prepare for future stressors.

In a related way, during the termination planning phase, the patient and therapist plan methods for the patient to seek help if needed and for the therapist systematically to provide supportive and preventive assistance during the post-therapy period. This latter element of treatment planning is of sufficient importance that we will give it special attention shortly.

In applying the procedures for termination planning, the same general principles that govern treatment selection during the change phase should be emphasized. Thus, the therapist should continue to concentrate on the focal theme, although its limits must be made more directly applicable to the patient's daily functioning and more interpersonal in form. It should be noted that one effect of treatment may be an alteration of the patient's dominant coping style. If this is true, the type of experience addressed by treatment procedures should also accommodate to this change.

Maintenance and Relapse Prevention

It is becoming increasingly obvious that treatment termination should not imply an end to treatment as much as it does a change of treatment intensity. Approximately 16 percent of patients will require consistent and ongoing maintenance (Howard, 1988). Approximately 40 percent of depressed patients relapse (Beutler et al., 1987; Jacobson, 1988; Rush, 1988) within two years of treatment, suggesting that some form of continuing maintenance or aftercare should be provided for patients after active treatment phase has been completed.

The importance of post-termination treatment contact has been recognized by Prochaska and colleagues (Prochaska, Velicer, DiClemente & Fava, 1988) by adding "relapse" to the list of behavior change stages (i.e., precontemplation, contemplation, action, maintenance, and relapse). Research has also turned to defining risk factors for relapse (e.g., Hooley & Teasdale, in press), thus paving the way for treatment aimed at interrupting problem recurrence.

Efforts to provide maintenance treatment and relapse prevention have focused either on booster sessions or social support assistance. It appears that a great many risk factors reflect on disturbed family or marital patterns of interaction (Marlatt et al., 1988; Hooley & Teasdale, in press). Thus, concentration on developing family and social support systems appears to be desirable in relapse prevention.

Accordingly, it is our recommendation that therapists reestablish contact with patients and family members on a regular basis. Some of the structured follow-up procedures that have been found to be effective in preventing relapse among alcohol abusers (Marlatt & George, 1984; Marlatt & Gordon, 1985) and depressed patients (Klerman et al., 1984) could reasonably guide the structuring of these follow-up efforts. By and large, follow-up plans should be designed to maximize patient access to social resources. Family systems, social groups, and the development of supportive activities can help avoid relapse for a variety of conditions.

We recommend planned follow-up for two years after active treatment ends. Regularly scheduled appointments at two weeks, one month, three months, six months, and the two annual posttreatment anniversaries help facilitate the introduction of prevention efforts when they are needed. Postcards to help patients remember these appointments and to invite additional contact as well as comment may also provide a level of support that is helpful.

Follow-up appointments might be designed to gather information about the patient's current level of coping. Booster sessions may be designed to review and to reinforce those skills that the patient initially found to be helpful during treatment. Within these sessions, the therapist can then help the patient apply these principles to current activities.

There are a variety of reasons for placing the responsibility for follow-up on the therapist rather than on the patient. Follow-up with our own patients suggests that some patients are reluctant to recontact their therapist when problems reoccur after successful treatment because they don't want a favored therapist to feel like a failure. Other patients have had no recurrence of difficulties and see no reason for calling their therapist. Still others experience a reoccurrence of symptoms, but having developed the expectation that they would remain symptom-free, are angry at and disappointed in their therapist. In any of these cases, when the therapist takes the responsibility for maintaining regular follow-up contact, an opportunity is provided to catch problems before they become serious.

SUMMARY AND COMMENT

The second step in our multidimensional procedural analysis defines the levels of experience that are targeted by different therapeutic procedures. These levels of targeted experience have been defined along a continuum ranging from overt behavior to unconscious motivations and wishes. A rational analysis of different therapeutic systems suggests that these systems have been devoted to provoking changes at different levels of experience.

Beyond the types of experience to which interventions are directed, different procedures also are distinguished by the mediating processes that mark the phases of treatment. Step three of our decision model has defined four treatment phases which dictate the patterning of interventions across time. These tasks are modified to coincide with the depth of experience to which the treatment is addressed.

Following the lead of Beitman (1987), the four phases of treatment include: (1) engagement, (2) pattern search, (3) making changes, and (4) planning for termination. Engagement is associated with the acquisition of knowledge, insight, and emotional awareness; pattern search is associated with defining the nature of the focal goals, representing either symptomatic relationships or recurrent interpersonal conflicts; change is associated both with personal and interpersonal alterations of patterns; termination is associated with anticipation of problems and planning resolution strategies.

Throughout the application of the decisional processes required at each level of intervention and phase of treatment, the therapist's inferential judgment is an important element of success. If therapists fail to integrate the needs of patients with the characteristics or demands of therapy, they may lose the therapeutic focus. When the interventions applied are appropriate to the patient's problem complexity, coping style, and treatment phase objectives, it's likely that therapeutic gains will be enhanced.

Psychotherapeutic tasks are extremely complex. Technical skill must be combined with sound judgment, intuitive observation, well-founded assessment, and the willingness of patient and therapist to take collaborative risk. The effective therapist creates a model of the therapeutic processes and defines those mediating goals that are likely to enhance the focus of treatment at each treatment phase, and then responds to the moment-to-moment changes in the relationship in a way designed to provide an environment that safely allows and encourages the patient to move through the stages and phases of growth.

SUGGESTED READINGS

Beitman, B. D. (1987). *The Structure of individual psychotherapy*. New York: Guilford.

Gleser, G. C. & Ihlevich, D. (1969). An objective instrument to measure defense mechanisms. *Journal of Consulting and Clinical Psychology, 33,* 51–60.

Lazarus, R. S. & Folkman, S. (1984). *Stress, appraisal, and coping.* New York: Springer.

London, P. (1986). *The modes and morals of psychotherapy,* 2nd ed. Washington, DC: Hemisphere Publishing Co.

Millon, T. & Everly, G. S. (1981). *Personality and its disorders.* New York: John Wiley and Sons.

Shapiro, D. (1965). *Neurotic styles.* New York: Basic Books.

13

Conducting Therapeutic Work

and the sharing of the journey,
the unselfish giving of one gentle and kind heart.
And in that gesture you paid tribute
to the bridges in your life
and so, too, will I watch always
for the survivor on the shore.

(S.B., one year after termination of treatment)

An effective therapist intuitively is able to respond to the unique characteristics and needs of patients, and in this process to apply a variety of interventions that encourage movement and enhance the persuasive power of the interpersonal experience of psychotherapy.

But what of the therapist who lacks intuitive ability? Who is to judge when the multitude of moment-to-moment decisions made by the therapist reflect sound judgment? Unfortunately, therapists are probably not the most accurate judges of their own effectiveness, and the least effective therapists may be among the most inaccurate when asked to assess their own effectiveness rates (e.g., Beutler, Dunbar & Baer, 1980).

The focus of treatment depends upon a large number of patient, therapist, and interactional factors. This complexity is reflected in the four-step model for achieving psychotherapy specificity that we have been discussing in the previous two chapters. It is inevitable that the decisional alternatives become more complex with each step in this model; approaching the decision process sequentially is designed to ease this complexity. We are now ready to address the fourth step of our model, that relating to the moment-to-moment decisions that one must make in order to conduct therapeutic work.

Consistent with the two previous chapters, we will begin with a review of current concepts, concluding with a set of dimensions that seem adequately to capture the variety of treatment procedure represented in different approaches. We then will direct our attention to outlining the

265

procedures for matching these dimensions to the patient dimensions described in earlier chapters.

THE DIMENSIONS OF SPECIFIC PROCEDURES

The fourth level in our analysis of psychotherapy procedures represents the most discrete and procedurally specific of the various steps in our conceptual model. This level of our analysis will classify and catalogue the dimensions of activity that characterize specific procedures. It would be possible, of course, to provide an exhaustive list of psychotherapy procedures broken down by the interactions among treatment requirements.

It potentially is more helpful to define the fundamental dimensions along which procedures can be distinguished and that are related to their differential effectiveness than simply to itemize all of the specific procedures now available. Hence, in this section, we propose to outline the dimensions of implementation to which therapists should be sensitive and to provide some samples of the discrete procedures that attend to these various dimensions.

At this level of specificity, we must depart somewhat from the rational analysis that has characterized our descriptions of therapeutic decisions in the three preceding steps. Only from observing specific therapy transactions can we develop a list of the types of therapeutic procedures that might be distinguished in application to different patients.

Either direct or indirect observations can provide the bases from which a list of relevant procedural dimensions can be obtained. Indirect methods assess what therapists within different theoretical systems say they would do in given situations, while direct approaches observe, catalogue, and rate the in-treatment behaviors of these therapists. Indirect methods provide a set of therapist beliefs about what they do, while direct methods are designed to derive less subjective lists of the dimensions that distinguish among procedures. These two approaches result in complementary dimensions by which therapist behaviors can be differentiated.

Indirect Observations

The best known series of indirect investigations on therapist behaviors culminated in a 1977 report by Donald Sundland. The factorial structure of a lengthy questionnaire that was designed to reflect both theoretical beliefs and treatment predelictions revealed that the practices of therapists could be described and differentiated by reference to the degree of adherence to 11 characteristic beliefs about what constitutes good practice:

(1) Use of body sensations, nonverbal cues, guided daydreams, and emotional release procedures

(2) Exploration of childhood experiences, the development of dynamic formulations, emphasis on the therapeutic transference, and belief in intensive or long-term therapy

(3) Belief in the importance of planning for change and learning to adapt to societal rules

(4) Therapist directiveness and activity level as well as a willingness to interrupt the patient or to provide instruction and information

(5) Belief in the importance of feeling awareness as an avenue to improvement and/or growth

(6) A tendency to become personally committed, caring, and responsive to the patient

(7) Belief or disbelief in the presence of an innate drive toward mental health

(8) The sense of security and freedom from countertransference feelings toward the patient

(9) Belief in the importance of the therapist's personality and intuitive ability in facilitating the healing nature of psychotherapy

(10) Belief in verbal and conceptual learning as the avenue to successful change

(11) Use of encounter and sensitivity exercises or physical touch as techniques for enhancing psychotherapeutic change

The relative standing of therapists in relation to these 11 dimensions was found to distinguish among those whose theoretical adherences led them to value intrapsychic (psychodynamic), experiential, or cognitive-behavioral procedures. Not surprisingly, experiential therapists tended to emphasize an informal therapeutic stance with emphasis on nonverbal treatment techniques that included exercises designed to enhance interpersonal sensitivity and contact. Psychodynamic therapists adopted a formal and nonconfrontive stance which explored childhood experiences, but they avoided using exercises to enhance arousal and either nonverbal or physical interventions. Cognitive and behavioral therapists adopted an impersonal stance from which they advocated learning and conditioning procedures to accomplish predetermined treatment goals.

In spite of their ability to distinguish among the adherents of different broad theories, these 11 categories of technique reflect a relatively small number of separate dimensions, some of which have little apparent relationship to the implementation of specific procedures.

The preponderance of variables presented in this formulation are really aspects of the therapist's philosophy and beliefs rather than aspects of psychotherapy behavior. There are only three factors that represent procedural distinctions. These patterns include the degree to which the therapist (1) uses nonverbal interventions, (2) explores childhood experiences, and/or (3) implements strategies designed to enhance interpersonal contact and sensitivity.

In an effort to make the foregoing findings more reflective of actual practice, Beutler (1983) contrasted the results of over a dozen comparative studies of psychotherapy processes. From this analysis, he found that psychodynamic, interpersonal, experiential, behavioral, and cognitive psychotherapists could be distinguished by cross-matching the long-term goals of the specific interventions (i.e., symptomatic or conflictual—step one in our analysis) and two aspects of their implementation. Implementation characteristics included continua ranging from (1) evocative to directive and (2) intratherapy to extratherapy attentional focus.

Evocative interventions allow maximal patient freedom of response and are designed to stimulate a deepening exploration by the patient. They do not require a specific response from the patient, but do invite responses through the use of reflections, questions, interpretations, and the like. The form of the patient's response is left open-ended, but is characteristically verbal and exploratory.

Directive interventions, on the other hand, are those that limit patient response in some way. The response by the therapist typically entails the performance of some activity or reporting some specific information. Directive interventions take the form of focused or closed questions, statements, homework suggestions, or guided experience. In each case, the responses may be either verbal or behavioral and the form of the response desired by the therapist is known in advance.

Procedures having an *intratherapy attentional focus* are those that direct attention to activities, thoughts, and feelings that are occurring within the session. These experiences may include evocative discussions of the patient-therapist relationship or explorations of current thoughts and feelings. Alternatively, they may include directed activities such as relaxation exercises, hypnosis, and reporting present images and fantasies.

Finally, procedures with an *extratherapy attentional focus* are those that direct attention to experiences that have occurred or will occur outside of the office. Discussing external relationships, changes in the therapeutic relationship, parental injunctions, past feelings, and expectations of the future are some examples of activities and topics that may be suited to an evocative intervention. Directed activities with an extratherapy focus include dream recall, homework assignments, and requests to describe early experiences and memories.

Direct Observations

As a supplement to indirect methods of observing therapeutic procedures, direct observational methods have expanded the list of therapeutic activities. A number of different systems have been developed for classifying and coding therapeutic transactions that are directly observed. These systems differ in the unit of interaction used for defining a relevant or meaningful intervention. For example, Stiles (1978, 1979) defined eight exclusive categories within which a meaningful intervention could be classed. The category assigned to the intervention represented an interface between the literal meaning of the words used and the meaning intended by the communication between the therapist and patient. The response categories ranged from questions to edification, advice, and personal disclosure. In a different fashion, Elliott (1985) defined 10 overlapping dimensions which he thought were required to describe the nature of the exchange between patient and therapist.

A still more extensive list of interventions was developed by Goldberg et al. (1984) to fit the theoretical model of therapy originally outlined by Hobson (1985). This system describes the functional nature of the therapist's interventions by assigning each therapist response to one of 11 mutually exclusive categories. Similarly, Hill (1978) defined 14 mutually exclusive categories of therapist intervention, based upon the functional intent of discrete sentences or phrases used by the therapist (Hill, Helms, Spiegel & Tichenor, 1988).

At the furthest extreme, Mahrer (1983) defined 35 highly specific and mutually exclusive categories of therapist intervention. Even these very specific categories of therapist response could not solely be based upon the form of the therapist's intervention, however. They also incorporated implied intentions such as the establishment of *therapy structure, descriptive clarifications,* and *therapist approval and reassurance.*

The range of categories and the distinctions among the foregoing classification systems suggest both that there is overlap among systems and that the relevant dimensions by which technical procedures may be described can be usefully reduced. In an effort to accomplish this latter task, Elliott, Hill, Stiles, Friedlander, Mahrer and Margison (1987) systematically compared six systems for classifying therapist procedure, based upon a common sample of seven psychotherapy sessions. In spite of the variability of procedures and units of analysis used by the different systems, six distinguishing verbal interventions were identified by all systems: (1) questions, (2) providing information, (3) advising, (4) reflecting, (5) interpreting and (6) self-disclosing.

Interactive Dimensions

Collectively, the distinguishing elements of discrete procedures can be adequately captured as interactions among directly and indirectly observed dimensions, as presented in Table 13.1. Directly observed and indirectly reported observations yield different types of information that together may provide an interactive network for describing the nature of specific therapeutic procedures. Each category of directly observed activity can be constructed to fit within any of several positions along the dimensions of reported activity. For example, questions can be directive and externally focused:

T: "Will you monitor your handwashing rituals this week—see how often they occur?"

Or, they can be evocative and intrasession focused:

T: "Can you sense that conflict between wanting to get angry at your father and your fear of him right now?"

In the same way, the other *observed* dimensions also can be varied to fit the demands of each of the *reported* dimensions.

Table 13.1
Dimensions of Therapeutic Work

Global Dimension	*Type of Procedure*
Reported Activity	Ranging from Directed interventions, controlled by the therapist to Evocative interventions, controlled by the patient.
	Ranging from focus upon Extratherapy experience and behavior to Intratherapy experience and behavior.
Verbal Activity	Questions
	Providing information
	Advising
	Reflecting
	Interpreting patient meanings/motives
	Self Disclosing

In addition, the various verbal behaviors of the therapist may direct attention to one of several levels of experience (unconscious, emotional, cognitive, and behavioral) and at the same time direct change efforts either to symptoms or conflicts. The significance of this observation is in the fact that correspondence between interventions and formulations or guiding objectives tends to facilitate patient productive response (e.g., Silberschatz, Fretter & Curtis, 1986; Crits-Christoph, Cooper & Luborsky, 1988; Hill et al., 1988).

Table 13.2 illustrates how specific verbal procedures may vary in their reliance on evocative and directive implementation. Though not explicitly illustrated, one can either find or imagine among the partial list of procedures presented some that may be implemented to draw attention variously to intratherapy activity or to extratherapy activities. Similarly, one can easily think of procedures that can be presented in a way that focuses either upon specific symptoms or upon inferred conflicts.

Table 13.2
Representative Techniques by
Depth of Intervention and Directiveness

Level of Experience	Nature of Procedure	
	Evocative (E)	Directed (D)
(1) Unidentified Feelings	Reflection	Two-Chair Splits Sensate Focus Flooding
(2) Unconscious Motives	Interpretation	Free Association Dream Recall
(3) Cognitive Content	Questions	Evidence Gathering Thought Stopping
(4) Behavioral Events	Advising	Role Enactment Self Monitoring

The list presented in the foregoing table can be extended to whatever level of specificity one desires and can be constructed to reflect permutations among these several dimensions. Analysis of dreams, for example, is a directed activity typically aimed at conflict resolution, but may be implemented in such a way as to make dream reporting an intratherapy experience in the manner of Gestalt therapists (i.e., recreating the dream as an expression of a person's conflicts in the here and now), or as an extratherapy experience in the manner of psychoanalytic therapists (i.e., associating dream content to early experiences in the there and then). More than the specific procedure itself, the characteristics of its implementation are of importance when matching the demands of treatment to the needs of the patient.

Step #4—Conducting Therapeutic Work

The fourth and most specific level of psychotherapy matching defines the dimensions on which the therapist responds to moment-to-moment demands of the treatment process, selecting interventions, targets of conversation, and methods of communication. We propose that there are three patient dimensions, the recognition of which will allow the therapist to selectively use treatment menus in order to respond to these moment-to-moment changes in the therapeutic process: *problem severity, reactance level* and *problem-solving phase*. Sensitivity to the first two of these dimensions will help the therapist optimally maintain patient arousal. Specifically, problem severity, as indexed by patient distress, serves as an indicator of whether increased arousal or decreased arousal is indicated, and patient reactance level is a marker for determining how directive or evocative the therapist should be. Sensitivity to the patient's problem-solving cycle will help the therapist maintain a helpful balance between addressing intrasession and extratherapy issues.

Maintaining Therapeutic Arousal.   Previously we have seen that the focal goals of therapeutic activity can be either symptomatic (narrow band) or conflictual (broad band), the prescription of one over the other being dependent upon the complexity of the patient's problem. Now, we desire to refine the implementation of this recommendation by drawing to the reader's attention the value also of adjusting the intervention to fit the patient's level of problem severity as manifested in distress and arousal.

All varieties of psychotherapy are devoted to managing the level of patient arousal or distress in order to keep these experiences within a range that is conducive to effective work (Arkowitz & Hannah, in press). If arousal level is optimal, it will facilitate self observation, disconfirmation of pathognomic beliefs, and cognitive change. While different theories may value these latter consequences to a greater or lesser degree, virtually all theories acknowledge the reciprocal nature of these processes as the therapist appropriately manages patient arousal level and therapy activity.

As a general formulation and in order to maintain progress, the therapist attempts to ascertain *what* experiences a patient is avoiding and *how* that avoidance is occurring. The *"what is avoided"* constitutes either precipitating, symptom-contingent events or the conflicted want or impulse; the *"how it is avoided"* constitutes the patient's coping style.

In the case of J.I., for example, we can see both symptomatic and conflict-driven coping styles. It will be recalled that the patient presented with acute anxiety symptoms after a traumatic automobile accident. Her efforts to avoid physical danger (i.e., the "what," content or object of her symptomatic avoidance) consisted of becoming hypervigilant and phobic of cars and travel (i.e., the "how" or coping style that typified her symptomatic avoidance). At the same time, her conflict-driven coping style consisted of efforts to repress and deny (i.e., the "how" of her avoidance) the helplessness that she experienced both at the time when she was stabbed and subsequently in intimate relationships (i.e., the "what" or object of her conflictual avoidance). Her coping style, in other words, consisted of repressing memories and denying vulnerable feelings such as sexuality and dependence.

In all models of psychotherapy, the therapist introduces arousal by *exposure*. Arousal can be created either by confronting a patient with those aspects of experience, behavior, and sensation that are being avoided or by preventing the exercise of usual coping strategies. In either case, the process increases the patient's arousal level through cognitive dissonance. Exposure to avoided experience necessitates that the patient reorganize conceptual systems and respond differently. Indeed, it is important to induce the selective increases in arousal levels that accompany exposure in order to allow the workings of extinction, insight, and new learning.

On the other hand, some procedures are designed specifically to decrease arousal. A very high distress level may indicate that the patient's defenses are not working well. If this is a continuing aspect of the patient's condition, the process of psychotherapy may be impeded and susceptibility to other illnesses is even likely to increase (Coyne & Holroyd, 1982; Beutler, Engle et al., 1986; Brownlee-Duffeck, Peterson, Simonds, Goldstein, Kilo & Hoette, 1987). Since extreme distress impedes the process of maintaining attentional focus, increases defensive activities, and reduces behavioral flexibility, reduction of distress in such cases may advantageously precede selective arousal induction around specific issues. Procedures such as breathing control, attention to somatic sensations, cognitive control strategies, and managed exposure (e.g., Rapee, 1987) can reduce arousal levels to manageable limits.

In the case of J.I.'s symptomatic anxiety symptoms, for example, the first therapeutic task would be to decrease arousal level regarding travel. *In vivo* or *in vitro* desensitization, along with relaxation instructions, breath control, and cognitive rehearsal, would be appropriate treatments for these acute, reactive symptoms.

After the symptomatic phase of treatment was completed, J.I.'s conflictual patterns could be addressed by exposing her to the unwanted memories and sexual intimacy that are associated with physical danger and the avoidance of which drives her repressive coping style. She would be encouraged to directly confront the emotional distance present in her marriage and to move toward sources of anxiety.

The same basic rules apply whether the patient is assigned to long-term or time-limited treatment. The distinction between treatments of different intensities is in the degree to which one narrows the number and variety of symptoms or conflicts. In symptom-focused, time-limited treatment, only a few symptoms and circumstances may be addressed; in conflict-focused, time-limited treatment, a circumscribed type of conflicts form the objectives of change.

Patient arousal levels should reach a peak some time before the end of the treatment hour (Beutler, 1983). In those instances when a patient comes to the session in a state of extreme distress, the necessary time should be committed to reducing symptomatic distress before more conflict-oriented procedures can be utilized to advantage. Procedures that tend to reduce immediate distress levels include:

(1) Ventilation,

(2) Reassurance,

(3) Relaxation and distraction,

(4) Reflection,

(5) Advice and teaching,

(6) Hypnosis aided pleasant images,

(7) Breath control,

(8) Focus on sensations, and

(9) Counterconditioning.

On the other hand, some patients may come to the session with too little arousal to maintain productive levels of motivation. The induction of arousal may be necessary in order effectively to motivate change. The procedures that are useful for increasing arousal levels include:

(1) Confrontation,

(2) Encounters with significant others,

(3) Two-chair dialogues around unfinished relationships,

(4) Directed fantasies,

(5) Analysis of transference and defense,

(6) Interpretation,

(7) Silence, and

(8) Questions.

It should be observed that some patients respond to therapy procedures with a paradoxical effect. For example, most behavioral clinicians will recall patients who have become aroused and anxious when being taught to relax and those who feel quite relaxed when imagining their most feared events (e.g., Heide & Borkovec, 1983; Barlow & Waddell, 1985; Borkovec et al., 1987). These paradoxical responses identify a patient as having *high reactance* when faced with loss of perceived control or freedom, and invoke decisions about the degree of directiveness to utilize in the therapeutic process.

Selecting Directive and Evocative Treatments. The experienced clinician will recognize that patient arousal level also varies as a function of how the responsibilities for therapy tasks are distributed. Therapist directiveness alters the responsibility for session activity in favor of the therapist, while evocative therapy procedures, including silence, place responsibility for the session on the patient. Concomitantly, for most patients, reducing the amount of therapist directiveness will be reflected in corresponding increases in patient arousal level (cf. Beutler, 1983; Beutler, Crago & Arizmendi, 1986; Tracey, 1987). However, patient "resistance" to therapist interventions is an important consideration in selecting the amount of directiveness to utilize when implementing procedures.

"Reactance" reflects patient resistance at an interpersonal level, in the way that "coping style" reflects patient resistance at an intrapsychic level. "Reactance" refers to defense against external threat, while "coping style" reflects efforts to avoid internal experience.

When it was originally presented as a concept of clinical significance, *reactance* was described as a universal state that was induced by threat of losing personal choice (Brehm, 1976). Only later was it expanded to include a characteristic and enduring response trait of significance in selecting treatments (Beutler, 1979a, 1983; Dowd & Pace, in press).

We propose three working assumptions to govern therapist directiveness in response to patient reactance level. First, we propose that therapeutic effects will be enhanced if evocative procedures are emphasized over directive ones among patients with high levels of reactance, and conversely, if directive procedures are emphasized among patients who present with low levels of reactance. Indeed , there is some evidence that treatment may be affected negatively by mismatching patient reactance levels and therapist directiveness (cf. Forsyth & Forsyth, 1982; Weary & Mirels, 1982; Beutler, Crago & Arizmendi, 1986).

A second and related assumption is that momentary changes of patient reactance levels occurring during the course of a session will respond well if a therapist shifts in counterpoint between directive and evocative procedures. That is, as the patient exhibits high reactance, the therapist utilizes evocative and nondirective procedures; as the patient exhibits low reactance, the therapist assumes more direction.

Both of the foregoing points have been illustrated quite well by Blau (1988). Emphasizing the need to differentiate among *"unintrusive," "moderately intrusive,"* and *intense or probative* interventions, Blau asserts that relatively unintrusive interventions such as acceptance, empathy, encouragement, restatement, and the use of metaphor and analogy are most appropriate for the patient who exhibits—by disposition or by situation—high levels of resistance to the therapist's influence. In contrast, moderately intrusive interventions, including such therapist acts as structuring, asking direct questions, clarifying patient feelings, setting limits, and providing guidance and advice are used to advantage among moderately reactant patients who, by trait or state, have come to trust the level of safety and support provided by the therapist.

Blau emphasizes that "intense and probative" (p. 126) interventions should be used only when the patient is very secure with the therapist and when patients' own strong and positive self attitudes protect them from the need to resist the therapist's efforts. Such directed and interpretive activities as analysis of resistance and transference, the use of guided fantasy, dream analysis, magnification of patient or therapist gestures, and confrontation of behaviors and fears tend to evoke reactance and should be employed carefully and slowly by the therapist in order to preserve the therapeutic attachment. Even therapist humor can evoke resistance and should be applied cautiously (e.g., Saper, 1987).

Blau also emphasizes that patients usually begin treatment (i.e. during the stage of engagement) in a stance of fear and distrust, thus responding better to nonintrusive than to intrusive and probative treatment events. As the treatment relationship strengthens through the stages of pattern search and change, increasingly intrusive interventions can be used. The therapist must ensure that the strength of the relationship is always sufficient to help the patient through the resistance and arousal that characteristically accompany directive and intrusive interventions, however.

The third assumption that guides the use of directive procedures applies to the case of paradoxical interventions. Dowd and Pace (in press) have suggested that paradoxical interventions should not be used unless more straightforward procedures are ineffective. We accept this proposal, at least as applied to some types of paradoxical strategies. In describing the differential uses of paradoxical procedures, Seltzer (1986) emphasizes a distinction that we find to be particularly helpful. He distinguishes between *compliance-* and *defiance-*based paradoxical interventions.

Compliance-based paradoxical interventions are those that rely upon patient cooperation for effectiveness. These are the first-order change procedures identified by Dowd and Pace which are used in most psychotherapy. For example, asking a patient to identify and experience a state of anxiety rather than to continue in a pattern of overcontrol is a suggestion, the compliance with which may facilitate the process of extinction. Frequently, the use of these procedures includes an explanation or philosophy from which to think about one's behavior (i.e., what has been called "reframing"). A high correspondence between the therapist's interpretations and the theory that the therapist is using to guide treatment tends to facilitate therapeutic movement (e.g., Silberschatz et al., 1986; Crits-Christoph et al., 1988).

On the other hand, defiance-based paradoxical interventions include symptom prescription, countermanded change (i.e., suggesting that change will not or should not occur during a designated period of time), and magnifying or exaggerating symptoms (Dowd & Pace, in press). For example, in symptom prescription one might direct a patient with initial insomnia to avoid sleep or even to get worse, or suggest that a patient with performance anxiety intentionally fail during sexual intercourse.

While compliance-based paradoxical injunctions are designed to provide a new framework within which the patient observes a pattern of ongoing behavior, the defiance-based injunction assumes that the motivational force behind the symptom is reactance—the patient's need to resist the therapist's influence. Prescribing the symptom, in this case, motivates the patient to give up the symptom rather than to maintain it.

In concert with our proposal here, Shoham-Salomon and colleagues (Shoham-Salomon & Rosenthal, 1987; Shoham-Salomon, Avner & Zevlodever, 1988) have demonstrated that defiance-based paradoxical interventions have their most desirable effects among patients who exhibit high levels of reactance. Among such highly reactant patients, paradoxical strategies are likely to be considerably more effective than those that rely on patient cooperation.

In spite of their effectiveness, when defiance-based paradoxical interventions are used with highly reactant patients, the therapist should exercise care to provide a suitable rationale in order to establish the motivational forces upon which such procedures rely. Moreover, the therapist should be aware of the potential for abuse in these procedures. For example, Fremont and Anderson (1988) have observed that therapist annoyance (i.e., negative countertransference) is easily evoked by patients who exhibit highly reactant behaviors. Issues of countertransference should be considered carefully before employing any directive intervention, particularly paradoxical ones.

Some of the principles of implementing defiance-based interventions can be illustrated with a case description. N.K., a 38-year-old professor at a major eastern university, requested assistance for problems of sleep initiation and maintenance insomnia. His symptoms had begun to occur coincidentally with family problems in which his marital relationship was threatened. His family physician prescribed an anxiolytic and a sedative, but the patient responded paradoxically, becoming more anxious and experiencing an increase of sleep disruption. He attributed his further impaired sleep to the "addictive" effects of the medication and became very angry at his doctors. In the months prior to his seeking treatment in the current program, the patient had been treated by several mental health professionals, and had become steadily worse. His wife, while very distressed by her husband's sleep difficulty, had paradoxically become increasingly committed to trying to preserve the relationship, accepting his assertion that the problem was the poor treatment provided by his doctors.

When initial evaluation revealed that the patient was highly reactant but had no discernible medical problem, he was given a brief course of symptomatic treatment utilizing defiance-based paradoxical interventions. Longer treatment was not possible because of the patient's need to return to his home. It was suggested to the patient that the medication had upset his biological clock and that he would continue to sleep poorly until his normal sleeping cycle was reset. He was told that if he found himself unable to initiate or reinitiate sleep within 20 minutes on any given night, he should help his body reset its cycle by intentionally not sleeping at all until the next night. He was told that this might take several nights and recur from time to time. He was instructed to remain in bed with his eyes closed and to occupy his mind with anything that would keep him awake until morning, but to rest his body as much as he could.

The next day the patient reported unhappily that when he found himself unable to sleep, he had tried to stay awake but had been unable to do so in spite of his best efforts. He was assured that his failure intentionally to remain awake was indeed unfortunate. When he slept well the second night as well, he was sent home with a treatment plan that included marital therapy to help him find ways of expressing his fear and anger at his wife in more direct ways than that offered by his sleep problem. A two-month follow-up indicated that the patient had experienced no reoccurrence of sleep disturbance.

Two considerations went into the decision to apply a paradoxical, symptom-focused treatment for this patient. The first consideration was the amount of time permitted for treatment by virtue of the patient's limited availability. His employment required his immediate return to his home state. Second, the patient's unstable, externalized defenses resulted in poor motivation for other than a symptomatic focus at the outset. He had tried and failed at several efforts to work within a more conflict-oriented framework, and was suspicious of any efforts to suggest a goal other than symptomatic change.

Intratherapy versus Extratherapy Processes.   Therapeutic arousal can be increased by attention to the "here and now" of therapy experiences—those occurring within the session and between patient and therapist. Conversely, arousal ordinarily can be reduced by establishing distance between feelings and environments, as is done by discussing things "there and then."

Although this is a valuable guiding rule, there are other guidelines to govern the use of intratherapy and extratherapy experience as well. As a general rule, the further along the patient is in the problem-solving process, the more the focus of therapy will be upon extratherapy experience. During the action and maintenance phases of behavior change that are described by Prochaska (1984), for example, discussion is often of social support systems and the interpersonal reinforcements available for maintaining change. During the precontemplative and contemplative phases, on the other hand, the therapy focus is more heavily balanced toward in-therapy experiences.

A second guideline for directing the attentional focus of interventions pertains to changes over the session itself. The first portion of the session, for example, is usually controlled by the patient's desire to report on changes and problems arising over the course of the week. The therapist ordinarily allows this attentional focus and gradually encourages more intratherapy attention in order to manage arousal levels effectively. As the session draws to a close, attention may be redirected to extratherapy activity as the therapist seeks to establish a homework assignment.

While homework assignments are valuable tools to facilitate and consolidate treatment gains, their nature must be altered to accommodate the patient's reactance level. In order to reinforce their own sense of control, highly reactant patients ordinarily are asked to design their own homework assignments (i.e., behavioral contracts), or are assigned tasks that require no external performance by which they might express defiance (e.g., "Think about what we've talked about" rather than "See if you can make some notes about what you remember from today's session"), or are given defiance-based paradoxical assignments on which they cannot fail (e.g., "If you attempt to perform sexually this week, try to lose your erection and pay attention to how you are able to do so").

In contrast, the patient with a low reactance level can tolerate and respond well to extratherapy assignments that are constructed largely by the therapist. However, these assignments, too, must be adjusted to accommodate the level of experience being addressed, the phase of treatment, and the nature of the therapeutic task. One assigns to an overcontrolled, internalizing patient tasks of observing sensations (in accordance with the stage of pattern search) or expressing affect (in accordance with the task of interpersonal change), for example. An externalizing patient at similar stages of therapy may be asked to monitor patterns of reinforcement or to practice social skills.

TREATMENT MANUALS AND THE FOUR STEPS

Some of the principles discussed in the last three chapters can be summarized by our reflecting on how the procedures described by the five treatment manuals discussed in earlier chapters apply to the four steps in our prescriptive psychotherapy model. In reference to each, it will be instructive to classify the interventions used according to our four-step decisional scheme. A summary of the variations among these manuals is provided in Table 13.3.

Table 13.3
Dimensions of Therapeutic Technique and Treatment Manuals

	Breadth	Level	Therapy Structure
Behavioral	Sym	Beh.Ch.	D and Ex
Cognitive	Sym	Cog.Ch.	Ev, D, and Ex
IPT	Con	Uncs./Beh.Ch.	Ev, D, and Ex
TLDP	Con	Uncs.Ch.	Ev, I, and Ex
Minuchin	Con	Beh.Ch.	D, I, and Ex
Gestalt	Con	Aff.Ch.	Ev, D, and I

Sym = Symptomatic Focus
Con = Conflictual Theme Focus
Beh.Ch. = Behavioral Level of Experience
Cog.Ch. = Cognitive Level of Experience
Aff.Ch. = Affective Level of Experience
Uncs.Ch. = Unconscious Motives Level of Experience
D = Directive
Ev = Evocative
I = Intratherapy Focus
Ex = Extratherapy Focus

Behavioral Treatment of Agoraphobia. The outcome goal of Barlow and Waddell's (1985) behavioral treatment is a relatively specific and narrow one: the reduction or elimination of the phobic symptom. The focal theme (Step one) consists of the evoking environment and associated reinforcers assumed to support the symptom. In turn, the level of experience (Step two) addressed is patient behavior. Specifically, treatment is designed to change behavior (i.e., to approach feared objects) in order to achieve the intermediate goals (Step three) of altering cognitions and reducing anxiety. Specific strategies (Step four) designed to achieve mediating goals include successive movements toward the feared areas and the development of coping thoughts to facilitate behavioral change.

The majority of specific treatment techniques will be directive in nature, and include providing information about the nature of anxiety, advice in the use of coping statements, and encouragement to approach the feared areas. The sessions will maintain an extratherapy focus, including homework assignments to increase exposure. Coping statements and relaxation instruction will be used to lower nonspecific anxiety; graduated exposure will be used both to keep the patient targeted on the focal object and to maintain optimal intensity of arousal.

Cognitive Therapy. The ultimate treatment goal in Cognitive Therapy (Beck et al., 1979) is the elimination or reduction of depressive symptoms. The therapeutic focus (Step one) consists of the A-B-C formulation comprising the relationship among situation, belief and automatic thought, and feeling. The patient experiences (Step two) that are given most attention are habitual cognitive patterns, especially those automatic processes that relate to self-evaluation. Intermediate tasks (Step three) include learning the theoretical rationale, identifying the nature of one's cognitive distortions, and learning to adopt a questioning and reflective attitude in regard to one's automatic assumptions.

In Cognitive Therapy, both directive and evocative techniques (Step four) are used to specify, explore, and test the validity of the patient's cognitions. Questions have been a particularly favorite verbal technique for clarifying patient assumptions and facilitating collaborative learning without raising patient resistance. In addition, advising and providing information is encouraged.

In recent years cognitive theorists have given considerable attention to "hot cognitions" (Freeman, Beutler, Arkowitz & Simon, in press) emphasizing an increasing awareness on the part of cognitive therapists of the importance of maintaining an optimal level of arousal. This concern permeates other therapeutic activities as well.

Though the principal focus is on extratherapy experiences, intratherapy contacts with the therapist are used to identify "hot cognitions." Failure to address emotionally charged interpersonal relationships in cognitive therapy may result in diminished outcomes (Gaston, Marmar & Ring, in press). Homework assignments, in turn, are designed to facilitate the testing of these cognitive habits and to practice new cognitive patterns.

Focused Expressive Psychotherapy (FEP). The goal of FEP (Daldrup et al., 1988) is to help the patient develop an awareness of and the ability to express unwanted affect, such as anger. Hence, the therapeutic focus (Step one) is conflictual rather than symptomatic and centers on unrecognized feelings (Step two) as well as the parental injunctions that prevent their acknowledgement and expression.

The mediating goals (Step three) of FEP treatment include identifying sensory expressions of unwanted emotions in unfinished interpersonal relationships, and practice in the expression of affect around emotionally charged incidents in the patient's past.

FEP relies both on evocative and directive techniques (Step four) to elicit patient response. Verbal interventions are principally in the form of questions and reflections, but direct instruction is used to implement therapeutic experiments. Emotional and cognitive experiments are designed to reintegrate disowned emotional experience within the session.

Arousal levels are specifically monitored, with effort to increase patient arousal rather than to symptomatically reduce it. It is assumed that only when the emotional component of occluded experiences is reintegrated with one's memory of that experience will benefit occur.

With the hope that intratherapy experience will become translated to more integrated relationships outside of the treatment, homework assignments are employed. The usual homework experiment is designed to intensify the feelings arising from one's relations with others.

Interpersonal Psychotherapy (IPT). The primary treatment goal in IPT (Klerman et al., 1984) is the alteration of an interpersonal event that underwrites the symptom of depression. The symptom is viewed as an expression of interpersonal loss or conflict, including unrealistic and unmet expectations and grief. Hence, the nature of the patient's interpersonal conflicts serves as the therapeutic focus (Step one) rather than the symptom of depression per se. Changes in affect are viewed as indicators that interpersonal difficulties are resolving, either spontaneously or as a product of the therapeutic intervention.

The level of experience (Step two) addressed by IPT varies between behavior change and awareness of unconscious processes. Mediating goals (Step three) include the development of knowledge about the nature of depression, especially its cyclical pattern (i.e., the stage of pattern search), and the development of new interpersonal skills (i.e., the stage of interpersonal change). In the service of these objectives, the therapist provides (Step four) support through reflection, questions the patient about history and feelings, provides information, and gives direct advice. These procedures involve an array that extends from evocative to directive and intrasession to extratherapy. Homework assignments are included in the intervention and skills are taught in the service of reducing interpersonal conflict.

Time-Limited Dynamic Psychotherapy (TLDP). The treatment goals of TLDP (Strupp & Binder, 1984) are decidedly conflictual in nature, extending beyond the reduction of a specific symptom. The therapeutic focus (Step one) is on the unconscious determinants of recurrent interpersonal interactions that are thought to index disturbed early relationships. Within this core theme or conflict, the therapist identifies the cognitive and affective experiences (Step two) comprising the steps in the repeated pattern, independent of the symptomatic form in which the conflict is expressed.

The mediating goals (Step three) of the therapy are to achieve insights about the driving forces behind repetitive interpersonal patterns and, concomitantly, to achieve insight into how these patterns are enacted in the patient's relationship with the therapist (i.e., the stage of pattern search).

In the service of these ends, aspects of the conflictual theme are explored as they become manifest in the patient-therapist relationship (Step four). Thus, the therapist draws attention to the reenactment of the patient's early experience within interpersonal relationships generally, and especially within the therapy session.

The predominant interventions are evocative. Reflections, questions, and indirect provision of information in the form of interpretations are the dominant techniques used to attain insight. While the sessions focus on both extrasession and intrasession material, the emphasis is on translation of intrasession experiences to extratherapy relationships.

Family Therapy. The goal of structural family therapy (Minuchin, 1974; Minuchin & Fishman, 1984) is the alteration of rigid and malfunctioning family roles. The treatment focus (Step one) is not the "symptoms" that may be manifest in one family member, but rather a patterned relationship that is supported by all family members.

The level of experience (Step two) addressed by this form of family therapy is behavioral, but includes all family members. The mediating goals (Step three) are interpersonal in nature and include awareness (i.e., the stage of pattern search) of family interaction patterns and the upsetting of interpersonal alliances (i.e., the stage of change). These mediating and final goals do not involve insight in the traditional sense, but attempt to induce behavioral change in the repetitive, failing interaction patterns.

In implementing the therapeutic procedures (Step four), directive techniques are used to elicit in-therapy behaviors that are reenactments of the problem behaviors occurring at home. Advising and instructing are among the procedures used, while homework is utilized to build upon and strengthen the behavioral changes that are stimulated and started in the therapy sessions.

SUMMARY AND COMMENT

In the last three chapters we have reviewed four basic steps through which patient presentations can be matched to characteristics of the psychotherapy intervention. At the first step, we have pointed out that the complexity of the presenting problem is an indicator for the use either of conflict- or symptom-oriented treatment goals. The specific nature of those goals will depend upon a careful analysis of the presenting complaints and circumstances that give rise to them. Whether symptomatic or conflictual, the formulation of the problem embodied in defining the goals of treatment constitutes the therapeutic focus. This focus, in turn, can be described from a number of viewpoints, the preference among which depends jointly upon the symptomatic versus conflictual focus and the therapist's own preferred theory of psychological distress.

At the second and third steps of decision making, the selection of treatment activities, respectively, can be designed to accommodate to the patient's coping style by adjusting the level of experience toward which the intervention is aimed, and by ordering the mediating treatment objectives to the stage of therapy achieved.

Finally, as a fourth step, we have suggested that considerable specificity of technique selection comes from an awareness of the moment-to-moment psychotherapy transactions. Indirect observations have revealed variations in therapist directiveness and in the use of external versus internal structuring or focus. Direct observations, on the other hand, have emphasized the structure of the therapist's speech, including the use of questions, reflections, advice, interpretations, providing information, and self disclosing. The patient's motivation, compliance, and achievement can be enhanced by matching these procedures to patient distress (problem severity), reactance, and problem-solving phase.

Collectively, the process of controlling the in-therapy experience of the patient is one of managing arousal level and therapeutic focus. If the therapist is successful in keeping the patient within the range of therapeutic arousal and is able to maintain focus upon the intrasession or extratherapy experiences that are significant to the symptomatic or conflictual dynamic of the problem, success is likely. If, on the other hand, the therapist fails to retain the focus and allows arousal to exceed or remain beneath a level that will maintain motivation, progress will be hampered. The most powerful tool that the therapist has for maintaining arousal and focus is his or her own powers of persuasion and inference.

The persuasive potency of the therapist is enhanced by his or her maintaining a sense of empathic resonance, affirming the patient's worth, and adhering to promised roles (Orlinsky & Howard, 1987). The persuasive therapist is not a dominant or manipulative one (e.g., Zook & Sipps, 1987). Not infrequently, specific efforts to attune to the patient's feelings and to become open to hearing the patient's pain and concern may result in moments of empathic resonance that contribute to an expanded awareness and growth for both patient and therapist (Larson, 1987). From the resulting bond, the therapist provides information, suggestions, and interpretations that can have a persuasive and positive influence.

SUGGESTED READINGS

Blau, T. H. (1988). *Psychotherapy tradecraft: The technique and style of doing therapy.* New York: Brunner/Mazel.

Polster, E. & Polster, M. (1973). *Gestalt therapy integrated.* New York: Brunner/ Mazel.

Seltzer, L. F. (1986). *Paradoxical strategies in psychotherapy: A comprehensive overview and guidebook.* New York: John Wiley and Sons.

Yost, E., Beutler, L. E., Corbishley, M. A. & Allender, J. R. (1986). *Group cognitive therapy: A treatment approach for depressed older adults.* New York: Pergamon Press.

PART VI

Training Directions

The final section of this volume discusses the future of eclectic theories for training. We appreciate the contribution of Dr. John C. Norcross to this final chapter. We have come to value the perspective that he has acquired about training practitioners who are creatively integrative in thought and practice.

To this point, we have been talking primarily to the seasoned practitioner who wants to hone his or her treatment skills in order to reach a broader range of patients, and to the emerging clinical practitioner who seeks to learn a consistent way of planning treatment. In this final section, we will turn our attention to the interests of the teacher and students.

Chapter 14 presents our collective thoughts on how to ensure competency among psychotherapy practitioners. The role of theoretical versus practical training, sequencing courses, and quality assurance are all addressed in this chapter.

14

Training in Differential
Treatment Selection

with John C. Norcross, Ph.D.

Abraham Maslow is said to have once remarked that if you only have
a hammer you treat everything like a nail. The history of psychotherapy
has repeatedly confirmed Maslow's observation. Sad to say, the preponderance of contemporary clinicians still reach for their favorite tool when
confronted with puzzling or unsettling situations. It is not uncommon for
our inveterate colleagues to recommend the identical treatment (i.e., their
treasured proficiency) to virtually every patient who crosses their paths.

The approach to differential treatment selection presented in this book
requires discriminating craftworkers who selectively draw on training, experience, and research to meet the multivaried challenges of clinical reality.
Discriminating clinicians go beyond subjective preference, institutional
custom, and immediate availability to predicate their treatment selection
on patient need and comparative outcome research. That is to say, they
develop and employ an expanded toolbox instead of senselessly "hammer-
ing away" at anything remotely similar to a nail (Norcross, 1985).

The introduction of an integrative and prescriptive approach to clinical
work compounds the training enterprise. Single, "pure" systems of psychotherapy markedly reduce the range of clinical observations and treatment
possibilities. Now, with these perceptual blinders loosened, a broader
range of formulations and interventions must be carefully considered (cf.
Group for the Advancement of Psychiatry, 1987). Not only must students
become aware of the relative indications for matching patient and treatment but they, in many cases, must also become competent in offering

multiple therapy modalities. Both are unprecedented training objectives in the history of psychotherapy.

Moreover, if the current practice of training in a single psychotherapy model does so little to ensure competence, how can competency be ensured if we attempt to teach practitioners several intervention models? To contemplate such issues is to understand why systematic approaches to psychotherapy integration are not taught in most mental health programs (Beutler, 1986; Norcross, 1986). Indeed, in a survey of 58 prominent integrationists and eclectics (Norcross & Thomas, 1988), the second most severe impediment confronting integrative psychotherapy was inadequate commitment to training in more than one psychotherapy system.

Still, as formidable as the challenge is, the future of psychotherapy rests heavily on instruction and dissemination. This chapter explores various training models for enhancing therapist effectiveness and presents a recommended model for training which allows both the development of individual style and the application of treatment procedures that are responsive to patient needs. In the process, we identify recurrent obstacles in conventional as well as integrative psychotherapy training and suggest a prescriptive approach to clinical supervision.

CRITIQUE OF CONVENTIONAL TRAINING

Throughout our professional careers we have been singularly impressed by the immense responsibilities and collective failures in training competent practitioners. We are hardly alone in arriving at this conclusion; numerous studies in the past decade have underscored the inadequacy or irrelevancy of clinical training with respect to preparing skilled psychotherapists (e.g., Kalafat & Neigher, 1983; Stern, 1984; Robertson, 1986). Psychotherapy training in an academic environment is often just that— academic— long on exposition and short on experience (Robertson, 1984). This "erosion of excellence" (Strupp, 1975) can be attributed to distorted institutional contingencies and confused personal priorities, but these do not excuse the training system, nor us, the trainers, from dereliction of duty.

The indictment against conventional clinical training is lengthy and growing. Below we enumerate a small number of these concerns in an effort to outline corrective steps one would take in an ideal training program.

Inadequate Experience

Experience in applied settings is often optional, at least prior to internship or residency training. The principal complaint of psychotherapists surveyed following graduation is inadequate clinical experience (e.g., Garfield & Kurtz, 1976; Rachelson & Clance, 1980; Norcross & Prochaska, 1982; Tibbits-Kleber & Howell, 1987; Watkins et al., 1987). The consistent recommendation is to increase the instruction of clinical skills and the provision of sophisticated supervision (Robertson, 1986; Group for the Advancement of Psychiatry, 1987).

Exposure Rather Than Competence

It appears that psychotherapy training programs believe in the "germ theory" of education (Beutler, 1988)—If you're exposed to the theory and procedures you will "catch" them, thereafter being and remaining competent and skilled. Training therapists to achieve a stated criterion of competence has seldom been attempted (Matarazzo & Patterson, 1986; Dobson & Shaw, 1988). Rather, we rely on a host of criteria—most academic or temporal—that bear, at best, a negligible relationship to clinical skills (cf. Ford, 1986). Beutler (1986) somberly concludes that training and licensing procedures tacitly assume "that practice makes perfect, regardless of what one practices, how imperfectly one does so, or how difficult the task to be learned" (p. 73).

Insufficient Evaluation

The competence of our graduates and, indeed, the adequacy of clinical training typically are assumed rather than verified. Most clinical training programs have not evaluated systematically their impact on trainees, nor their trainees' impact on clients (cf. Garfield, 1977; Edelstein & Brasted, 1983; Norcross & Stevenson, 1984; Stevenson & Norcross, 1986). Korman (1974) notes that "considering the financial cost and human effort represented by professional education, there has been a curious lack of concern over product and program evaluation. . . . Its absence is all the more remarkable in a discipline that prides itself on its expertise in evaluation research" (p. 445).

Strupp, Butler, and Rosser (1988) emphasize that, to date, we have not defined the criteria by which to judge competence. They observe that defining such criteria is a critically important need in order for training issues to come under the purview of research. In turn, they emphasize the difference between technical skill and precision of application, concluding that both must be assessed in criteria-based definitions of "competence." With the development of psychotherapy manuals, competence is being defined in increasingly specific and meaningful ways but with still little systematic incorporation into psychotherapy training programs (Luborsky

& DeRubeis, 1984; Dobson & Shaw, 1988; Rounsaville, O'Malley, Foley & Weissman, 1988).

Superficial Multitheory or Single Theory

Trainees are traditionally taught either in the isolated single-theory approach to treatment or the multiple competing-theory approach. The single-theory concentration suggests that "this" is the one and only truth, while the multitheory comparison suggests that no truth exists. The result is frequently the production of either narrow adherents to rigid orthodoxy or a cohort of broadly based and "flexible" practitioners who possess a confused hodgepodge of half facts (Frances, Clarkin & Perry, 1984).

Disjointed Training Process

The acquisition of psychotherapy skills tends to be a poorly coordinated, if not chaotic, process in many training programs. It is not unusual to encounter interns whose entire clinical experience rests on one theory or one modality. Few training programs offer an articulated and systematic curriculum designed to ensure competence in multiple theories and formats (cf. Group for the Advancement of Psychiatry, 1987).

This lamentable state of affairs is partly due to a corresponding paucity of evidence on critical training content and method. However, as Matarazzo and Patterson (1986) note, knowledge about the value of training is limited by our knowledge about the effectiveness of the particular forms of psychotherapy that are likely to be most helpful for a particular type of client. Hence, as the reliable evidence on treatment matching increases, so too should the coordination of psychotherapy training.

Comment

The foregoing problems become particularly problematic for psychotherapists who advocate differential therapeutics and integrative psychotherapy. These practitioners must acquire theoretical and practical mastery of multiple treatment combinations and then adjust their therapeutic approach to fit the needs of the client. This "ideal" training outcome may well necessitate an "ideal" psychotherapy training model.

Before considering ideal training models, clinical trainers must be willing to address a critical decision with respect to training objectives. The major choice is whether the program's objective will be to train students in assessment geared toward referral of the client to the most appropriate treatment and/or whether its avowed mission will be for students to accommodate most of these patients themselves by virtue of the students' competence in multimethod, multimodality psychotherapy.

Either alternative would represent, in our view, a vast improvement over current training paradigms. A program combining both objectives would be the ideal solution, but probably beyond the existing resources of most facilities. Each choice raises unique training needs and prospects. Of critical importance to the decision to train integrative practitioners is the assumption that students can learn to practice several models competently. While it still is uncertain whether all or even most mental health trainees are capable of acquiring such skill, at least some evidence is accumulating to suggest that it is possible for a given therapist to selectively apply in an effective way methods drawn from different perspectives (e.g., Hardy & Shapiro, 1985).

In the following pages we will present suggested training models for teaching both systematic referral and technical application.

IDEAL TRAINING MODELS

Differential Referral

In order to make thoughtful decisions about referral, the clinician should have knowledge of available community resources. Since many students are trained in a geographically different location than that in which they are ultimately employed, this needed information cannot readily translate from training programs. Instead of teaching specific resources, therefore, training programs are well advised to ensure that students know how to seek and find resources in a community.

Ideally, a clinical training program will provide several specific types of experience in order to assure the student's ability to develop community knowledge. First, specific instruction and course work might be provided to emphasize the value of community support services. To complement this specific instruction, the value of such services should be emphasized as the student studies theories of psychopathology, learns methods of psychological assessment, is taught the principles of psychological consultation, and begins practicum training.

Along with specific lectures on the value of social support services, students routinely can be provided with names, addresses, and phone numbers both of national resource groups and local referral services. A number of national directories are available that allow referral both to specific practitioners and to service agencies. For example, referral to specific practitioners can be facilitated by reference to the *Biographical Directory of the American Psychiatric Association* (APA, 1983), the *National Register of Health Service Providers in Psychology* (Council for the National Register of Health Service Providers in Psychology, 1987), the *Directory of Diplomates* (American Board of Professional Psychology, 1980), the *Register of Clinical Social Workers* (National Association of Social Workers, 1987), and the *National Directory of Medical Psychotherapists* (American Board of Medical Psychotherapists, 1987).

All of these directories provide information about areas of training and some provide additional information about areas of special interest and/or training. Similarly, *The National Directory of Mental Health* (Neal-Schuman Publishers, 1980) provides a listing of all state mental health associations, national hot line numbers for mental health information and support services (e.g., Veterans Administration Information Service, National Clearinghouse for Drug Abuse Information, National Clearinghouse for Mental Health Information), and a description both of public and private mental health facilities and services broken down by state.

In addition to national listings, local resources include telephone information and referral services that are supported by psychological and psychiatric societies, directories of community services supported by such agencies as the United Way, listings published through the local Chamber of Commerce, membership lists of local and state organizations, and special publications by local special interest groups. Regional chapters of the American Group Psychotherapy Association, for example, often publish in-house organs describing the types of psychotherapy groups being conducted by their membership, along with information about fees, times, etc.

Beyond giving trainees information about where they can locate information about resources, visits to community housing projects, community mental health clinics, family counseling agencies, foster placement agencies, child protective services, and substance abuse programs may give a sampling of the variety of services and resources available. Practice exercises also might systematically be incorporated both into coursework and practica. Trainees might be assigned, for example, the task of locating a list of treatment resources and preparing an integrated treatment plan based upon potential referral sources for an actual problem presented in either a case conference or prepared as a vignette for class illustration.

In addition to course work and knowledge of referral sources, trainees should have extensive experience in actually evaluating a range of patients and participating under close supervision in differential referral and treatment assignment.

The kind of experience described here is most easily obtained in a setting where different treatment programs are available. In such a setting, the trainee can practice assessing the patient and environmental characteristics and making differential treatment recommendations concerning treatment setting, format and mode, duration and frequency, and potential strategies and techniques. In an evaluation clinic like this, the trainee is free to consider a whole range of therapies in selecting those that might be optimal for the individual patient.

Integrative Psychotherapy

An ideal psychotherapy education would encompass an interlocking sequence of training experiences predicated on the crucial therapist-mediated and therapist-provided determinants of psychotherapy outcome. Our suggested training program would consist of five steps.

The first step would entail training in fundamental relationship and communication skills, such as active listening, nonverbal communication, empathy, modeling, respect, and regard for patient problems. The primacy of these skills for psychotherapy progress is underscored by robust research findings.

Acquisition of these generic interpersonal skills would follow one of the systematic modules that have empirically demonstrated significant training effects compared to controls or less specified programs (Matarazzo & Patterson, 1986). Promising candidates would include human relations training (Truax & Carkhuff, 1967), microcounseling (Ivey & Authier, 1978), and structured learning therapy (Goldstein, 1973).

In general, the most efficient way of maximizing learning of facilitative psychotherapy skills and attitudes is to structure their acquisition systematically (Lambert & Arnold, 1987). The standard sequence involves instruction, demonstration (modeling), practice, evaluation (feedback), and more practice. With such practice, students do seem to acquire increasing levels of sensitivity, become more willing to confront difficult emotions, and develop greater flexibility (e.g., Tracey, Hays, Malone & Herman, 1988).

In our proposed program, students would be retained in this foundations course until a predefined level of competence was achieved in the expression of therapeutic warmth and understanding. Criterion-referenced situational tests, expert ratings, and demonstration experiments could conceivably be utilized to confirm such effectiveness.

The second interlocking step in training would be an exploration of various models of human behavior. At a minimum, the courses would explore in some depth psychoanalytic, humanistic-existential, cognitive-behavioral, interpersonal-systems, and social-anthropological theories of human function and dysfunction. Students would be exposed to all approaches without judgment being made as to their relative contributions to truth. Theoretical paradigms would be introduced as tentative and explanatory notions, varying in level of analysis and methodology.

The third step in our ideal training model would be a course on theories of psychotherapy. The focus in this course would be on applying the models of human function and dysfunction to methods of behavioral change. At the outset, multiple systems of psychotherapy would be presented critically but within a paradigm of comparison and integration.

The conceptual underpinnings of change processes would be examined in the context of understanding the human values and cultural norms which are used to explain change. At this point students would be encouraged to adopt tentatively that perspective which is most harmonious with their own values and which engenders their own individual clinical preferences.

The fourth step in the training sequence would entail a series of practica. Neophyte psychotherapists would be expected to become competent in the use of at least four systems that vary in therapeutic objectives (conflict resolution and symptomatic change) and levels of experience (see Chapters 11 and 12). In each case, completion of the practicum would depend on specific criteria to ensure acquisition of the skills associated with a given approach. Relevant psychotherapy handbooks and treatment manuals would be used specifically to outline criteria for implementing specific interventions.

Compliance with competency criteria based upon treatment manuals has been found to relate to treatment processes that are considered to be therapeutic and to a lesser extent has been found to relate to treatment efficacy (e.g., Luborsky et al., 1983; Shaw, 1983; Rounsaville et al., 1987; Dobson & Shaw, 1988; Strupp, Butler & Rosser, 1988).

We suggest that competency standards based upon various psychotherapy models may be used to establish standards of trainee performance even in those situations where determination of competency on the basis of outcome may be impractical or difficult (e.g., long-term psychoanalytic psychotherapy). At the level of specific skills, Silberschatz and associates (Silberschatz, Fretter & Curtis, 1986) have developed a methodology for identifying "suitable" interpretations and Crits-Christoph, Cooper, and Luborsky (1988) have explored ways of identifying the "accuracy" of dynamic interpretations. Similarly, both Greenberg (1980; Greenberg & Clarke, 1979; Greenberg & Sarkissian, 1984; Greenberg & Goldman, 1988) and Davis et al. (1985) have described effective role playing methods for training students to intervene at the affective level of experience. The limitations of experience and expertise could be delineated for each student, utilizing standardized dimensions and criteria outlined for each approach. Approached in this way, students would know their strengths and their limits.

Following satisfactory completion of these competency-based courses, the fifth and final interlocking step in this ideal training sequence would be the integration of disparate models and methods. The emerging consensus is that the sophisticated adoption of an integrative perspective occurs after the learning of specific therapy systems and techniques (see Norcross, 1986; Robertson, 1986; Beutler et al., 1987; Guest & Beutler, 1988; Halgin, 1988).

The formal course on psychotherapeutic integration would provide a decisional model for selecting the procedures from various therapeutic orientations to be applied in given circumstances and with given clients. Concomitantly, an intensive practicum experience, such as an internship or residency, with a wide variety of patients representing different problems, coping styles, and interpersonal sensitivities would allow therapists to practice systematic integration and to evaluate their technical skills.

These training experiences are the beginning and, in our view, the critical steps in the development of competent psychotherapists. But genuine education continues far after the internship or residency. Students would be encouraged—nay, expected—to go forth to receive additional training in specialized methods and preferred populations as well as to keep abreast of professional developments.

RECURRENT OBSTACLES IN INTEGRATIVE TRAINING

Clinical programs committed to multidimensional and prescriptive training can expect to encounter resistance. These recurring obstacles, drawn largely from two special sections of the *Journal of Eclectic and Integrative Psychotherapy* on training of integrative/eclectic psychotherapists (Norcross, 1986; Beutler et al., 1987), can be organized around three broad categories: the content itself, faculty, and students.

Content

One of the most prevalent complaints heard about integration is that there is "just too much to know." Faculty complain of insufficient time to present the material and students complain of the resulting information overload. Indeed, a literal computation of all treatment possibilities staggers the imagination. With conservative estimates of 10 major psychotherapy metatheories, 100 established interventions, and at least three formats (individual, marital/family, group), the resulting combinations would be 3,000 possible treatments!

The historical absence of compelling methods of integration complicate the picture. The recent development of sophisticated models of integrative psychotherapy, which articulate treatments of choice, delineate a finite set of change principle, or enumerate transtheoretical interventions, has reduced the magnitude of this enterprise dramatically.

Nonetheless, there remains in any training program an inherent conflict between depth and breadth. An indisputable disadvantage of aiming to establish competence in multiple psychotherapy systems is that it requires more and longer training than if competency were established only in a single system. Integrative psychotherapists, similar to bilingual children and switch hitters in baseball, may be delayed initially in the acquisition of skills and, consequently, are more apt to feel frustrated. The future promises of increased efficacy, efficiency, and applicability seem to exercise little influence in relation to the urgent daily needs of clients and students (Norcross, 1988).

On a positive note, there is some evidence to suggest that exposing students to many different models rather than to a single point of view increases rather than decreases interest in psychotherapy (Fisher, 1987). Perhaps the issue is how to keep students interested and hopeful rather than leaving them overwhelmed and pessimistic.

Faculty

The number one obstacle to psychotherapy integration, according to responding members of the Society for the Exploration of Psychotherapy Integration (SEPI), is the intrinsic investment of individuals in their private perceptions and theories (Norcross & Thomas, 1988). Various therapy systems thrive on their differences and practitioners are invested in their uniqueness. This partisan zealotry and ideological warfare appear, too, as the most intransigent impediments to integrative training. The root problem with our inveterate colleagues is not ignorance but prejudice—willful ignorance (Suedfeld in Norcross, 1986).

The narrow and inflexible curricula of most psychotherapy training programs reflect their progenitors' prejudices. Private allegiances lead to overrepresentation, if not domination, of one or two models of psychotherapy at the expense of integration. An integrative training program requires substantial support from the faculty, especially from those faculty supervisors with a strong affinity for a given point of view. It is, therefore, highly desirable that the faculty in integrative programs be pluralistic and versatile, as against recruiters selecting like-minded and homogeneous fellow travelers (Frances, Clarkin & Perry, 1984).

Students

One frustration for many psychotherapy students is that the process of professionalization in graduate programs often consists of indoctrination rather than education. Success in such programs is too frequently incumbent on the trainee adopting, or appearing to adopt, the prevailing viewpoint. Students indoctrinated in one system can experience considerable difficulty in overcoming their loyalty and lethargy. Deviations are experienced, both by them and by their mentors, as betrayal, confusion, or vulnerability.

Having located their comfortable niche in the psychotherapy morass (Halgin, 1986), students may be satisfied with their treasured proficiencies and are less than motivated, for the most part, to expand their therapeutic repertoires (Woody & Robertson, 1988). This separation anxiety can be reduced by acknowledging the validity of individual theoretical preferences and the principle that integrative training is intended to build on clinicians' strengths rather than replace their preferential approaches (cf. pages 306-307 in Beutler et al., 1987, for specific suggestions).

A premature affiliation with a discrete, "pure" therapy model may occur for a variety of reasons. On one level, this affiliation may be part of a common developmental sequence through which beginning therapists often pass (Loganbill, Hardy & Delworth, 1982; Halgin, 1986); they find a native comfort and strong institutional support via a single theoretical identity (Goldfried, 1980). On another level, such affiliations may actually be attributable to the failure of educators to articulate the value of informed pluralism in courses, in curriculum, and in supervision.

In a related way, avoidance of an integrative stance may be driven by its inchoate identity and demanding nature. Until quite lately, to be "eclectic" was to have a marginal professional existence and to espouse dissatisfaction with orthodox schoolism. Further, the ability or willingness to perform at a competent level in a variety of modalities and to integrate these modalities is certainly demanding of experienced practitioners and an uncertain possibility for fledgling psychotherapists. Should students be unable or unwilling to develop proficiency in a desirably broad range of procedures, then we believe this should be accepted openly. They should then be encouraged to generate guidelines for directing their referral patterns and implementing adjunctive treatments as indicated.

One final obstacle in integrative training is the tendency of students to be confused or disheartened by multiplicity. Analogous to the cognitive-developmental model of intellectual development described by Perry (1970) for college students, many psychotherapy trainees regularly struggle with their own needs to eradicate the ambiguity in an unavoidably ambiguous craft. They may well reach a relativistic position without attaining a sense of commitment or conviction to a given approach. Appropriate role modeling and open inquiry into the need to identify a single "right" perspective, both by themselves and their clients, can attenuate the problem significantly.

A Final Clarification

The intention of integrative training is not necessarily to produce card-carrying, flag-waving "eclectic" or "integrative" psychotherapists. Instead, our goal is to educate therapists to think and, perhaps, to behave integratively—openly, synthetically, but critically—in their clinical pursuits. Our aim is to prepare students to develop, if they possess the motivation and ability, into knowledgeable prescriptive therapists.

We firmly believe that it is *in*appropriate to demand that students adopt any single metatheoretical perspective, integrative or otherwise. We are equally convinced that each practitioner should develop an individual clinical style within his or her chosen perspective. The goal of every training program should be graduates who are widely knowledgeable, broad as well as deep in their interests, and sufficiently curious to keep learning and growing professionally (Frances et al., 1984). The hope is that, in Halleck's (1978) words, our students will "approach our patients with open minds and a relentless commitment to study and confront the complexities of human behavior" (p. 501).

CLINICAL SUPERVISION

Clinical supervision, integrative or otherwise, is a complex and demanding task. Supervisors are expected to attend to diverse and frequently conflicting objectives, despite the fact that relatively few supervisors have ever received formal training in the activity (Hess, 1987). Supervision must incorporate and balance multiple foci: the patient's need for competent treatment, the student's immediate comfort, the student's long-term development, the training program's need for evaluation of the student, and not least of all, "the supervisor's personal needs to be viewed favorably by supervisees and to be respected by colleagues" (Tyler & Weaver, 1981, p. 434).

Insomuch as psychotherapy is learned primarily through experience and supervision, an intensive apprenticeship is needed—all the more so for treatment selection. Clinical supervision is generally rated the single most important contribution to one's professional development (Henry, Sims & Spray, 1973). In forecasting the future directions of converging trends in psychotherapy, Goldfried and Padawer (1982) concluded that, "The only effective way of learning the art of psychotherapy is through an apprenticeship undertaken with a skilled clinician" (p. 29). Clinical supervision thus constitutes one of our most formidable challenges and promising opportunities.

Needs Assessment

We have been singularly impressed by the failure of supervisors to assess their students' expressed desires and genuine needs. Trainees invariably present with multiple agendas—some manifest and some latent—and diverse needs, some of which are quite out of their awareness. However, many supervisors assume that their students all present with identical needs and thus subscribe to a variant of the "uniformity myth" (Kiesler, 1966).

As in clinical work, supervision should ideally begin with a needs assessment: What do they want and/or need from the supervisory experience? Are they here to facilitate personal growth? To ventilate about therapy frustrations? To validate their theoretical allegiances? To evaluate technical weaknesses? To analyze countertransferential reactions? To achieve all of these (e.g., "to become a better therapist") or none of these (e.g., "because I was assigned to you")?

It is likely that students need and seek different things at different points in their training experiences (e.g., Loganbill et al., 1982; Worthington, 1984, 1987). Early in training they tend to be rigid and inflexible (Tracey, Hays, Malone & Herman, 1988). They look to valued and status-endowed supervisors to set their theoretical perspectives (Beutler & McNabb, 1981; Guest & Beutler, 1988). Moreover, the viewpoints of valued supervisors become more solidified, albeit more integrated, in the years after professional training (Guest & Beutler, 1988), and the integrative influence of experience tends to result in former trainees coming to value those experiences most highly that have served to solidify both theoretical positions and technical competence. Indeed, Guest and Beutler (1988) suggest that supervisors who focus on the establishment of proficiency may not be as highly valued during training as they are some years later.

Because of such patterns, initial and continual redefinition of supervision objectives is required. Supervisees come with a panoply of preconceptions and needs, many unrecognized, and it is best to examine these at the outset and to modify them as the trainee obtains experience. In addition to the assessment of needs and clarifying expectations, both our experience and supervision research highlight the importance of sharing perceptions of the supervision relationship. Hassenfeld and Sarris (1978) attribute mutual failure in a supervisory relationship to discrepant perceptions of each other and their appropriate roles.

There are occasions, of course, when the supervisee's preferences are in conflict with the supervisor's judgment as to legitimate needs. For example, when asked how he best handled negative feedback in supervision, one advanced trainee seriously replied, "By ignoring it" [!]. However, as in this case, the disparities sometimes are uncovered early by tactful inquiry and can become a focus of supervision. Supervisees' desires should be elicited, articulated, and considered, but will not necessarily commit the supervisor to that tack.

Prescriptive Supervision

This volume is centrally concerned with tailoring treatment interventions and interpersonal stances to client needs. Just as we ask our students to be prescriptive in their clinical work, we too should match our supervision to their unique needs and clinical strategies. The determinants of therapist behavior are too numerous and supervisee needs too heterogeneous to provide the identical supervisory experience to each and every student. The prescriptive nature of supervision will obviously take into account numerous trainee variables, three of which will be addressed here: therapy approach, level of clinical experience, and cognitive style.

Therapy Approach. Within certain limits, the "how" of supervision (method) should parallel the "what" of supervision (content). In other words, the supervision approach should mirror the therapeutic approach (Frances & Clarkin, 1981). When the supervisee's treatment approach entails verbal, insight-oriented work, supervision profitably explores the student's countertransference reactions to both patient and supervisor. Similarly, didactic instruction and role playing in the supervision hour are especially congruent with more behavioral, action-oriented approaches. However, there may also be some value to conceptualizing supervision as a complement to treatment. Work on countertransference, for example, would not be limited to the supervision of insight-oriented treatment but also extended to students who are prone to ignore it in treatment (Stricker, 1988).

Interpersonally, the supervisor may need to adapt his/her stances across supervisees and even within supervisees when their patients are treated with divergent interventions. As Hess (1980) points out, a supervisor can flexibly and fruitfully vary amongst lecturer, teacher, case reviewer, collegial peer, monitor, and therapist throughout the course of one supervision or over many supervision contacts.

Level of Clinical Experience. The developmental needs of clinical supervisees shift over the course of their training (Worthington, 1987). General experience in supervision (e.g., Hess, 1980; Blumenfield, 1982; Hart, 1982) and developmental models of supervision (e.g., Hogan 1964; Stoltenberg, 1981; Loganbill et al., 1982; Yogev, 1982) suggest that different supervisory styles are differentially effective for trainees at varying levels of experience. Beginning students are most interested in the acquisition of specific interviewing and therapy techniques; advanced practicum students are more inclined toward the development of alternative formulations; interns tend to be most intrigued by examination of personal dynamics affecting therapy.

Likewise, Heppner and Roehlke (1984) observed that beginning practicum students sought skills and support, moderately advanced trainees sought to expand their conceptual skills and theoretical knowledge while even more advanced students expressed the desire to explore personal issues that might affect their ability to provide treatment (cf. Nelson, 1978; Worthington, 1984; Wiley & Ray, 1986). As with any "stage model," the steps obviously overlap and the emphases are relative rather than absolute.

Freud captured this progression within the context of supervision in the following quote attributed to him by one of his analysands (Blanton, 1971):

I do not believe that one can give the method of technique through papers. It must be done by personal teaching. Of course, beginners probably need something to begin with. Otherwise they would have nothing to go on. But if they follow the directions conscientiously, they will soon find themselves in trouble. They then must learn to develop their own technique. (p. 48)

From such literature, we conclude that the goals of supervision should reflect the developmental stage of the trainee (Guest & Beutler, 1988). Supervisory goals should begin with support and training in technical skill and progress to considering more complex theoretical concepts and finally endeavor to solidify and integrate theory and technique with personal response patterns. These later skills include special focus on interpersonal dynamics, particularly transference and countertransference. In oversimplified terms, students move from techniques to knowledge to self. It is no small coincidence that most psychotherapy patients evidence a similar pattern, particularly those engaged in long-term treatment.

Cognitive Style. A nascent body of research indicates that the conceptual level of the trainee is an important consideration in fitting the supervision to the student. One aspect of "conceptual level" refers to students' level of conceptual complexity and includes the degree of self-initiative, ability to generate concepts, and tolerance for ambiguity (Handley, 1982). Students high in conceptual development benefit more from a self-directed instructional approach, while those lower in conceptual development perform better with externally oriented and externally controlled training programs (e.g., Hunt & Sullivan, 1974; Rosenthal, 1977).

With this observation, it is apparent that another aspect of cognitive style is conceptually related to "interpersonal reactance," a concept we have discussed at length as a patient variable. Like the high-reactant patient who is resistant to therapist directiveness, the high-reactant student is likely to be resistant to a directive and authoritarian supervisor. This student is likely to do best with a reflective and evocative supervisor who focuses upon the student's experience and is less direct in recommending technical procedures. This student is contrasted to the low-reactant (externally focused) student who is likely to respond well to supervisor directives.

Coherent Framework

Although clinical supervision should be sensitive and tailored to the needs of the student and to the particulars of the case, it must also operate from a coherent conceptual framework. The presence of a systematic schema determines in large part whether supervision is experienced as intelligible or bewildering.

A recent study by Allen, Szollos, and Williams (1986) found that integrative supervision within a superordinate framework is associated positively with the quality of the learning experience. Conversely, relatively less valued integrative or eclectic supervisors neglected this need by failing to ground their interventions and decisions within a larger, guiding perspective. "Atheoretical" supervisors may lack the big picture—an encompassing structure that organizes the case formulations and prioritizes clinical intervention.

There are several coherent frameworks now available that offer a glimpse of the "big picture." Whereas the choice of a particular framework may be an individual student decision, the underlying rationale for differential treatment selection should not be discarded without ample proof of the alternative. Psychotherapy should be predicated primarily on client need and secondarily on clinician preference. We do not denigrate personal preferences; we need to feel comfortable with our favorite methods, to be convinced of their validity, and to communicate this conviction to patients. Our conceptual and ethical framework, however, does object to personal preferences dictating treatment when they are in stark contrast to and override the extant clinical and research knowledge. To put it bluntly: The psychotherapist's theoretical narcissism should not be placated at the client's expense (Norcross, 1988).

CONCLUSIONS AND RECOMMENDATIONS

One reason for the relative paucity of empirical research and of our recommendations on training methods is that technology assumes a secondary position to the interpersonal relationship in clinical supervision. The supervisory relationship, in our opinion, is paramount to the acquisition of interpersonal and technical competence in psychotherapy. After all, clinical supervision—like psychotherapy itself—is essentially a dyadic human interaction with the intent of modifying the behaviors, affects, and cognitions of supervisees in ways that enable them to provide more effective services to their patients (Hess, 1980). We ask our trainees on occasion to recognize their undue preoccupation with technology at the expense of the relationship, a propensity that Mahoney (1986) has labeled the "tyranny of technique." Psychotherapy techniques are most adequately construed as strategies for structuring and communicating the therapeutic message, but they should not be confused with it.

In the supervisory relationship, the importance of modeling open-mindedness and synthetic thinking cannot be overemphasized. Not unlike our children, our students learn to emulate what we do more closely than what we say (cf. Beutler et al., 1987). But too often, therapy trainers teach eclecticism in the form of value *statements* instead of value *actions* (Robertson, 1986). Supervisors should reliably model the curiosity and incisiveness central to psychotherapy success as well as to psychotherapy integration.

At the same time, we are careful to distinguish between informed open-mindedness and uninformed empty-headedness. Uncritical acceptance is not prized. As the Maharani of Jaipus was once reported to have said: "Keep an open mind; an open mind is a very good thing, but don't keep your mind so open that your brains fall out."

The emphasis of training should be placed squarely on *"how* to think" rather than on *"what* to think." This modified focus engenders informed pluralism and self-evolving clinical styles, in contrast to young disciples or mindless imitators. The training process can then progress from imitative learning to creative learning (Fleming, 1953), a transition from therapy skills to skilled therapists (Grater, 1985).

With experienced supervisees, an appropriate goal for psychotherapy supervision is what Phillips and Kanter (1984) have termed "mutuality." The exchange is a process of mutual exploration and bidirectional exchanges with an "inquiring colleague" (Kagan, 1980). Supervisors should not abdicate their professional responsibilities nor deny disparities in knowledge and power between themselves and students, of course. However, supervisors can create a collaborative relationship and a "holding environment" that encourage trainees to express their insecurities and to disagree respectfully. A critical question (Norcross, 1988) that guides us is, "Will trainees be able to present what makes them look bad or only what makes them look good?"

An authoritarian style appears to be particularly detrimental to student esteem and competence (Rosenblatt & Mayer, 1975; Allen, Szollos & Williams, 1986). Demanding conformity and punishing divergence from the "party line" jeopardize the supervisory relationship and subvert central tenets of psychotherapy integration (Cherniss & Equatios, 1977; Moskowitz & Rupert, 1983).

Recommendations

It follows logically that just as psychotherapists are guided by data, so supervisors should be primarily guided by available evidence in their selection of supervision methods. Unfortunately, empirical research to date has not generated substantive direction in this regard (Lambert, 1980; Matarazzo & Patterson, 1986; Lambert & Arnold, 1987). Nonetheless, a few sprinkles of evidence and many years of experience in supervision concerning treatment selection lead us to offer a few recommendations.

First, despite their initial anxiety, supervisees appreciate our reliance on more than their edited verbal reports about what transpired during psychotherapy contacts. The research (e.g., Stein, Karasu, Charles & Buckley, 1975; Nelson, 1978; Allen et al., 1986) suggests verbatim recordings and direct observation are superior methods to reconstructed tales of therapy "heroics."

Second, we heartily recommend a wide variety of pedagogical methods in the supervision of diverse psychotherapy methods and formats. Structure should follow function. As the situation dictates, supervision might involve didactic presentations, reading assignments, open-ended discussions, personal modeling, experiential activities, video demonstrations, case examples, and mini-case conferences. Two techniques that have proven quite effective in expanding our own theoretical horizons are, first, formulation of the same case from disparate theoretical perspectives and, second, co-supervision with an invited colleague (Norcross, 1988).

Third, we have found it useful—as have other supervisors (e.g., Ekstein & Wallerstein, 1972; Doehrman, 1976; Dasberg & Winokur, 1984)—to examine the recurrence of parallels between supervision and psychotherapy. These parallel processes can take many forms. In one manifestation, trainees may behave in supervision in a way that is similar to how their patient behaves in psychotherapy. In another manifestation, the dynamics between supervisee and supervisor may mimic those of the therapeutic relationship. Trainees bring similar interpersonal and defensive patterns to all relationships, psychotherapy and supervision included. When these repetitive relationship patterns are addressed in supervision, the trainee's awareness and performance can be enhanced in all interpersonal pursuits, including but not limited to psychotherapy.

Fourth, we recommend that supervision goals and contracts, like those in therapy itself, be explicit. Attendance, interpersonal roles, and expectations should be shared at the outset, with both parties entering into the agreement. The acquisition of objectives should also be reviewed periodically with the trainee in a two-way dialogue, rather than simply as a critique of the student by the supervisor. Unlike much of psychotherapy, however, the supervisor can and probably should share personal experience and philosophy.

Fifth, we believe that the acquisition of technical competency can be enhanced by incorporating into the supervisory process formal methods of assessing therapeutic skill that have evolved from psychotherapy manuals. Criteria-based rating scales for assessing the skill of psychotherapists have been developed for cognitive therapy (e.g., Beck et al., 1979; Vallis, Shaw & Dobson, 1986), Time-Limited Psychodynamic Therapy (Butler, Strupp & Lane, 1987), Gestalt therapy (Greenberg & Sarkissian, 1984; Daldrup et al., 1988), Interpersonal Psychotherapy (DeRubeis, Hollon, Evans & Bemis, 1982; Chevron & Rounsaville, 1983; Rounsaville, Chevron, Weissman, Prusoff & Frank, 1986), and long-term psychodynamic psychotherapy (Koenigsberg, Kernberg, Haas, Lotterman, Rockland & Selzer, 1985) among others. These scales can be applied to the audio and videotapes on which supervision is often based, not only defining the procedures that are considered to be of value to the particular manual but also describing the behaviors that comprise their effective utilization. By applying different scales to the same series of psychotherapy sessions, a good deal of discussion can evolve to form the basis of exploring both differences and similarities among therapeutic approaches.

SUGGESTED READINGS

Beutler, L. E., Mahoney, M. J., Norcross, J. C., Prochaska, J. O., Sollod, R. M. & Robertson, M. (1987). Training integrative/eclectic psychotherapists II. *Journal of Integrative and Eclectic Psychotherapy, 6,* 296–332.

Guest, P. D. & Beutler, L. E. (1988). The impact of psychotherapy supervision on therapist orientation and values. *Journal of Consulting and Clinical Psychology, 56,* 653–658.

Hess, A. K. (Ed.) (1980). *Psychotherapy supervision.* New York: John Wiley.

Shaw, B. F. & Dobson, K. S. (1988). Competency judgments in the training and evaluation of psychotherapists. *Journal of Consulting and Clinical Psychology, 56,* 666–672.

Strupp, H. H., Butler, S. F. & Rosser, C. L. (1988). Training in psychodynamic therapy. *Journal of Consulting and Clinical Psychology, 56,* 689–695.

References

Abramowitz, S. I. & Murray, J. (1983). Race effects in psychotherapy. In J. Murray & P. R. Abramson (Eds.), *Bias in psychotherapy* (pp. 215–255). New York: Praeger.

Ackerman, N. W. (1958). *The psychodynamics of family life.* New York: Basic Books.

Agras, W. S. & Berkowitz, R. (1980). Clinical research in behavior therapy: Halfway there? *Behavior Therapy, 11,* 472–487.

Aldwin, C., Folkman, B., Schaefer, C., Coyne, J. & Lazarus, R. S. (1980, August). *Ways of coping: A process measure.* Presented at the annual meeting of the American Psychological Association, Montreal.

Alexander, J. F., Barton, C., Schiavo, R. S. & Parsons, B. V. (1976). Systems-behavioral interventions with families of delinquents: Therapist characteristics, family behavior, and outcome. *Journal of Consulting and Clinical Psychology, 17* 656–664.

Allen, G. J., Szollos, S. J. & Williams, B. E. (1986). Doctoral students' comparative evaluations of best and worst psychotherapy supervision. *Professional Psychology: Research and Practice, 17,* 91–99.

Allen, J., Coyne, L., Beasley, C. & Spohn, H. (1987). A conceptual model for research on required length of psychiatric hospital stay. *Comprehensive Psychiatry, 28,* 131–140.

American Board of Medical Psychotherapists (1987). *The national directory of medical psychotherapists.* Nashville, TN: ABMP Press.

American Board of Professional Psychology, Inc. (1980). *Directory of diplomates.* Washington, DC: American Board of Professional Psychology, Inc.

American Medical Association, Department of Drugs, Division of Drugs and Technology. (1986). *Drug evaluations,* 6th ed. Chicago, IL: American Medical Association.

American Psychiatric Association (1980). *Diagnostic and statistical manual of mental disorders,* 3rd ed. Washington DC: Author.

American Psychiatric Association (1983). *Biographical directory.* Washington DC: American Psychiatric Press.

American Psychiatric Association (1987). *Diagnostic criteria: DSM-IIIR.* Washington, DC: American Psychiatric Press.

American Psychiatric Association Commission on Psychotherapies (1982). *Psychotherapy research: Methodological and efficacy issues.* Washington, DC: American Psychiatric Association.

Anderson, M. P. (1980). Imaginal processes: Therapeutic applications and theoretical models. In M. J. Mahoney (Ed.), *Psychotherapy process: Current issues and future directions*, (pp. 211–248). New York: Plenum.

Andrews, G., Tennant, C., Hewson, D. & Vaillant, G. (1978). Life stress, social support, coping style, and risk of psychological impairment. *Journal of Nervous and Mental Disease, 166*, 307–316.

Aneshensel, C. S. & Stone, J. D. (1982). Stress and depression: A test of buffering model of social support. *Archives of General Psychiatry, 39*, 1392–1396.

Argyle, M., Bryant, B. & Trower, P. (1974). Social skills training and psychotherapy: A comparative study. *Psychological Medicine, 4*, 435–443.

Arizmendi, T. G., Beutler, L. E., Shanfield, S., Crago, M., & Hagaman, R. (1985). Client-therapist value similarity and psychotherapy outcome: A microscopic approach. *Psychotherapy: Theory, Research and Practice, 22*, 16–21.

Arkowitz, H. & Hannah, M. T. (in press). Cognitive, behavioral, and psychodynamic therapies: Converging or diverging pathways to change? In A. Freeman, H. Arkowitz, L. E. Beutler, and K. Simon (Eds.), *Comprehensive Handbook of Cognitive Therapy*, New York: Plenum.

Arkowitz, H., Holliday, S. & Hutter, M. (1982, November). *Depressed women and their husbands: A study of marital interaction and adjustment.* Paper presented at the meeting of the Association for the Advancement of Behavior Therapy, Los Angeles.

Arkowitz, H. & Messer, S. B. (Eds.) (1984). *Psychoanalytic and behavior therapy: Is integration possible?* New York: Plenum.

Ashinger, P. A. G. (1981). Social networks related to counseling interventions. *Dissertation Abstracts International, 42*, 2495–A.

Azrin, N. H., Naster, B. J., & Jones, R. (1973). Reciprocity counselling: A rapid learning-based procedure for marital counselling. *Behaviour Research and Therapy, 11*, 365–382.

Bachrach, L. L. (1988). Defining chronic mental illness: A concept paper. *Hospital and Community Psychiatry, 39*, 383–388.

Baekeland, F. & Lundwall, M. A. (1975). Dropping out of treatment: A critical review. *Psychological Bulletin, 82*, 738–783.

Bandura, A. (1977). *Social learning theory.* Englewood Cliffs NJ: Prentice-Hall.

Barlow, D. H. (Ed.) (1985). *Clinical handbook of psychological disorders: A step-by-step treatment manual.* New York: Guilford.

Barlow, D. H. (1988). *Anxiety and its disorders: The nature and treatment of anxiety and panic.* New York: Guilford.

Barlow, D. H., O'Brien, G. T. & Last, C. G. (1984). Couples treatment of agoraphobia. *Behavior Therapy, 15*, 41–58.

Barlow, D. H. & Waddell, M. T. (1985). Agoraphobia. In D. H. Barlow (Ed.), *Clinical handbook of psychological disorders: A step-by-step treatment manual* (pp. 1–68). New York: Guilford.

Barnett, P. A. & Gotlib, I. H. (1988). Psychosocial functioning and depression: Distinguishing among antecedents, concomitants, and consequences. *Psychological Bulletin, 104*, 97–126.

Barrett-Lennard, G. T. (1972). Dimensions of therapist response as causal factors in therapeutic change. *Psychological Monographs, 76*, (43, Whole no. 562).

Beck, A. T. (1982). Cognitive therapy of depression: New perspectives. In P. Clayton (Ed.), *Depression*. New York: Raven Press.

Beck, A. T. & Emery, G. (1985). *Anxiety disorders and phobias: A cognitive perspective*. New York: Basic Books.

Beck, A. T., Rush, A. J., Shaw, B. F. & Emery, G. (1979). *Cognitive therapy of depression*. New York: Guilford Press.

Beck, A. T., Ward, C. H., Mendelson, M., Mock, J. & Erbaugh, J. (1961). An inventory for measuring depression. *Archives of General Psychiatry, 4,* 561–569.

Beck, A. T. & Weishaar, M. (in press). Cognitive therapy. In A. Freeman, H. Arkowitz, L. E. Beutler & K. Simon (Eds.),*Comprehensive handbook of cognitive therapy*. New York: Plenum.

Bednar, R. L., Burlingame, G. M. & Masters, K. S. (1988). Systems of family treatment: Substance or semantics: In M. R. Rosenzweig & L. W. Porter (Eds.), *Annual Review of Psychology*, Vol. 39 (pp. 401–434). Palo Alto: Annual Reviews, Inc.

Beidel, D. C. & Turner, S. M. (1986). A critique of the theoretical bases of cognitive-behavioral theories and therapy. *Clinical Psychology Review, 6,* 177–197.

Beitman, B. D. (1987). *The structure of individual psychotherapy*. New York: Guilford.

Bell, P. A., Fisher, J. D. & Loomis, R. J. (1978). *Environmental psychology*. Philadelphia: W. B. Saunders Co.

Bellack, A. (1985). Psychotherapy research in depression: An overview. In E. Beckham & W. Leber (Eds.), *Handbook of depression: Treatment, assessment and research* (pp. 204–219). Homewood, IL: Dorsey Press.

Bellack, A. S., Hersen, M. & Himmelhoch, J. M. (1980). Social skills training for depression: A treatment manual. *Journal Supplement Abstract Service Catalog of Selected Documents in Psychology, 10,* 92 (Ms. No. 2156).

Bellack, A. S., Hersen, M. & Himmelhoch, J. M. (1981). Social skills training compared with pharmacotherapy in the treatment of unipolar depression. *American Journal of Psychiatry, 138,* 1562–1567.

Bellack, A. S., Hersen, M. & Himmelhoch, J. M. (1983). A comparison of social skills training, pharmacotherapy and psychotherapy for depression. *Behaviour Research and Therapy, 21,* 101–107.

Bennun, I. (1984). Marital therapy with one spouse. In K. Hahlweg & N. S. Jacobson (Eds.), *Marital interaction: Analysis and modification*. New York: Guilford Press.

Bergin, A. E. (1980). Psychotherapy and religious values. *Journal of Consulting and Clinical Psychology, 48,* 95–105.

Bergin, A. E. & Lambert, M. J. (1978). The evaluation of psychotherapeutic outcomes. In S. L. Garfield & A. E. Bergin (Eds.), *Handbook of psychotherapy and behavior change: An empirical analysis*. New York: John Wiley.

Berman, J. S., Miller, R. C. & Massman, P. J. (1985). Cognitive therapy versus systematic desensitization: Is one treatment superior? *Psychological Bulletin, 97,* 451–461.

Berry, D. S. & McArthur, L. Z. (1986). Perceiving character in faces: The impact of age-related craniofacial changes on social perception. *Psychological Bulletin, 100,* 3–18.

Berzins, J. I. (1977). Therapist-patient matching. In A. S. Gurman & A. M. Razin (Eds.), *Effective psychotherapy: A handbook of research* (pp. 222–251). New York: Pergamon.

Beutler, L. E. (1979a). Toward specific psychological therapies for specific conditions. *Journal of Consulting and Clinical Psychology, 47,* 882–897.

Beutler, L. E. (1979b). Values, beliefs, religion and the persuasive influence of psychotherapy. *Psychotherapy: Theory, Research and Practice, 16,* 432–440.

Beutler, L. E. (1981). Convergence in counseling and psychotherapy: A current look. *Clinical Psychology Review, 1,* 79–101.

Beutler, L. E. (1983). *Eclectic psychotherapy: A systematic approach.* New York: Pergamon.

Beutler, L. E. (1986). Systematic eclectic psychotherapy. In J. C. Norcross (Ed.), *Handbook of eclectic psychotherapy* (pp. 94–131). New York: Brunner/Mazel.

Beutler, L. E. (1988). Introduction: Training to competency in psychotherapy. *Journal of Consulting and Clinical Psychology, 56,* 651–652.

Beutler, L. E. (in press). Differential treatment selection: The role of diagnosis in psychotherapy. *Psychotherapy.*

Beutler, L. E., Arizmendi, T. G., Crago, M., Shanfield, S. & Hagaman, R. (1983). The effects of value similarity and clients' persuadability on value convergence and psychotherapy improvement. *Journal of Social and Clinical Psychology, 1,* 231–245.

Beutler, L. E. & Crago, M. (1983). Self-report measures of psychotherapy outcome. In M. J. Lambert, E. R. Christensen & S. S. DeJulio (Eds.), *The assessment of psychotherapy outcome* (pp. 453–497). New York: John Wiley and Sons.

Beutler, L. E. & Crago, M. (1987). Strategies and techniques of prescriptive psychotherapeutic intervention. In R. E. Hales & A. J. Frances (Eds.), *American Psychiatric Association: Annual Review* (Vol. 6) (pp. 378–397), Washington, DC: American Psychiatric Association.

Beutler, L. E., Crago, M. & Arizmendi, T. G. (1986). Therapist variables in psychotherapy process and outcome. In S. L. Garfield & A. E. Bergin (Eds.), *Handbook of psychotherapy and behavior change,* 3rd ed. (pp. 257–310), New York: John Wiley and Sons.

Beutler, L.E., Daldrup, R., Engle, D., Guest, P. & Corbishley, A. (1988). Family dynamics and emotional expression among patients with chronic pain and depression. *Pain, 32,* 65–72.

Beutler, L. E., Daldrup, R. J., Engle, D., Oro'-Beutler, M. E., Meredith, K. & Boyer, J. T. (1987). Effects of therapeutically induced affect arousal on depressive symptoms, pain, and beta-endorphins among rheumatoid arthritis patients. *Pain, 29,* 325–334.

Beutler, L. E., Dunbar, P. W. & Baer, P. E. (1980). Individual variation among therapists' perceptions of patients, therapy process and outcome. *Psychiatry, 43,* 205–210.

Beutler, L. E., Engle, D., Oro'-Beutler, M. E., Daldrup, R. & Meredith, K. (1986).

Inability to express intense affect: A common link between depression and pain? *Journal of Consulting and Clinical Psychology, 54,* 752–759.

Beutler, L. E., Frank, M., Scheiber, S. C., Calvert, S. & Gaines, J. (1984). Comparative effects of group psychotherapies in a short-term inpatient setting: An experience with deterioration effects. *Psychiatry, 47,* 66–76.

Beutler, L. E., & Guest, P. D. (in press). The role of cognitive change in psychotherapy. In A. Freeman, L. E. Beutler, H. Arkowitz & K. Simon (Eds.), *Handbook of cognitive therapy.* New York: Plenum.

Beutler, L. E. & Hamblin, D. L. (1986). Individual outcome measures of internal change: Methodological considerations. *Journal of Consulting and Clinical Psychology* (special edition), *54,* 48–53.

Beutler, L. E., Jobe, A. M. & Elkins, D. (1974). Outcomes in group psychotherapy: Using persuasion theory to increase treatment efficiency. *Journal of Consulting and Clinical Psychology, 42,* 547–553.

Beutler, L. E., Mahoney, M. J., Norcross, J. C., Prochaska, J. O., Sollod, R.M. & Robertson, M. (1987). Training integrative/eclectic psychotherapists II. *Journal of Integrative and Eclectic Psychotherapy, 6,* 296–332.

Beutler, L. E. & McNabb, C. (1981). Self-evaluation for the psychotherapist. In C.E. Walker (Ed.), *Clinical practice of psychology* (pp. 397–440). New York: Pergamon.

Beutler, L. E. & Mitchell, R. (1981). Psychotherapy outcome in depressed and impulsive patients as a function of analytic and experiential treatment procedures. *Psychiatry, 44,* 297–306.

Beutler, L. E., Pollack, S. & Jobe, A. M. (1978). "Acceptance," values and therapeutic change. *Journal of Consulting and Clinical Psychology, 46,* 198–199.

Beutler, L. E., Scoggin, F., Kirkish, P., Schretlen, D., Corbishley, M. A., Hamblin, D., Meredith, K., Potter, R., Bamford, C. R. & Levenson, A. I. (1987). Group cognitive therapy and alprazolam in the treatment of depression in older adults. *Journal of Consulting and Clinical Psychology, 55,* 550–556.

Biglan, A., Hops, H., Sherman, L., Friedman, L. S., Arthur, J. & Osteen, V. (1985). Problem-solving interactions of depressed women and their spouses. *Behavior Therapy, 16,* 431–451.

Billings, A. G., Cronkite, R. C. & Moos, R. H. (1983). Social-environmental factors in unipolar depression: Comparisons of depressed patients and nondepressed controls. *Journal of Abnormal Psychology, 92,* 119–133.

Billings, A. G. & Moos, R. H. (1982). Psychosocial theory and research on depression: An integrative framework and review. *Clinical Psychology Review, 2,* 213–237.

Billings, A. G. & Moos, R. H. (1982). Social support and functioning among community and clinical groups: A panel model. *Journal of Behavioral Medicine, 5,* 295–311.

Billings, A. G. & Moos, R. H. (1985). Psychosocial stressors, coping, and depression. In E. E. Beckham & W. R. Leber (Eds.), *Handbook of depression: Treatment, assessment, and research* (pp. 940–974). Homewood, IL: Dorsey Press.

Biondo, J. & MacDonald, A. P., Jr. (1971). Internal-external locus of control and response to influence attempts. *Journal of Personality, 39,* 407–419.

Blackburn, I. M., Bishop, S., Glen, A. I. M., Whalley, L. J. & Christie, J. E. (1981). The efficacy of cognitive therapy in depression: A treatment trial using cognitive therapy and pharmacotherapy, each alone and in combination. *British Journal of Psychiatry, 139,* 181–189.

Blanchard, E. B. & Andrasik, F. (1985). *Management of chronic headaches: A psychological approach.* New York: Pergamon Press.

Bland, R. C., Parker, J. H. & Orn, H. (1978). Prognosis in schizophrenia. *Archives of General Psychiatry, 35,* 72–77.

Blanton, S. (1971). *Diary of my analysis with Sigmund Freud.* New York: Hawthorn Books.

Blase, J. J. (1979). A study of the effects of sex of the client and sex of the therapist on clients' satisfaction with psychotherapy. *Dissertation Abstracts International, 39,* 6107B–6108B.

Blashfield, R. K. (1984). *The classification of psychopathology: Neo-Kraepelinian and qualitative approaches.* New York: Plenum Press.

Blau, T. H. (1988). *Psychotherapy tradecraft: The technique and style of doing therapy.* New York: Brunner/Mazel.

Blier, M. J., Atkinson, D. R. & Geer, C. A. (1987). Effect of client gender and counselor gender and sex roles on willingness to see the counselor. *Journal of Counseling Psychology, 34,* 27–30.

Blumenfield, M. (Ed.). (1982). *Applied supervision in psychotherapy.* New York: Grune & Stratton.

Bond, J. A., Hansell, J. & Shevrin, H. (1987). Locating transference paradigms in psychotherapy transcripts: Reliability of relationship episode location in the Core Conflictual Relationship Theme (CCRT) method. *Psychotherapy, 24,* 736–749.

Bootzin, R. R. & Ruggill, J. S. (1988). Training issues in behavior therapy. *Journal of Consulting and Clinical Psychology, 56,* 703–709.

Bordin, E. S. (1976). The generalizability of the psychoanalytic concept of the working alliance. *Psychotherapy: Theory, Research, and Practice, 16,* 252–260.

Borkovec, T., Mathews, A. M., Chambers, A., Ebrahimi, S., Lytle, R. & Nelson, R. (1987). The effects of relaxation training with cognitive therapy or nondirective therapy and the role of relaxation-induced anxiety in the treatment of generalized anxiety. *Journal of Consulting and Clinical Psychology, 55,* 883–888.

Boster, F. J. & Mongeau, P. (1984). Fear-arousing persuasive messages. In R. N. Bostrom (Ed.), *Communication Yearbook 8* (pp. 330–375). Beverly Hills, CA: Sage Publications.

Brehm, S. S. (1976). *The application of social psychology to clinical practice.* New York: John Wiley and Sons.

Brehm, S. S. & Brehm, J. W. (1981). *Psychological reactance: A theory of freedom and control.* New York: Academic Press.

Brehm, S. S. & Smith, T. (1986). Social psychological approaches to psychotherapy and behavior change. In S. L. Garfield & A. E. Bergin (Eds.), *Handbook of psychotherapy and behavior change,* 3rd ed. (pp. 69–115). New York: John Wiley and Sons.

Breuer, J. & Freud, S. (1955). *Studies on hysteria*. In *Standard Edition* (Vol. 2). London: Hogarth Press (First German edition, 1895).

Brickman, P., Rabinowitz, V. C., Karuza, J., Coates, D., Cohn, E. et al. (1982). Models of helping and coping. *American Psychologist, 37,* 368–384.

Broderick, C. B. & Schrader, S. S. (1981). The history of professional marriage and family therapy. In A. S. Gurman & D. P. Kniskern (Eds.), *Handbook of family therapy* (pp. 5–35). New York: Brunner/Mazel.

Brody, C. M. (1987). White therapist and female minority clients: Gender and culture issues. *Psychotherapy, 24,* 108–113.

Brown, G. W., Bhrolchain, M. N. & Harris, T. (1975). Social class and psychiatric disturbance among women in an urban population. *Sociology, 9,* 225–254.

Brown, G. W., Birley, J. L. T. & Wing, J. K. (1972). Influence of family life on the course of schizophrenic disorders: A replication. *British Journal of Psychiatry, 121,* 241–258.

Brown, G. W. & Harris, T. O. (1978). *Social origins of depression: A study of psychiatric disorder in women.* New York: Free Press.

Brown, G. W., Monck, E. M., Carstairs, G. M. & Wing, J. K. (1962). The influence of family life on the course of schizophrenic illness. *British Journal of Preventive and Social Medicine, 16,* 55.

Brown, J. (1987). A review of meta-analyses conducted on psychotherapy outcome research. *Clinical Psychology Review, 7,* 1–23.

Brownlee-Duffeck, M., Peterson, L., Simonds, J. F., Goldstein, D., Kilo, C. & Hoette, S. (1987). The role of health beliefs in regimen adherence and metabolic control of adolescents and adults with diabetes mellitus. *Journal of Consulting and Clinical Psychology, 55,* 139–144.

Bruch, H. (1975). The constructive use of ignorance. In E. J. Anthony (Ed.), *Explorations in child psychiatry* (pp. 247–264). New York: Plenum Press.

Brunink, S. & Schroeder, H. (1979). Verbal therapeutic behavior of expert psychoanalytically oriented, gestalt and behavior therapists. *Journal of Consulting and Clinical Psychology, 47,* 567–574.

Buchanan, D. R., Goldman, M. & Juhnke, R. (1977). Eye contact, sex, and the violation of personal space. *Journal of Social Psychology, 103,* 19–25.

Budman, S. H. (Ed.) (1981). *Forms of brief therapy.* New York: Guilford.

Budman, S. H., Demby, A., Redondo, J. P., Hannan, M., Feldstein, M., Ring, J. & Springer, T. (1988). Comparative outcome in time-limited individual and group psychotherapy. *International Journal of Group Psychotherapy, 38,* 63–86.

Budman, S. H. & Gurman, A. S. (1983). The practice of brief therapy. *Professional Psychology: Research and Practice, 14,* 277–292.

Budman, S. H. & Springer, T. (1987). Treatment delay, outcome, and satisfaction in time-limited group and individual psychotherapy. *Professional Psychology: Research and Practice, 18,* 647–649.

Buglass, D., Clarke, J., Henderson, A. S., Kreitman, N. & Presley, A. S. (1977). A study of agoraphobic housewives. *Psychological Medicine, 7* (1), 73–86.

Burgoon, J. K., Buller, D. B., Hale, J. L. & de Turck, M. A. (1984). Relational messages associated with nonverbal behaviors. *Human Communication Research, 10,* 351–378.

Burgoon, M., Burgoon, J. K. & McCroskey, J. C. (1974). *Small group communication: A functional approach.* New York: Holt, Rinehart & Winston.

Burgoon, M. & Miller, G. R. (1971). Prior attitude and language intensity as predictors of message style and attitude change following counterattitudinal advocacy. *Journal of Personality and Social Psychology, 20,* 240–253.

Burgoon, M. & Ruffner, M. (1978). *Human communication.* New York: Holt, Rinehart & Winston.

Burlingame, G. M. & Behrman, J. A. (1987). Clinician attitudes toward time-limited and time-unlimited therapy. *Professional Psychology: Research and Practice, 18,* 61–65.

Butcher, J. N. & Koss, M. P. (1978). Research on brief and crisis-oriented psychotherapies. In S. L. Garfield & A. E. Bergin (Eds.), *Handbook of psychotherapy and behavior change,* 2nd ed. (pp. 725–768). New York: John Wiley and Sons.

Butler, S. F., Strupp, H. H. & Lane, T. W. (1987, June). *The time-limited dynamic psychotherapy therapeutic strategies scale: Development of an adherence measure.* Paper presented at the meetings of the Society of Psychotherapy Research, Ulm, West Germany.

Byrne, D. & Sheffield, J. (1965). Responses to sexually arousing stimuli as a function of repressing and sensitizing defenses. *Journal of Abnormal Psychology, 70,* 114–118.

Calhoun, K. S. & Atkeson, B. M. (1986). *Treatment of victims of sexual assault.* New York: Pergamon Press.

Calvert, S. J., Beutler, L. E., & Crago, M. (1988). Psychotherapy outcome as a function of therapist-patient matching on selected variables. *Journal of Social and Clinical Psychology, 6,* 104–117.

Cannon, D. S., Baker, T. B., Gino, A. & Nathan, P. E. (1986). Alcohol-aversion therapy: Relation between strength of aversion and abstinence. *Journal of Consulting and Clinical Psychology, 54,* 825–830.

Caplan, G. (1974). Support systems. In G. Caplan (Ed.), *Support systems and community mental health.* New York: Basic Books.

Caplan, G. & Killilea, M. (Eds.) (1976). *Support systems and mutual help: Multidisciplinary explorations.* New York: Grune & Stratton.

Carkhuff, R. R. & Pierce, R. (1967). Differential effects of therapist race and social class upon patient depth of self-exploration in the initial clinical interview. *Journal of Consulting Psychology, 31,* 632–634.

Carpenter, W. T. & Heinrichs, D. W. (1981) Treatment-relevant subtypes of schizophrenia. *Journal of Nervous and Mental Disease, 169,* 113–119.

Carpenter, W. T. & Strauss, J. S. (1973). Are there pathognomonic symptoms in schizophrenia? An empirical investigation of Schneider's first rank symptoms. *Archives of General Psychiatry, 28,* 847–852.

Carpenter, W. T., Strauss, J. S. & Bartko, J. J. (1973). Flexible system for diagnosis of schizophrenia: Report from the WHO International Pilot Study of Schizophrenia. *Science, 182,* 1275–1278.

Carr, D. B. & Sheehan, D. V. (1984). Panic anxiety: A new biological model. *Journal of Clinical Psychiatry, 45,* 323–330.

Carson, R. C. & Heine, R. W. (1962). Similarity and success in therapeutic dyads. *Journal of Consulting Psychology, 26,* 38–43.

Carson, R. C. & Llewellyn, C. E., Jr. (1966). Similarity in therapeutic dyads. *Journal of Consulting Psychology, 30,* 458.

Chambless, D. L. & Mason, J. (1986). Sex, sex role stereotyping, and agoraphobia. *Behaviour Research and Therapy, 24,* 321–325.

Charone, J. K. (1981). Patient and therapist treatment goals related to psychotherapy outcome. *Dissertation Abstracts International, 42,* 365B.

Cherniss, C. & Equatios, E. (1977). Styles of clinical supervision in community mental health programs. *Journal of Consulting and Clinical Psychology, 45,* 1195–1196.

Chevron, E. & Rounsaville, B. J. (1983). Evaluating the clinical skills of psychotherapists: A comparison of techniques. *Archives of General Psychiatry, 40,* 1129–1132.

Childress, R. & Gillis, J. S. (1977). A study of pretherapy role induction as an influence process. *Journal of Clinical Psychology, 33,* 540–544.

Christensen, H., Hadzi-Pavlovic, D., Andrews, G., & Mattick, R. (1987). Behavior therapy and tricyclic medication in the treatment of obsessive-compulsive disorder: A quantitative review. *Journal of Consulting and Clinical Psychology, 55,* 701–711.

Clark, D. M. & Bemis, K. M. (1982). A cognitive-behavioral approach to anorexia nervosa. *Cognitive Therapy and Research, 6,* 123–150.

Clarkin, J. F. (1989). Family education. In A. Bellack (Ed.), *A clinical guide for the treatment of schizophrenia.* New York: Plenum.

Clarkin, J. F., Haas, G. L. & Glick, I. D. (Eds.) (1988). *Affective disorders and the family: Assessment and treatment.* New York: Guilford Press.

Clarkin, J. F., Widiger, T., Frances, A., Hurt, S. W. & Gilmore, M. (1983). Prototypic typology and the borderline personality disorder. *Journal of Abnormal Psychology, 92,* 263–275.

Coates, B. (1978). Consistency of attachment behavior in the human infant: A multivariate approach. *Child Study Journal, 8,* 131–148.

Cobb, J., McDonald, R., Marks, I. & Stern, R. (1980). Marital versus exposure therapy: Psychological treatments of co-existing marital and phobic-obsessive problems. *Behavioral Analysis Modification, 4* (1), 3–16.

Cobb, S. (1976). Social support as a moderator of life stress. *Psychosomatic Medicine, 38,* 300–313.

Cohen, C. I. & Sokolovsky, J. (1978). Schizophrenia and social networks: Ex-patients in the inner city. *Schizophrenia Bulletin, 4,* 546–560.

Cole, J. K. & Magnussen, M. (1966). Where the action is. *Journal of Consulting and Clinical Psychology, 30,* 539–545.

Conn, D. & Crowne, D. (1964). Instigation to aggression, emotional arousal and defensive emulation. *Journal of Personality, 32,* 163–179.

Connors, G. J. & Tarbox, A. R. (1985). Macroenvironmental factors as determinants of substance use and abuse. In M. Galizio & S. A. Maisto (Eds.), *Determinants of substance abuse treatment: Biological, psychological, and environmental factors* (pp. 283–316). New York: Plenum.

Corrigan, J. D. (1978). Salient attributes of two types of helpers: Friends and mental health professionals. *Journal of Counseling Psychology, 25,* 588–590.

Corrigan, J. D., Dell, D. M., Lewis, K. N. & Schmidt, L. D. (1980). Counseling as a social influence process: A review. *Journal of Counseling Psychology Monograph, 27,* 395–441.

Corsini, R. J. (1981). *Handbook of innovative psychotherapies.* New York: John Wiley and Sons.

Costello, C. G. (1982). Social factors associated with depression: A retrospective community study. *Psychological Medicine, 12,* 329–339.

Council for the National Register of Health Service Providers in Psychology (1987). *National register of health service providers in psychology.* Washington, DC: Council for the National Register of Health Service Providers in Psychology.

Covi, L., Lipman, R. S., Derogatis, L. R., Smith, J. E. & Pattison, J. H. (1974). Drugs and group psychotherapy in neurotic depression. *American Journal of Psychiatry, 131,* 191–198.

Coyne, J. C. (1976). Depression and the response of others. *Journal of Abnormal Psychology, 85,* 186–193.

Coyne, J. C. (in press). Thinking post-cognitively about depression. In A. Freeman, H. Arkowitz, L. E. Beutler & C. Simon (Eds.), *Comprehensive handbook of cognitive therapy.* New York: Plenum.

Coyne, J. C., Aldwin, C. & Lazarus, R. S. (1981). Depression and coping in stressful episodes. *Journal of Abnormal Psychology, 90,* 439–447.

Coyne, J. C. & DeLongis, A. M. (1986). Getting beyond social support: The role of social relationships in adaptational outcomes. *Journal of Consulting and Clinical Psychology, 54,* 454–460.

Coyne, J. C. & Holroyd, K. (1982). Stress, coping, and illness. In T. Millon, C. Green & R. Meagher (Eds.), *Handbook of clinical health psychology* (pp. 103–127). New York: Plenum Press.

Coyne, J. C., Kahn, J. & Gotlib, I. H. (1986). Depression. In T. Jacob (Ed.), *Family interaction and psychotherapy* (pp. 509–533). New York: Plenum.

Cramer, P. (1987). The development of defense mechanisms. *Journal of Personality, 51,* 78–94.

Cramer, P., Blatt, S. J. & Ford, R. Q. (1988). Defense mechanisms in the anaclitic and introjective personality configuration. *Journal of Consulting and Clinical Psychology, 56,* 610–616.

Crits-Christoph, P., Cooper, A. & Luborsky, L. (1988). The accuracy of therapists' interpretations and the outcome of dynamic psychotherapy. *Journal of Consulting and Clinical Psychology, 56,* 490–495.

Dahlstrom, W. G., Welsh, G. S. & Dahlstrom, L. E. (1972). *An MMPI handbook. Volume I: Clinical interpretations.* Minneapolis: University of Minnesota Press.

Daldrup, R. J., Beutler, L. E., Engle, D. & Greenberg, L. S. (1988). *Focused expressive psychotherapy: Freeing the overcontrolled patient.* New York: Guilford Press.

Dangler, R. F. & Polster, R. A. (1985). *Teaching child management skills.* New York: Pergamon Press.

Dasberg, H. & Winokur, M. (1984). Teaching and learning short-term dynamic psychotherapy: Parallel processes. *Psychotherapy, 21,* 184–188.

Davenport, Y. B. & Adland, M. L. (1988). Family therapy intervention in the management of manic episodes. In J. F. Clarkin, G. Haas & I. D. Glick (Eds.), *Affective disorders and the family* (pp. 173–195). New York: Guilford.

Davenport, Y. B., Ebert, M. H., Adland, M. L. & Goodwin, F. K. (1976). Couples group therapy as an adjunct to lithium maintenance of the manic patient. *American Journal of Orthopsychiatry, 47,* 496–502.

Davidson, S. & Packard, T. (1981). The therapeutic or friendship between women. *Psychology of Women Quarterly, 5,* 495–510.

Davis, J. D. & Skinner, A. E. G. (1974). Reciprocity of self-disclosure in interviews: Modeling or social exchange? *Journal of Personality and Social Psychology, 29,* 779–784.

Davis J. M. (1976). Overview: Maintenance therapy in psychiatry: II. Affective disorders. *American Journal of Psychiatry, 133,* 1–13.

Davis, K. L., Hector, M. A., Meara, N. M., King, J. W., Tracy, D. C. & Wycoff, J. P. (1985). Teaching counselor trainees to respond consistently to different aspects of anger. *Journal of Counseling Psychology, 32,* 580–588.

Deci, E. L. (1980). *The psychology of self-determination.* Lexington, MA: D. C. Heath.

Derogatis, L. R., Rickels, K. & Rock, A. F. (1976). The SCL-90 and the MMPI: A step in the validation of a new self-report scale.*British Journal of Psychiatry, 128,* 280–289.

DeRubeis, R. J., Hollon, S. E., Evans, M. D., & Bemis, K. M. (1982). Can psychotherapies for depression be discriminated? A systematic investigation of cognitive therapy and interpersonal therapy. *Journal of Consulting and Clinical Psychology, 50,* 744–756.

Dickey, B. A. (1964). *Intra-staff conflict, morale, and treatment effectiveness in a therapeutic community setting.* Paper presented at the annual meeting of the American Psychological Association.

Dicks, H.V. (1967). *Marital tensions.* London: Routledge and Kegan Paul.

DiMascio, A., Weissman, M. M., Prusoff, B. A., Neu, C., Zwilling, M. & Klerman, G. L. (1979). Differential symptom reduction by drugs and psychotherapy in acute depression. *Archives of General Psychiatry, 36,* 1450–1456.

DiNardo, P. A., O'Brien, G. T., Barlow, D. H., Waddell, M. T. & Blanchard, E. B. (1983). Reliability of DSM-III anxiety disorder categories using a new structured interview. *Archives of General Psychiatry, 40,* 1070–1074.

Dobson, K. S. & Shaw, B. F. (1988). The use of treatment manuals in cognitive therapy: Experience and issues. *Journal of Consulting and Clinical Psychology, 56,* 673–680.

Doehrman, M. (1976). Parallel processes in supervision and psychotherapy. *Bulletin of the Menninger Clinic, 40*(1).

Dohrenwend, B. S. & Dohrenwend, B. P. (1981). Hypotheses about stress processes linking social class to various types of psychopathology. *American Journal of Community Psychology, 9,* 146–159.

Dollard, J. & Miller, N. E. (1950). *Personality and psychotherapy: An analysis in terms of learning, thinking and culture.* New York: McGraw-Hill.

Dooley, D. & Catalano, R. (1980). Economic change as a cause of behavioral disorder. *Psychological Bulletin, 87,* 450–468.

Dowd, E. T. & Pace, T. F. (in press). The relativity of reality: Second order change in psychotherapy. In A. Freeman, H. Arkowitz, L. E. Beutler & K. Simon (Eds.), *Comprehensive handbook of cognitive therapy.* New York: Plenum.

DuBrin, J. R. & Zastowny, T. R. (1988). Predicting early attrition from psychotherapy: An analysis of a large private-practice cohort. *Psychotherapy, 25,* 393–408.

Dubro, A. F., Wetzler, S. & Kahn, M. (1987, May). *A comparison of three self-report questionnaires for the diagnosis of DSM-III personality disorders.* A paper presented at the annual meeting of the American Psychiatric Association, Chicago.

Edelstein, B. A. & Brasted, W. S. (1983). Clinical training. In M. Hersen, A. E. Kazdin & A. S. Bellack (Eds.), *The clinical psychology handbook* (pp. 35–56). New York: Pergamon.

Edinger, J. A. & Patterson, M. L. (1983). Nonverbal involvement and social control. *Psychological Bulletin, 93,* 30–56.

Edwards, D. J. A. (in press). Restructuring early memories through guided imagery: A contribution to cognitive therapy. In A. Freeman, H. Arkowitz, L. E. Beutler & K. Simon (Eds.). *Comprehensive handbook of cognitive therapy.* New York: Plenum.

Edwards, G. (1986). The alcohol dependence syndrome: A concept as stimulus to inquiry. *British Journal of Addiction, 81,* 171–183.

Ekman, P. (1964). Body position, facial expression and verbal behavior during interviews. *Journal of Abnormal and Social Psychology, 68,* 295–301.

Ekman, P. (Ed.). (1982). *Emotion in the human face* (2nd ed.). New York: Cambridge University Press.

Ekstein, R. & Wallerstein, R. S. (1972). *The teaching and learning of psychotherapy.* 2nd edition. New York: International University Press.

Elkin, I. (moderator) (1986, June). *NIMH treatment of depression collaborative research program: Part I.* Panel presented at the meeting of the Society for Psychotherapy Research, Wellesley, Massachusetts.

Elkin, I. E., Parloff, M. B., Hadley, S. W. & Autry, J. H. (1985). NIMH treatment of depression collaborative research program. *Archives of General Psychiatry, 42,* 305–316.

Ellenbogen, G. C. (1986). Oral sadism and the vegetarian personality. In G. C. Ellenbogen (Ed.), *Oral sadism and the vegetarian personality* (pp. 65–70). New York: Brunner/Mazel.

Elliott, R. (1985). Helpful and nonhelpful events in brief counseling interviews: An empirical taxonomy. *Journal of Counseling Psychology, 32,* 307–322.

Elliott, R., Hill, C. E., Stiles, W. B., Friedlander, M. L., Mahrer, A. R. & Margison, F. R. (1987). Primary therapist response modes: A comparison of six rating systems. *Journal of Consulting and Clinical Psychology, 55,* 218–223.

Ellsworth, P. C. (1975). Direct gaze as a social stimulus: The example of aggression. In P. Pliner, L. Krames & T. Alloway (Eds.), *Nonverbal communication of aggression* (pp. 53–76). New York: Plenum.

Ellsworth, R. (1983). Characteristics of effective treatment milieu. In J. Gunderson, O. Will & L. Mosher (Eds.), *Principles and practice of milieu therapy* (pp. 87–123). New York: Jason Aronson.

Ellsworth, R. B., Collins, J. F., Casey, N. A., Hickey, R. H., Twemlow, S. W., Schoonover, R. A., Hyer, L. & Nesselroade, J. R. (1979). Some characteristics of effective psychiatric treatment programs. *Journal of Consulting and Clinical Psychology, 47,* 799–817.

Ellsworth, R. B., Dickman, H. R. & Maroney, R. J. (1972). Characteristics of productive and unproductive unit systems in VA psychiatric hospitals. *Hospital & Community Psychiatry, 23,* 261–271.

Emmelkamp, P. (1986). Behavior therapy with adults. In S. L. Garfield & A. E. Bergin (Eds.), *Handbook of psychotherapy and behavior change,* 3rd ed. (pp. 385–442). New York: John Wiley and Sons.

Endicott, N.A. & Endicott, J. (1963). "Improvement" in untreated psychiatric patients. *Archives of General Psychiatry, 9,* 575–585.

Ersner-Hershfeld, R. & Kopel, S. (1979). Group treatment of preorgasmic women: Evaluation of partner involvement and spacing of sessions. *Journal of Consulting and Clinical Psychology, 47,* 750–759.

Exline, R. V. (1963). Explorations in the process of person perception: Visual interaction in relation to competition, sex, and need for affiliation. *Journal of Personality, 31,* 1–20.

Eysenck, H. J. & Eysenck, S. B. G. (1969). *Personality structure and measurement.* San Diego: Knapp Press.

Eysenck, H. J., Wakefield, J. A. & Friedman, A. F. (1983). Diagnosis and clinical assessment: The DSM-III. *Annual Review of Psychology, 34,* 167–193.

Fairweather, G. (Ed.) (1964). *Social psychology in treating mental illness: An experimental approach.* New York: John Wiley and Sons.

Fairweather, G., Simon, R., Gebhard, M. E., Weingarten, E., Holland, J. L., Sanders, R., Stone, G. B. & Reahl, J. E. (1960). Relative effectiveness of psychotherapeutic programs: A multicriteria comparison of four programs for three different patient groups. *Psychological Monographs: General and Applied, 74* (5, Whole No. 492).

Falloon, I. R. H. (1985). *Family management of schizophrenia.* Baltimore: Johns Hopkins University Press.

Falloon, I. R. H., Boyd, J. L. & McGill, C. W. (1984). *Family care of schizophrenia.* New York: Guilford.

Falloon, I. R. H., Boyd, J. L., McGill, C. W., Razani, J., Moos, H. B. & Gilderman, A. M. (1982). Family management in the prevention of exacerbations of schizophrenia. *New England Journal of Medicine, 306,* 1437–1440.

Fankhauser, M. P. & German, M. L. (1987). Understanding the use of behavioral rating scales in studies evaluating the efficacy of antianxiety and antidepressant drugs. *American Journal of Hospital Pharmacy, 44,* 2087–2100.

Farrell, A. D., Cjaplair, P. S. & McCullough, L. (1987). Identification of target complaints by computer interview: Evaluation of the computerized assessment system for psychotherapy evaluation and research. *Journal of Consulting and Clinical Psychology, 55,* 691–700.

Feighner, J. P., Robins, E., Guze, S. B., Woodruff, R. A., Winokur, G. & Munoz, R. (1972). Diagnostic criteria for use in psychiatric research. *Archives of General Psychiatry, 26,* 57–63.

Fiedler, F. E. (1950). The concept of an ideal therapeutic relationship. *Journal of Consulting Psychology, 14,* 239–245.

Fischer, C. S. & Oliker, S. J. (1983). A research note on friendship, gender, and the life cycle. *Social Forces, 62,* 124–133.

Fisher, D. C. (1987). Choice of therapeutic orientation and treatment effectiveness. *Psychotherapy, 24,* 260–265.

Flaherty, J. A. & Richman, J. A. (1986). Effects of childhood relationships on the adult's capacity to form social supports. *American Journal of Psychiatry, 143,* 851–855.

Fleming, J. (1953). The role of supervision in psychiatric training. *Bulletin of the Menninger Clinic, 17,* 157–169.

Fletcher, B. C. & Payne, R. L. (1980a). Stress at work: A review and theoretical framework, Part 1. *Personnel Review, 9* (1), 19–29.

Fletcher, B. C. & Payne, R. L. (1980b). Stress at work: A review and theoretical framework, Part 2. *Personnel Review, 9* (2), 5–8.

Flynn, H. & Henisz, J. (1975). Criteria for psychiatric hospitalization: Experience with a checklist for chart review. *American Journal of Psychiatry, 132,* 847–850.

Folkman, S. & Lazarus, R. S. (1980). An analysis of coping in a middle-aged community sample. *Journal of Health and Social Behavior, 21,* 219–239.

Folkman, S. & Lazarus, R. S. (1986). Stress processes and depressive symptomatology. *Journal of Abnormal Psychology, 95,* 107–113.

Foon, A. E. (1986). Locus of control and clients' expectations of psychotherapeutic outcome. *British Journal of Clinical Psychology, 25,* 161–171.

Ford, J. D. (1986). Research on training counselors and clinicians. *Review of Educational Research, 49,* 87–130.

Foreman, S. A. & Marmar, C. R. (1984, June). *Therapist actions which effectively address initial poor therapeutic alliances.* Paper presented at the Society for Psychotherapy Research, Lake Louise, Ontario, Canada.

Forer, B. R. (1969). The taboo against touching in psychotherapy. *Psychotherapy: Theory, Research and Practice, 6,* 229–231.

Forsyth, N. L. & Forsyth, D. R. (1982). Internality, controllability, and the effectiveness of attributional interpretation in counseling. *Journal of Counseling Psychology, 29,* 140–150.

Frances, A. & Clarkin, J. F. (1981). No treatment as the prescription of choice. *Archives of General Psychiatry, 38,* 542–545.

Frances, A., Clarkin, J. F. & Marachi, J. (1980). Selection criteria for group therapy. *Hospital and Community Psychiatry, 31,* 245–250.

Frances, A., Clarkin, J. & Perry, S. (1984). *Differential therapeutics in psychiatry.* New York: Brunner/Mazel.

Frank, J. D. (1973). *Persuasion and healing: A comparative study of psychotherapy* (rev. ed.). Baltimore: Johns Hopkins University Press.

Frank, J. D. (1987). Psychotherapy, rhetoric, and hermeneutics: Implications for practice and research. *Psychotherapy, 24,* 293–302.

Frankel, A. S. & Barrett, J. (1971). Variations in personal space as a function of authoritarianism, self esteem, and racial characteristics of a stimulus situation. *Journal of Consulting and Clinical Psychology, 37,* 95–98.

322   SYSTEMATIC TREATMENT SELECTION

Freebury, M. B. (1984). The prescription of psychotherapy. *Canadian Journal of Psychiatry, 29,* 499–503.

Freeman, A., Arkowitz, H., Beutler, L. E. & Simon, K. E. (Eds.). (In press). *Comprehensive handbook of cognitive therapy.* New York: Plenum.

Fremont, S. K. & Anderson, W. (1988). Investigation of factors involved in therapists' annoyance with clients. *Professional Psychology: Research and Practice, 19,* 330–335.

Fretz, B. R. (1966). Postural movements in a counseling dyad. *Journal of Counseling Psychology, 13,* 335–343.

Freud, S. (1955). The Ego and the Id. *Standard edition.* London: Hogarth Press.

Friedlander, M. L. (1982). Counseling discourse as a speech event: Revision and extension of the Hill Counselor Verbal Response Category System. *Journal of Counseling Psychology, 29.* 425–429.

Fuchs, C. Z. & Rehm, L. P. (1977). A self-control behavior therapy program for depression. *Journal of Consulting and Clinical Psychology, 45,* 206–215.

Fuhriman, A., Paul, S. C., & Burlingame, G. M. (1986). Eclectic time-limited therapy. In J. C. Norcross (Ed.), *Handbook of eclectic psychotherapy* (pp. 226–259). New York: Brunner/Mazel.

Gadow, K. D. (1985). Relative efficacy of pharmacological, behavioral, and combination treatments for enhancing academic performance. *Clinical Psychology Review, 5,* 513–533.

Gallagher, D. & Thompson, L. W. (1981). *Depression in the elderly: A behavioral treatment manual.* Los Angeles: University of Southern California Press.

Garfield, S. L. (1977). Research on the training of professional psychotherapists. In A. S. Gurman & A. M. Razin (Eds.), *Effective psychotherapy: A handbook of research* (pp. 63–83). New York: Pergamon.

Garfield, S. L. (1978). Research on client variables in psychotherapy. In S. L. Garfield & A. E. Bergin (Eds.), *Handbook of psychotherapy and behavior change,* 2nd ed. (pp. 191–232). New York: John Wiley and Sons.

Garfield, S. L. (1980). *Psychotherapy: An eclectic approach.* New York: John Wiley.

Garfield, S. L. (1986a). Problems in diagnostic classification. In T. Millon & G. L. Klerman (Eds.), *Contemporary directions in psychopathology: Toward the DSM-IV* (pp. 99–114). New York, Guilford Press.

Garfield, S. L. (1986b). Research on client variables in psychotherapy. In S. L. Garfield & A. E. Bergin (Eds.), *Handbook of psychotherapy and behavior change,* 3rd ed. (pp. 213–256). New York: John Wiley and Sons.

Garfield, S. L. & Bergin, A. E. (1986). Introduction and historical overview. In S. L. Garfield & A. E. Bergin (Eds.), *Handbook of psychotherapy and behavior change,* 3rd ed. (pp. 3–22). New York: John Wiley and Sons.

Garfield, S. L. & Kurtz, R. (1976a). Clinical psychologists in the 1970s. *American Psychologist, 31,* 1–9.

Garfield, S. L. & Kurtz, R. (1976b). Personal therapy for the psychotherapist: Some findings and issues. *Psychotherapy: Theory, Research and Practice, 13,* 188–192.

Garfield, S. L., Prager, R. A. & Begin, A. E. (1974). Some further comments on evaluation of outcome in psychotherapy. *Journal of Consulting and Clinical Psychology, 42,* 307–313.

Gaston, L., Marmar, C. R. & Ring, J. (in press). The difficult patient in cognitive therapy: Therapist and patient contributions to the therapeutic alliance. *American Journal of Psychiatry.*

Gaston, L., Marmar, C. R., Thompson, L. W. & Gallagher, D. (1988). Relation of patient pretreatment characteristics to the therapeutic alliance in diverse psychotherapies. *Journal of Consulting and Clinical Psychology, 56,* 483–489.

Gelder, M. G., Marks, I., Wolff, H. H. & Clarke, M. (1967). Desensitization and psychotherapy in the treatment of phobic states: A controlled inquiry. *British Journal of Psychiatry, 113,* 53–73.

Gendlin, E. T. (1969). Focusing. *Psychotherapy: Theory, Research, and Practice, 6,* 4–15.

Gillis, J. S. & Jessor, R. (1970). Effects of brief psychotherapy on belief in internal control: An exploratory study. *Psychotherapy: Theory, Research and Practice, 7,* 135–136.

Gillis, J. S., Lipkin, M. D., & Moran, T. J. (1981). Drug therapy decisions: A social judgement analysis. *The Journal of Nervous and Mental Disease, 169,* 439–447.

Gillis, J. S. & Moran, T. J. (1981). An analysis of drug decisions in a state psychiatric hospital. *Journal of Clinical Psychology, 37,* 32–42.

Gleser, G. C. & Ihlevich, D. (1969). An objective instrument to measure defense mechanisms. *Journal of Consulting and Clinical Psychology, 33,* 51–60.

Glick, I. D., Clarkin, J. F. & Kessler, D. R. (1987). *Marital and family therapy,* 3rd ed. New York: Grune & Stratton.

Glick, I. D. & Hargreaves, W. (1979). *Psychiatric hospital treatment for the 1980's.* Lexington, Mass.: Heath and Co.

Goldberg, A. (1973). Psychotherapy of narcissistic injuries. *Archives of General Psychiatry, 28,* 722–726.

Goldberg, D. P., Hobson, R. F., Maguire, G. P., Margison, F. R., O'Dowd, T., Osborn, M. & Moss, S. (1984). The clarification and assessment of a method of psychotherapy. *British Journal of Psychiatry, 144,* 567–580.

Goldfried, M. R. (1980). Toward the delineation of therapeutic change principles. *American Psychologist, 35,* 991–999.

Goldfried, M. R. (Ed.) (1982). *Converging themes in the practice of psychotherapy.* New York: Springer.

Goldfried, M. R. & Davison, G. C. (1976). *Clinical behavior therapy.* New York: Holt, Rinehart and Winston.

Goldfried, M. R. & Padawer, W. (1982). Current status and future directions in psychotherapy. In M. R. Goldfried (Ed.), *Converging themes in psychotherapy* (pp. 3–49). New York: Springer.

Goldstein, A. P. (1966). Psychotherapy research by extrapolation from social psychology. *Journal of Counseling Psychology, 13,* 38–45.

Goldstein, A. P. (1971). *Psychotherapeutic attraction.* New York: Pergamon.

Goldstein, A. P. (1973). *Structured learning therapy: Toward a psychotherapy for the poor.* New York: Academic Press.

Goldstein, A. P. & Stein, N. (1976). *Prescriptive psychotherapies.* New York: Pergamon Press.

Goldstein, M. J. & Strachan, A. M. (1987). The family and schizophrenia. In T. Jacob (Ed.), *Family interaction and psychopathology: Theories, methods, and findings* (pp. 481–508). New York: Plenum.

Gottlieb, B. H. (1978). The development and application of a classification scheme of informal helping behaviors. *Canadian Journal of Behavioral Science, 10,* 105–115.

Goulding, M. & Goulding, R. (1979). *Changing lives through redecision therapy.* New York: Brunner/Mazel, Inc.

Grater, H. A. (1985). Steps in psychotherapy supervision: From therapy skills to skilled therapist. *Professional Psychology: Research and Practice, 16,* 605–610.

Greenberg, L. S. (1980). Training counselors in gestalt methods. *Canadian Counselor, 14,* 174–180.

Greenberg, L. S. & Clarke, K. M. (1979). Differential effects of the two-chair experiment and empathic reflections at a conflict marker. *Journal of Counseling Psychology, 26,* 1–8.

Greenberg, L. S. & Goldman, R. L. (1988). Training in experiential therapy. *Journal of Consulting and Clinical Psychology, 56,* 696–702.

Greenberg, L. S. & Pinsoff, W. M. (1986). *The psychotherapeutic process: A research handbook.* New York: Guilford.

Greenberg, L. S. & Safran, J. (1986). *Emotion in psychotherapy.* New York: Guilford.

Greenberg, L. S. & Sarkissian, M. G. (1984). Evaluation of counselor training in gestalt methods. *Counselor Education and Supervision, 24,* 328–340.

Greene, L. R. (1976). Body image boundaries and small group seating arrangements. *Journal of Consulting and Clinical Psychology, 44,* 224–249.

Grigg, A. E. & Goodstein, L. D. (1957). The use of clients as judges of the counselor's performance. *Journal of Counseling Psychology, 4,* 31–36.

Group for the Advancement of Psychiatry (1987). *Teaching psychotherapy in contemporary psychiatric residency training.* New York: Brunner/Mazel.

Guest, P. D. & Beutler, L. E. (1988). The impact of psychotherapy supervision on therapist orientation and values. *Journal of Consulting and Clinical Psychology, 56,* 653–658.

Gunderson, J. G. (1978). Defining the therapeutic processes in psychiatric milieus. *Psychiatry, 41,* 327–335.

Gunderson, J. G. (1985). Hospital care of borderline patients. In J. G. Gunderson (Ed.), *Borderline personality disorder* (pp. 131–152). Washington DC: American Psychiatric Press.

Gurel, L. (1964). *An assessment of psychiatric hospital effectiveness* (intramural report 64–5). Washington DC: Veterans Administration.

Gurman, A. S. (1977). Therapist and patient factors influencing the patient's perception of facilitative therapeutic conditions. *Psychiatry, 40,* 16–24.

Gurman, A. S. (1981). Integrative marital therapy: Toward the development of an interpersonal approach. In S. H. Budman (Ed.), *Forms of brief therapy* (pp. 415–457). New York: Guilford Press.

Gurman, A. S., Kniskern, D. P. & Pinsof, W. M. (1986). Research on marital and family therapies. In S. L. Garfield & A. E. Bergin (Eds.), *Handbook of psychotherapy and behavior change* (pp. 565–624). New York: John Wiley.

Guy, W., Gross, M., Hogarty, G. & Dennis, H. (1969). A controlled evaluation of day hospital effectiveness. *Archives of General Psychiatry, 20,* 329–338.

Haas, G. L. & Clarkin, J. F. (1987). Differential therapeutics and treatment format. In R. E. Hales & A. J. Frances (Eds.), *American Psychiatric Association: Annual Review,* Vol. 6 (pp. 353–377). Washington DC: American Psychiatric Press.

Haase, R. F. & Tepper, D. T., Jr. (1972). Nonverbal components of empathic communication. *Journal of Counseling Psychology, 19,* 417–424.

Hadley, S. W. & Autry, J. H. (1984). DSM-III and psychotherapy. In S. Turner & M. Hersen (Eds.), *Adult psychopathology and diagnosis* (pp. 465–484). New York: John Wiley.

Hafner, R. J. & Ross, M. W. (1984). Agoraphobia in women: Factor analysis of symptoms and personality correlates of factor scores in a clinical population. *Behavior Research and Therapy, 22,* 441–445.

Hafner, R. R. (1979). Agoraphobic women married to abnormally jealous men. *British Journal of Medical Psychology, 52,* 99–104.

Hahlweg, K. & Goldstein, M. J. (Eds.) (1987) *Understanding major mental disorder: The contribution of family interaction research.* New York: Family Process Press.

Haley, J. (1973). *Uncommon therapy: The psychiatric techniques of Milton H. Erickson, M.D.* New York: Norton.

Haley, J. (1984). *Ordeal therapy: Unusual ways to change behavior.* San Francisco: Jossey-Bass.

Halgin, R. P. (1985). Teaching integration of psychotherapy models to beginning therapists. *Psychotherapy, 22,* 555–563.

Halgin, R. P. (Ed.) (1988). Special section: Issues in the supervision of integrative psychotherapy. *Journal of Integrative and Eclectic Psychotherapy, 7,* 152–180.

Halleck, S. L. (1978). *The treatment of emotional disorders.* New York: Jason Aronson.

Hamblin, D. L., Beutler, L. E., Scogin, F. R. & Corbishley, A. (1988, June). *Patient responsiveness to therapist values and outcome in group cognitive therapy.* Paper presented at the annual meeting of the Society for Psychotherapy Research, Santa Fe, N.M.

Hamilton, D. (1969). Responses to cognitive inconsistencies: Personality, discrepancy level, and response stability. *Journal of Personality and Social Psychology, 11,* 351–362.

Hamilton, E. W. & Abramson, L. Y. (1983). Cognitive patterns and major depressive disorder: A longitudinal study in a hospital setting. *Journal of Abnormal Psychology, 92,* 173–184.

Hamilton, M. (1967). Development of a rating scale for primary depressive illness. *British Journal of Social and Clinical Psychology, 6,* 278–296.

Handley, P. (1982). Relationship between supervisors' and trainees' cognitive styles and the supervision process. *Journal of Counseling Psychology, 29,* 508–515.

Harding, C. M. & Strauss, J. S. (1984). How serious is schizophrenia? Comments on prognosis. *Biological Psychiatry, 19,* 1597–1600.

Harding, C. M. & Strauss, J. S. (1985). The course of schizophrenia: An evolving concept. In M. Alpert (Ed.), *Controversies in schizophrenic changes and constancies* (pp. 339–350). New York: Guilford Press.

Hardy, G. E. & Shapiro, D. A. (1985). Therapist response modes in prescriptive vs. exploratory psychotherapy. *British Journal of Clinical Psychology, 24,* 235–245.

Harper, R. G., Wiens, A. N. & Matararazzo, J. D. (1978). *Non-verbal communications: The state of the art.* New York: John Wiley & Sons.

Hart, G. M. (1982). *The process of clinical supervision.* Baltimore: University Park Press.

Harvey, J. H. & Weary, G. (Eds.) (1985). *Attribution: Basic issues and applications.* Orlando, FL: Academic Press.

Hassenfeld, I. & Sarris, J. (1978). Hazards and horizons of psychotherapy supervision. *American Journal of Psychotherapy, 32,* 393–401.

Hatcher, S. L., Huebner, D. A. & Zakin, D. F. (1986). Following the trail of the focus in time-limited psychotherapy. *Psychotherapy, 23,* 513–520.

Hautzinger, M., Linden, M. & Hoffman, N. (1982). Distressed couples with and without a depressed partner: An analysis of their verbal interaction. *Journal of Behavior Therapy and Experimental Psychiatry, 13,* 307–314.

Hay, W. & Nathan, P. E. (Eds.) (1982). *Clinical case studies in behavioral treatment of alcoholism.* New York: Plenum.

Hazelrigg, M. D., Cooper, H. M. & Borduin, C. M. (1987). Evaluating the effectiveness of family therapies: An integrative review and analysis. *Psychological Bulletin, 101,* 428–442.

Heide, F. J. & Borkovec, T. D. (1983). Relaxation-induced anxiety: Paradoxical anxiety enhancement due to relaxation training. *Journal of Consulting and Clinical Psychology, 51,* 171–182.

Heinrichs, D. W. & Carpenter, W. T., Jr. (1983). The coordination of family therapy with other treatment modalities for schizophrenia. In W. R. McFarlane (Ed.), *Family therapy in schizophrenia* (pp. 267–287). New York: Guilford.

Heitler, J. B. (1976). Preparatory techniques in initiating expressive psychotherapy with lower-class, unsophisticated patients. *Psychological Bulletin, 83,* 339–352.

Hellman, I. D., Morrison, T. L. & Abramowitz, S. I. (1987). Therapist flexibility/rigidity and work stress. *Professional Psychology, 18,* 21–27.

Henry, W. E., Sims, J. H. & Spray, S. L. (1973). *Public and private lives of psychotherapists.* San Francisco: Jossey-Bass.

Heppner, P. P. & Dixon, D. N. (1981). A review of the interpersonal influence process in counseling. *Personnel and Guidance Journal, 59,* 542–550.

Heppner, P. P. & Heesacker, M. (1982). Interpersonal influence process in real-life counseling: Investigating client perceptions, counselor experience level, and counselor power over time. *Journal of Counseling Psychology, 29,* 215–223.

Heppner, P. P. & Heesacker, M. (1983). Perceived counselor characteristics, client expectations, and client satisfaction with counseling. *Journal of Counseling Psychology, 30,* 32–39.

Heppner, P. P. & Roehlke, H. J. (1984). Difference among supervisees at different levels of training: Implications for a developmental model of supervision. *Journal of Counseling Psychology*, *31*, 76–90.

Hepworth, S. J. (1980). Moderating factors of the psychological impact of unemployment. *Journal of Occupational Psychology*, *53*, 139–145.

Herbert, D. L., Nelson, R. O. & Herbert, J. D. (1988). Effects of psychodiagnostic labels, depression severity, and instruction on assessment. *Professional Psychology: Research and Practice*, *19*, 496–502.

Hermansson, G. L., Webster, A. C. & McFarland, K. (1988). Counselor deliberate postural lean and communication of facilitative conditions. *Journal of Counseling Psychology*, *35*, 149–153.

Herz, M., Endicott, J. & Spitzer, R. (1976). Brief versus standard hospitalization: The families. *American Journal of Psychiatry*, *133*, 795–801.

Herz, M., Endicott, J., Spitzer, R. & Mesnikoff, A. (1971). Day versus inpatient hospitalization: A controlled study. *American Journal of Psychiatry*, *127*, 1371–1382.

Hess, A. K. (Ed.). (1980), *Psychotherapy supervision*. New York: John Wiley.

Hess, A. K. (1980). Training models and the nature of psychotherapy supervision. In A.K. Hess (Ed.), *Psychotherapy supervision* (pp. 15–25). New York: Wiley.

Hess, A. K. (1987). Advances in psychotherapy supervision: Introduction. *Professional Psychology: Research and Practice*, *18*, 187–188.

Higbee, K. L. (1969). Fifteen years of fear arousal: Research on threat appeals: 1953–1968. *Psychological Bulletin*, *72*, 426–444.

Hill, C. E. (1978). The development of a system for classifying counselor responses. *Journal of Counseling Psychology*, *25*, 461–468.

Hill, C. E., Helms, J. E., Spiegel, S. B. & Tichenor, V. (1988). Development of a system for categorizing client reactions to therapist interventions. *Journal of Counseling Psychology*, *35*, 27–36.

Hill, J. A., Howard, K. I. & Orlinsky, D. E. (1970). The therapist's experience of psychotherapy: Some dimensions and determinants. *Multivariate Behavioral Research*, *5*, 435–451.

Hobson, R. R. (1985). *Forms of feeling*. London: Tavistock.

Hodgson, R. & Stockwell, T. (1985). The theoretical and empirical basis of the alcohol dependence model: A social learning perspective. In N. Heather, I. Robertson & P. Davies (Eds.), *The misuse of alcohol* (pp. 17–34). London: Groom Helm.

Hoehn-Saric, R., Frank, J. D., Imber, S. D., Nash, E. H., Stone, A. R., & Battle, C. C. (1964). Systematic preparation of patients for psychotherapy: I. Effects of therapy on behavior and outcome. *Journal of Psychiatric Research*, *2*, 267–281.

Hogan, R. A. (1964). Issues and approaches in supervision. *Psychotherapy: Theory, Research, and Practice*, *1*, 139–141.

Holliday, P. B. (1979). Effects of preparation for therapy on client expectations and participation. *Dissertation Abstracts International*, *39*, 3517B.

Holroyd, J. C. & Brodsky, A. M. (1980). Does touching patients lead to sexual intercourse? *Professional Psychology*, *11*, 807–811.

Holt, R. R. (1982). Occupational stress. In L. Goldberger and S. Breznitz (Eds.),

Handbook of stress: Theoretical and clinical aspects (pp. 419–444). New York: Free Press.

Hooley, J. M. (1986). Expressed emotion and depression: Interactions between patients and high versus low EE spouses. *Journal of Abnormal Psychology, 95,* 237–246.

Hooley, J. M. & Teasdale, J. D. (in press). Predictors of relapse in unipolar depressives: Expressed emotion, marital quality and perceived criticism. *Journal of Consulting and Clinical Psychology.*

Horgan, C. M. (1985). Specialty and general ambulatory mental health services. *Archives of General Psychiatry, 42,* 565–572.

Horn-George, J. B. & Anchor, K. N. (1982). Perceptions of the psychotherapy relationship in long- versus short-term therapy. *Professional Psychology, 13,* 483–491.

Horowitz, L. M., Rosenberg, S. E., Ureno, G., Kalehzan, M. & Halloran, P. (1988). The psychodynamic formulation, the modal response method and interpersonal problems. Manuscript in preparation.

Horowitz, L. M. & Vitkus, J. (1986). The interpersonal basis of psychiatric symptoms. *Clinical Psychology Review, 6,* 443–469.

Horowitz, M. (1976). *Stress response syndromes.* New York: Jason Aronson.

Horowitz, M., Marmar, C., Krupnick, J., Wilner, N., Kaltreider, N. & Wallerstein, R. (1984). *Personality styles and brief psychotherapy.* New York: Basic Books, Inc.

Horwitz, A. (1977). Social networks and pathways to psychiatric treatment. *Social Forces, 56,* 86–105.

Houston, B. K. (1972). Control over stress, locus of control and response to stress. *Journal of Personality and Social Psychology, 21,* 249–255.

Howard, K. I. (1988, June). *The psychotherapeutic service delivery system.* A paper presented at the annual meeting of the Society for Psychotherapy Research, Santa Fe, N.M.

Howard, K. I., Kopta, S. Krause, M. & Orlinsky, D. (1986). The dose-effect relationship in psychotherapy. *American Psychologist, 41,* 159–164.

Howard, K. I., Rickels, K., Mock, J. E., Lipman, R. S., Covi, L. & Baumm, N. C. (1970). Therapeutic style and attrition rate from psychiatric drug treatment. *Journal of Nervous and Mental Disease, 150,* 102–110.

Hubble, M. A., Noble, F. C. & Robinson, S. E. (1981). The effect of counselor touch in the initial counseling session. *Journal of Counseling Psychology, 28,* 533–535.

Hughes, J. & Goldman, M. (1978). Eye contact, facial expression, sex, and the violation of personal space. *Perceptual and Motor Skills, 46,* 579–584.

Hunt, D. E. & Sullivan, E. V. (1974). *Between psychology and education.* Hinsdale, IL: Dryden.

Ittelson, W. H., Proshansky, H. M. & Rivlin, L. G. (1970). Bedroom size and social interaction. *Environment and Behavior, 2,* 255–270.

Ittelson, W. H., Proshansky, H. M. & Rivlin, L. G. (1972). Bedroom size and social interaction of the psychiatric ward. In J. Wohlwill & D. Carson (Eds.),

Environment and the social sciences (pp. 95–104). Washington, DC: American Psychological Association.

Ivey, A. E. & Authier, J. (1978). *Microcounseling,* 2nd ed. Springfield: IL: Charles C. Thomas.

Jacob, T. (1987). *Family interaction and psychopathology: Theories, methods, and findings.* New York: Plenum.

Jacob, T. & Leonard, K. E. (1988). Alcoholic-spouse interaction as a function of alcoholism subtype and alcohol consumption interaction. *Journal of Abnormal Psychology, 97,* 231–237.

Jacobs, M. K., Trick, O. L. & Withersty, D. (1976). Pretraining psychiatric inpatients for participation in group psychotherapy. *Psychotherapy: Theory, Research, and Practice, 13,* 361–367.

Jacobson, G. F., Wilner, D. M., Morley, W., Schneider, S., Strickler, M. & Sommer, G. (1965). The scope and practice of an early-access brief treatment psychiatric center. *American Journal of Psychiatry, 121,* 1176–1182.

Jacobson, N. S. (1988, August). *Efficacy of Psychotherapy: Fact or Fiction?* A paper presented at the annual meeting of the American Psychological Association, Atlanta, Ga.

Jacobson, N. S., Follette, W. C. & Pagel, M. (1986). Predicting who will benefit from behavioral marital therapy. *Journal of Consulting and Clinical Psychology, 54,* 518–522.

Jacobson, N. S. & Margolin, G. (1979). *Marital therapy: Strategies based on several learning and behavior exchange principles.* New York: Brunner/Mazel.

Jacobson, N. S., Schmaling, K. B., Salusky, S., Follette, V. & Dobson, K. (1987, November). Marital therapy as an adjunct treatment for depression. Paper presented at the annual meeting of the Association for the Advancement of Behavior Therapy, Boston, MA.

Jarrett, R. B. & Rush, A. J. (1987). Psychotherapeutic approaches for depression. In R. Michels & J. O. Cavenar, Jr. (Eds.), *Psychiatry,* Vol. 1 (pp. 1–35).

Johnson, S. M. & Greenberg, L. S. (1985). Differential effects of experiential and problem-solving interventions in resolving marital conflict. *Journal of Consulting and Clinical Psychology, 53,* 175–184.

Jones, E. E. (1978). Effects of race on psychotherapy process and outcome: An exploratory investigation. *Psychotherapy: Theory, Research and Practice, 15,* 226–236.

Jones, E. E., Cumming, J. D. & Horowitz, M. J. (1988). Another look at the nonspecific hypothesis of therapeutic effectiveness. *Journal of Consulting and Clinical Psychology, 56,* 48–55.

Jones, E. E., Krupnick, J. L. & Kerig, P. K. (1987). Some gender effects in brief psychotherapy. *Psychotherapy, 24,* 336–352.

Kagan, N. (1980). Influencing human interaction: Eighteen years with IPR. In A. K. Hess (Ed.), *Psychotherapy supervision* (pp. 262–283). New York: Wiley.

Kalafat, J. & Neigher, W. D. (1983). Can quality survive in public mental health programs? The challenge for training. *Professional Psychology, 14,* 90–104.

Kaplan, H. (1974). *The new sex therapy.* New York: Brunner/Mazel.

Karasek, R. A. (1979). Job demands, job decision latitude, and mental strain: Implications for job redesign. *Administrative Science Quarterly, 24,* 285–308.

Kasl, S. V. (1978). Epidemiological contributions to the study of work stress. In C. L. Cooper & R. L. Payne (Eds.), *Stress at work* (pp. 3–48). London: John Wiley and Sons.

Kaul, T. & Bednar, R. (1986). Research on group and related therapies. In S. Garfield & A. E. Bergin (Eds.), *Handbook of psychotherapy and behavior change,* 3rd ed. (pp. 671–714). New York: John Wiley and Sons.

Kazdin, A. E. (1981). Drawing valid inferences from case studies. *Journal of Consulting and Clinical Psychology, 41,* 183–192.

Kazdin, A. E. (1982). *Single-case research designs: Methods for clinical and applied settings.* New York: Oxford University Press.

Kazdin, A. E. (1984). Statistical analyses for single-case experimental designs. In D. H. Barlow & M. Hersen (Eds.), *Single-case experimental designs: Strategies for studying behavior change,* 2nd ed. (pp. 285–394). New York: Pergamon.

Kellam, S. G., Goldberg, S. C. & Schooler, N. (1967). Ward atmosphere and outcome of treatment of acute schizophrenia. *Journal of Psychiatric Research, 5,* 145–163.

Kendell, R. E., Brockington, I. F. & Leff, J. P. (1979). Prognostic implications of six alternative definitions of schizophrenia. *Archives of General Psychiatry, 36,* 25–31.

Kernberg, O. F. (1984). *Severe personality disorders: Psychotherapeutic strategies.* New Haven: Yale University Press.

Kernberg, O. F., Selzer, M., Koenigsberg, H., Carr, A. & Appelbaum, A. (1989) *Psychodynamic psychotherapy of borderline patients.* New York: Basic Books.

Kerr, B. A. & Dell, D. M. (1976). Perceived interviewer expertness and attractiveness: Effects of interviewer behavior and attire and interview setting. *Journal of Counseling Psychology, 23,* 553–556.

Kessler, R. C., Price, R. H. & Wortman, C. B. (1985). Social factors in psychopathology: Stress, social support and coping processes. In M. R. Rosenzweig & L. W. Porter (Eds.), *Annual review of psychology* (Vol. 36, pp. 531–572). Palo Alto, CA: Annual Reviews.

Kiesler, C. (1982). Mental hospitals and alternative care: Non-institutionalization as potential public policy for mental patients. *American Psychologist, 37,* 349–360.

Kiesler, D. J. (1966). Some myths of psychotherapy research and the search for a paradigm. *Psychological Bulletin, 65,* 110–136.

Kimble, C. E., Forte, R. A. & Yoshikawa, J. C. (1981). Nonverbal concomitants of enacted emotional intensity and positivity: Visual and vocal behavior. *Journal of Personality, 49,* 271–283.

Kingsley, R. G. & Wilson, G. T. (1977). Behavior therapy for obesity: A comparative investigation of long-term efficacy. *Journal of Consulting and Clinical Psychology, 45,* 288–298.

Kirschenbaum, D. S. & Flanery, R. C. (1984). Toward a psychology of behavioral contracting. *Clinical Psychology Review, 4,* 597–618.

Kirshner, L. A., Genack, A. & Hauser, S. T. (1978). Effects of gender on short-term psychotherapy. *Psychotherapy: Theory, Research and Practice, 15,* 158–167.

Klar, H., Frances, A. & Clarkin, J. F. (1982). Selection criteria for partial hospitalization. *Hospital and Community Psychiatry, 33,* 929–933.

Klein, D. F., Gittelman, R., Quitkin, F. & Rifkin, A. (1980). *Diagnosis and drug treatment of psychiatric disorders: Adults and children,* 2nd ed. Baltimore, MD: Williams & Wilkins.

Klein, D. N. (1982). Relation between current diagnostic criteria for schizophrenia and the dimensions of premorbid adjustment, paranoid symptomatology, and chronicity. *Journal of Abnormal Psychology, 91,* 319–325.

Kleinke, C. L. (1986). Gaze and eye contact: A research review. *Psychological Bulletin, 100,* 78–100.

Klerman, G. L. (1986). Drugs and psychotherapy. In S. L. Garfield & A. E. Bergin (Eds.), *Handbook of psychotherapy and behavior change,* 3rd ed. (pp. 777–818). New York: John Wiley.

Klerman, G. L. (1983). The efficacy of psychotherapy as the basis for public policy. *American Psychologist, 38,* 929–934.

Klerman, G. L., DiMascio, A., Weissman, M. M., Prusoff, B. & Paykel, E. S. (1974). Treatment of depression by drugs and psychotherapy. *American Journal of Psychiatry, 131,* 186–191.

Klerman, G. L., Weissman, M. M., Rounsaville, B. J. & Chevron, E. S. (1984). *Interpersonal psychotherapy of depression.* New York: Basic Books, Inc.

Koenigsberg, H. W., Kernberg, O. F., Haas, G., Lotterman, A., Rockland, L. & Selzer, M. (1985). Development of a scale for measuring techniques in the psychotherapy of borderline patients. *The Journal of Nervous and Mental Disease, 173,* 424–431.

Kohut, H. (1977). *The restoration of the self.* New York: International Universities Press.

Kohut, H. (1984). *How does analysis cure?* Chicago: University of Chicago Press.

Kolb, D. L., Beutler, L. E., Davis, C. S., Crago, M. & Shanfield, S. (1985). Patient personality, locus of control, involvement, therapy relationship, dropout and change in psychotherapy. *Psychotherapy: Theory, Research and Practice, 22,* 702–710.

Kolb, L. C. (1968). *Noyes' modern clinical psychiatry,* 7th ed. Philadelphia: W. B. Saunders Co.

Korman, M. (1974). National conference on level and patterns of professional training in psychology: The major themes. *American Psychologist, 29,* 441–449.

Koss, M. P. (1979). Length of psychotherapy for clients seen in private practice. *Journal of Consulting and Clinical Psychology, 47,* 210–212.

Koss, M. P. & Butcher, J. N. (1986). Research on brief psychotherapy. In S. L. Garfield & A. E. Bergin (Eds.), *Handbook of psychotherapy and behavior change,* 3rd ed. (pp. 627–670). New York: John Wiley and Sons.

Kovacs, M. (1980). The efficacy of cognitive and behavior therapies for depression. *American Journal of Psychiatry, 137,* 1495–1501.

Kovacs, M. (1983). Psychotherapies for depression. In L. Grinspoon (Ed.), *Psychi-*

atry update, Vol. 2 (pp. 511–528). Washington, DC: American Psychiatric Press.

Kovacs, M., Rush, A. J., Beck, A. T. & Hollon, S. D. (1981). Depressed outpatients treated with cognitive therapy or pharmacotherapy: A one-year follow-up. *Archives of General Psychiatry, 38,* 33–39.

Krause, N. (1986). Stress and coping: Reconceptualizing the role of locus of control beliefs. *Journal of Gerontology, 41,* 617–622.

Lachman, M. E. (1986). Locus of control in aging research: A case for multidimensional and domain-specific assessment. *Journal of Psychology and Aging, 1,* 34–40.

LaCrosse, M. B. (1980). Perceived counselor social influence and counseling outcomes: Validity of the Counselor Rating Form. *Journal of Counseling Psychology, 27,* 320–327.

Lambert, M. J. (1980). Research and the supervisory process. In A. K. Hess (Ed.), *Psychotherapy supervision* (pp. 423–450). New York: John Wiley.

Lambert, M. J. & Arnold, R. C. (1987). Research and the supervisory process. *Professional Psychology: Research and Practice, 18,* 217–224.

Lambert, M. J. & Bergin, A. E. (1983). Therapist characteristics and their contribution to psychotherapy outcome. In C. E. Walker (Ed.), *The handbook of clinical psychology,* Vol. 1 (pp. 205–241). Homewood, IL: Dow Jones-Irwin.

Lambert, M. J., Christensen, E. R. & DeJulio, S. S. (Eds.) (1983). *The assessment of psychotherapy outcome.* New York: John Wiley.

Lambert, M. J. & DeJulio, S. S. (1978, March). *The relative importance of client, therapist and technique variables as predictors of psychotherapy outcome: The place of "nonspecific" factors.* Paper presented at the mid-winter meeting of the Division of Psychotherapy, American Psychological Association.

Lambert, M. J., Shapiro, D. A., & Bergin, A. E. (1986). The effectiveness of psychotherapy. In S. L. Garfield & A. E. Bergin (Eds.), *Handbook of psychotherapy and behavior change,* 3rd ed. (pp. 157–211). New York: John Wiley and Sons.

Langer, E. J. & Abelson, R. P. (1974). A patient by any other name...: Clinician group difference in labeling bias. *Journal of Consulting and Clinical Psychology, 42,* 4–9.

Larson, D. G. (1980). Therapeutic styles and schoolism: A national survey. *Journal of Humanistic Psychology, 20,* 3–20.

Larson, V. A. (1987). An exploration of psychotherapeutic resonance. *Psychotherapy, 24,* 321–324.

LaTorre, R. A. (1977). Pretherapy role induction procedures. *Canadian Psychological Review, 18,* 308–321.

Lawton, M. P. & Cohen, J. (1975). Organizational studies of mental hospitals. In M. Guttentag & E. L. Struening (Eds.), *Handbook of evaluation.* Beverly Hills, CA: Sage.

Lazarus, A. A. (1967). In support of technical eclecticism. *Psychological Bulletin, 21,* 415–416.

Lazarus, A. A. (1971). *Behavior therapy and beyond.* New York: McGraw-Hill.

Lazarus, A. A. (1976). *Multimodal behavior therapy.* New York: Springer.

Lazarus, A. A. (1981). *The practice of multimodal therapy.* New York: McGraw-Hill.

Lazarus, R. S. (in press). Constructs of the mind in mental health and psychotherapy. In A. Freeman, H. Arkowitz, L. E. Beutler & K. Simon (Eds.), *Comprehensive handbook of cognitive therapy*. New York: Plenum.

Lazarus, R. S. & Folkman, S. (1984). *Stress, appraisal, and coping*. New York: Springer.

Leeman, C. P. (1986). The therapeutic milieu and its role in clinical management. In L. I. Sederer (Ed.), *Inpatient psychiatry: Diagnosis and treatment*, 2nd ed. (pp. 219–239). Baltimore: Williams & Wilkins.

Lefcourt, H. M. (1980). Personality and locus of control. In J. Garber & M. E. P. Seligman (Eds.), *Human helplessness: Theory and applications* (pp. 245–259). New York: Academic Press.

Leff, J., Kuipers, L., Berkowitz, R., Eberlein-Vries, R. & Sturgeon, D. (1982). A controlled trial of social intervention in the families of schizophrenic patients. *British Journal of Psychiatry, 141,* 121–134.

Leff, J. & Vaughn, C. (1985). *Expressed emotion in families*. New York: Guilford Press.

Levenson, A. J., Lord, C. J., Sermas, C. E., Thornby, J. I., Sullender, W., & Comstock, B. A. (1977, April). Acute schizophrenia: An efficacious outpatient treatment approach as an alternative to full-time hospitalization. *Diseases of the Nervous System,* 242–245.

Lewin, K. (1947). Frontiers in group dynamics. *Human Relations, 1,* 5.

Lewinsohn, P. M., Biglan, T. & Zeiss, A. (1976). Behavioral treatment of depression. In P. Davidson (Ed.), *The behavior management of anxiety, depression and pain*. New York: Brunner/Mazel.

Lewinsohn, P. M., Steinmetz, J. L., Larson, D. W. & Franklin, J. (1981). Depression-related cognitions: Antecedent or consequences? *Journal of Abnormal Psychology, 90,* 213–219.

Lewis, K. N. (1983, August). *The impact of religious affiliation on therapists' judgments of clients*. Paper presented at the American Psychological Association Convention, Anaheim, CA.

Lewis, J. M. & Usdin, G. (Eds.) (1982). *Treatment planning in psychiatry*. Washington, DC: American Psychiatric Association.

Lieberman, M. A. & Videka-Sherman, L. (1986). The impact of self-help groups on the mental health of widows and widowers. *American Journal of Orthopsychiatry, 56,* 435–449.

Lieberman, M. A., Yalom, I. D. & Miles, M. B. (1973). *Encounter groups: First facts*. New York: Basic Books, Inc.

Linehan, M. M. (1981). A social-behavioral analysis of suicide and parasuicide: Implications for clinical assessment and treatment. In J. F. Clarkin & H. I. Glazer (Eds.), *Depression: Behavioral and directive intervention strategies* (pp. 229–294). New York: Garland STPM Press.

Linehan, M. M. (1987). Dialectical behavioral therapy: A cognitive behavioral approach to parasuicide. *Journal of Personality Disorders, 1,* 328–333.

Linn, L. S. (1970). Measuring the effectiveness of mental hospitals. *Hospital & Community Psychiatry, 21,* 381–386.

Linn, M., Caffey, E., Klett, J., Hogarty, C. & Lamb, H. R. (1979). Day treatment and psychotropic drugs in the aftercare of schizophrenic patients. *Archives of General Psychiatry, 36,* 1055–1056.

Loevinger, J. (1966). The meaning and measurement of ego development. *American Psychologist, 21,* 195–206.

Loganbill, C., Hardy, E., & Delworth, U. (1982). Supervision: A conceptual model. *The Counseling Psychologist, 10,* 3–42.

London, P. (1986). *The modes and morals of psychotherapy,* 2nd ed. Washington, DC: Hemisphere Publishing Co.

Longabaugh, R., Stout, R., Kriebel, G., McCullough, L. & Bishop, D. (1986). DSM-III and clinically identified problems as a guide to treatment. *Archives of General Psychiatry, 43,* 1097–1103.

Lopez, S. & Nuñez, J. A. (1987). Cultural factors considered in selected diagnostic criteria and interview schedules. *Journal of Abnormal Psychology, 96,* 270–272.

LoPiccolo, J. & Lobitz, W. C. (1973). Behavior therapy of sexual dysfunction. In L. A. Hamerlynck, L. C. Handy & E. J. Mash (Eds.), *Behavior change: Methodology, concepts and practice.* Champaign, IL: Research Press.

Lorion, R. P. (1973). Socioeconomic status and traditional treatment approaches reconsidered. *Psychological Bulletin, 79,* 263–270.

Lorion, R. P. & Felner, R. D. (1986). Research on psychotherapy with the disadvantaged. In S. L. Garfield & A. E. Bergin (Eds.), *Handbook of psychotherapy and behavior change,* 3rd ed. (pp. 739–776). New York: John Wiley and Sons.

Luborsky, L. (1971). Perennial mystery of poor agreement among criteria for psychotherapy outcome. *Journal of Consulting and Clinical Psychology, 37,* 316–319.

Luborsky, L. (1984). *Principles of psychoanalytic psychotherapy: A manual for supportive-expressive treatment.* New York: Basic Books, Inc.

Luborsky, L., Crits-Christoph, P., Alexander, L., Margolis, M. & Cohen, M. (1983). Two helping alliance methods for predicting outcomes of psychotherapy: A counting signs vs. a global rating method. *Journal of Nervous and Mental Disease, 171,* 480–491.

Luborsky, L., Crits-Christoph, P., McLellan, A. T., Woody, G., Piper, W., Liberman, B., Imber, S. & Pilkonis, P. (1986). Do therapists vary much in their success? Findings from four outcome studies. *American Journal of Orthopsychiatry, 56,* 501–512.

Luborsky, L. & DeRubeis, R. J. (1984). The use of psychotherapy treatment manuals: A small revolution in psychotherapy research style. *Clinical Psychology Review, 4,* 5–14.

Luborsky, L., McLellan, A. T., Woody, G. E., O'Brien, C. P. & Auerbach, A. (1985). Therapist success and its determinants. *Archives of General Psychiatry, 42,* 602–611.

Luborsky, L., Mintz, J., Auerbach, A., Crits-Christoph, P., Bachrach, H., Todd, T., Johnson, M., Cohen, M. & O'Brien, C. P. (1980). Predicting the outcome of psychotherapy: Findings of the Penn Psychotherapy Project. *Archives of General Psychiatry, 37,* 471–481.

Luborsky, L., Singer, B. & Luborsky, L. (1975). Comparative studies of psychotherapies. *Archives of General Psychiatry, 32,* 995–1008.

Madanes, C. (1981). *Strategic family therapy.* San Francisco: Jossey-Bass.

Mahoney, M. J. (1986). The tyranny of technique. *Counseling and Values, 30,* 169–174.

Mahrer, A. R. (1983). *Taxonomy of procedures and operations in psychotherapy.* Unpublished manuscript, School of Psychology, University of Ottawa, Canada I1N 6N5.

Mahrer, A. R. (1986). *Therapeutic experiencing: The process of change.* New York: W. W. Norton & Co.

Malan, D. H. (1963). *A study of brief psychotherapy.* New York: Plenum.

Malan, D. H. (1976). *Toward the validation of dynamic psychotherapy.* New York: Plenum.

Mann, B. & Murphy, K. C. (1975). Timing of self-disclosure, reciprocity of self-disclosure, and reactions to initial interview. *Journal of Counseling Psychology, 22,* 304–308.

Mann, J. (1973). *Time-limited psychotherapy.* Cambridge, MA: Harvard University Press.

Marks, I. (1985). *Fears, phobias, rituals.* New York: Oxford University Press.

Marlatt, G. A., Baer, J. S., Donovan, D. M. & Kivlahan, D. R. (1988). Addictive behavior: Etiology and treatment. *Annual Review of Psychology, 39,* 223–252.

Marlatt, G. A. & George, W. H. (1984). Relapse prevention: Introduction and overview of the model. *British Journal of Addictions, 79,* 261–273.

Marlatt, G. A. & Gordon, J. R. (1985). *Relapse prevention: Maintenance strategies in the treatment of addictive behaviors.* New York: Guilford.

Marsden, D. & Duff, E. (1975). *Workless: Some unemployed men and their families.* Penguin: Harmondsworth.

Marshall, W. L. & Barbaree, H. E. (1984). Disorders of personality, impulse, and adjustment. In S. M. Turner & M. Hersen (Eds.), *Adult psychopathology and diagnosis* (pp. 406–449). New York: John Wiley.

Martelli, M. F., Auerbach, S. M., Alexander, J., & Mercuri, L. G. (1987). Stress management in the health care setting: Matching interventions with patient coping styles. *Journal of Consulting and Clinical Psychology, 55,* 201–207.

Martin, P. J. (1975). Prognostic expectations and treatment outcome. *Journal of Consulting and Clinical Psychology, 43,* 572–576.

Martin, P. J., Moore, J. E. & Sterne, A. L. (1977). Therapists as prophets: Their expectancies and treatment outcome. *Psychotherapy: Theory, Research and Practice, 14,* 188–195.

Martin, P. J., Sterne, A. L. & Hunter, M. L. (1976). Share and share alike: Mutuality of expectations and satisfaction with therapy. *Journal of Clinical Psychology, 32,* 677–683.

Matarazzo, R. G. & Patterson, D. (1986). Research on the teaching and learning of therapeutic skills. In S. L. Garfield & A. E. Bergin (Eds.), *Handbook of psychotherapy and behavior change* (pp. 821–843). New York: John Wiley.

Mattes, J., Klein, D., Millan, D. & Rosen, B. (1979). Comparison of the clinical effectiveness of "short" versus "long" stay psychiatric hospitalization. IV. Predictors of differential benefit. *Journal of Nervous and Mental Disease, 167,* 175–181.

Maurer, R. E. & Tyndall, J. H. (1983). Effect of postural congruence on client's perception of counselor empathy. *Journal of Counseling Psychology, 30,* 158–163.

Mavissakalian, M. (1988, June). *The mutual potentiating effects of imipramine and exposure in agoraphobia.* A paper presented at the annual meeting of the Society for Psychotherapy Research, Santa Fe, NM.

Mayerson, N. H. (1984). Preparing clients for group therapy: A critical review and theoretical formulation. *Clinical Psychology Review, 4,* 191–213.

McConnaughy, E. A. (1987). The person of the therapist in psychotherapeutic practice. *Psychotherapy, 24,* 303–314.

McCrady, B. S. (1985). Alcoholism. In D. H. Barlow (Ed.), *Clinical handbook of psychological disorders* (pp. 245–298). New York: Guilford.

McCrady, B. S., Noel, N. E., Abrams, D. B., Stout, R. L., Nelson, H. F. & Hay, W. M. (1986). Comparative effectiveness of three types of spouse involvement in outpatient behavioral alcoholism treatment. *Journal of Studies in Alcoholism, 47,* 459–467.

McCullough, L., Farrell, A. D. & Longabaugh, R. (1986). The development of a microcomputer-based mental health information system. *American Psychologist, 41,* 207–214.

McFarlane, W. R. & Beels, C. C. (1983). A decision-tree for integrating family therapies for schizophrenia. In W. R. McFarlane (Ed.), *Family therapy in schizophrenia* (pp. 325–335). New York: Guilford.

McGlashan, T. (1986). Schizophrenia: Psychosocial treatments and the role of psychosocial factors in its etiology and pathogenesis. In A. Frances & R. Hales (Eds.), *Psychiatry update: Annual review* Vol. 5 (pp. 96–111). Washington, DC: American Psychiatric Press.

McKnight, D. L., Nelson, R. O., Hayes, S. C. et al. (1984). Importance of treating individually-assessed response classes in the amelioration of depression. *Behavior Therapy, 15,* 315.

McLachlan, J. C. (1972). Benefit from group therapy as a function of patient-therapist match on conceptual level. *Psychotherapy: Theory, Research and Practice, 9,* 317–323.

McLean, P. D. & Hakstian, A. R. (1979). Clinical depression: Comparative efficacy of outpatient treatments. *Journal of Consulting and Clinical Psychology, 47,* 818–836.

McLellan, A. T., Luborsky, L., Woody, G. E., O'Brien, C. P. & Druley, K. A. (1983). Predicting response to alcohol and drug abuse treatments: Role of psychiatric severity. *Archives of General Psychiatry, 40,* 620–625.

McLemore, C. & Benjamin, L. S. (1979). Whatever happened to interpersonal diagnosis: A psychosocial alternative to DSM-III. *American Psychologist, 34,* 17–34.

Megargee, E. I., Cook, P. E. & Mendelsohn, G. A. (1967). Development and validation of an MMPI scale of assaultiveness in overcontrolled individuals. *Journal of Abnormal Psychology, 72,* 519–528.

Meichenbaum, D. J. (1977). *Cognitive-behavior modification.* New York: Plenum.

Meichenbaum, D. & Turk, D. (1976). The cognitive-behavioral management of anxiety, anger and pain. In P. O. Davidson (Ed.), *The behavioral management of anxiety, depression and pain.* New York: Brunner/Mazel.

Meichenbaum, D. J. & Turk, D. C. (1987). *Facilitating treatment adherence: A practitioner's guidebook.* New York: Plenum Press.

Mendelsohn, G. A. & Geller, M. H. (1963). Effects of counselor-client similarity on the outcome of counseling. *Journal of Counseling Psychology, 10,* 71–77.

Mendelsohn, G. A. & Geller, M. H. (1967). Similarity, missed sessions, and early termination. *Journal of Counseling Psychology, 14,* 210–215.

Michelson, L., Mavissakalian, M. & Marchione, K. (1985). Cognitive and behavioral treatments of agoraphobia: Clinical, behavioral, psychophysiological outcomes. *Journal of Consulting and Clinical Psychology, 53,* 913–925.

Miller, I. W., III & Norman, W. H. (1981). Effects of attributions for success on the alleviation of learned helplessness and depression. *Journal of Abnormal Psychology, 90,* 113–124.

Miller, P. A. & Eisenberg, N. (1988). The relation of empathy to aggressive and externalizing/antisocial behavior. *Psychological Bulletin, 103,* 324–344.

Miller, R. C. & Berman, J. S. (1983). The efficacy of cognitive behavior therapies: A quantitative review of the research evidence. *Psychological Bulletin, 94,* 39–53.

Miller, W. R. (1987). Techniques to modify hazardous drinking patterns. In M. Galanter (Ed.), *Recent developments in alcoholism,* Vol. 5 (pp. 425–438). New York: Plenum.

Miller, W. R. & Hester, R. K. (1986a). Inpatient alcoholism treatment: Who benefits? *American Psychologist, 41,* 794–805.

Miller, W. R. & Hester, R. K. (1986b). Matching problem drinkers with optimal treatments. In W. R. Miller & N. Heather (Eds.), *Addictive behaviors: Processes of change* (pp. 175–203). New York: Plenum.

Millon, T. (1969). *Modern psychopathology.* Philadelphia: W. B. Saunders.

Millon, T. (1977). *Millon Clinical Multiaxial Inventory Manual.* Minneapolis: National Computer Systems, Inc.

Millon, T. (1981). *Disorders of personality: DSM-III; axis II.* New York: John Wiley and Sons.

Millon, T. & Everly, G. S. (1981). *Personality and its disorders.* New York: John Wiley and Sons.

Mintz, E. E. (1969). On the rationale of touch in psychotherapy. *Psychotherapy: Theory, Research and Practice, 6,* 232–234.

Mintz, J. (1981). Measuring outcome in psychodynamic psychotherapy. *Archives of General Psychiatry, 38,* 503–506.

Minuchin, S. (1974). *Families and family therapy.* Cambridge, MA: Harvard University Press.

Minuchin, S. & Fishman, H. C. (1981). *Family therapy techniques.* Cambridge, MA: Harvard University Press.

Mischel, W. (1968). *Personality and assessment.* New York: John Wiley and Sons.

Mitchell, K. M. & Atkinson, B. (1983). The relationship between therapist and client social class and participation in therapy. *Professional Psychology, 14,* 310–316.

Mitchell, K. M. & Namenek, T. M. (1970). A comparison of therapist and client social class. *Professional Psychology, 1,* 225–230.

Mittelman, B. (1948). The concurrent analysis of married couples. *Psychoanalytic Quarterly, 17,* 182–197.

Monroe, S. M., Bromet, E. J., Connell, M. M. & Steiner, S. C. (1986). Social support, life events, and depressive symptoms: A one-year prospective study. *Journal of Consulting and Clinical Psychology, 54,* 424–431.

Montgomery, L. M., Shadish, W. R., Jr., Orwin, R. G. & Bootzin, R. R. (1987). Psychometric structure of psychiatric rating scales. *Journal of Abnormal Psychology, 96,* 167–170.

Moos, R. (1969). *Ward atmosphere scale: Preliminary manual.* Stanford, CA: Stanford University Medical Center.

Moos, R. (1973). *Ward atmosphere scale: Manual.* Stanford, CA: Department of Psychiatry, Stanford University.

Moos, R. & Schwartz, J. (1972). Treatment environment and treatment outcome. *Journal of Nervous and Mental Disease, 54,* 264–275.

Morey, L. & McNamara, T. P. (1987). Comments: On definitions, diagnosis and DSM-III. *Journal of Abnormal Psychology, 96*(3), 283–285.

Morey, L. & Skinner, H. (1986). Empirically derived classifications of alcohol-related problems. In M. Galanter (Ed.), *Recent developments in alcoholism: Volume VI* (pp. 145–168). New York: Plenum Press.

Morgan, R., Luborsky, L., Crits-Christoph, P., Curtis, H. & Solomon, J. (1982). Predicting the outcomes of psychotherapy by the Penn Helping Alliance Rating Method. *Archives of General Psychiatry, 39,* 397–402.

Mosher, L. R. & Menn, A. Z. (1978). Lowered barrier in the community: The soteria model. In L. I. Stein & M. A. Test (Eds.), *Alternatives to mental health treatment* (pp. 75–113). New York: Plenum.

Moskowitz, S. & Rupert, P. (1983). Conflict resolution within the supervisory relationship. *Professional Psychology: Research and Practice, 14,* 632–641.

Mowrer, O. H. (1953). Neurosis and psychotherapy as interpersonal processes: A synopsis. In O. H. Mowrer (Ed.), *Psychotherapy: Theory and research* (pp. 69–94). New York: Ronald Publishing Co.

Munby, M. & Johnston, D. W. (1980). Agoraphobia: The long-term follow-up of behavioral treatment. *British Journal of Psychiatry, 137,* 418–427.

Murry, H. A. (1938). *Explorations in personality.* New York: Oxford University Press.

Muzekari, L. H. & Kreiger, P. (1975). Effects of inducing body awareness in chronic schizophrenics: Body boundary changes. *Journal of Consulting and Clinical Psychology, 43,* 435–436.

Myers, J. D., Jacob, J. L., & Pepper, M. P. (1972). Life events and mental status: A longitudinal study. *Journal of Health and Social Behavior, 13,* 398–406.

National Association of Private Psychiatric Hospitals (1985). The NAPPH study on prospective payment for psychiatric hospitals: A summary report. *NAPPH Newsline, 4,* 1–11.

National Association of Social Workers (1987). *Register of clinical social workers,* 5th ed. Silver Springs, MD: National Association of Social Workers.

Neal-Schuman Publishers, Inc. (1980). *The national directory of mental health.* New York: John Wiley.

Neimeyer, G. J. & Gonzales, M. (1983). Duration, satisfaction, and perceived effectiveness of cross-cultural counseling. *Journal of Counseling Psychology, 30,* 91–95.

Nelson, G. (1978). Psychotherapy supervision from the trainees' point of view: A survey of preferences. *Professional Psychology, 9,* 539–550.

Newman, F., Heverly, M., Rosen, M., Kopta, S. & Bedell, R. (1983). Influences on internal evaluation data dependability: Clinicians as a source of variance. In A.J. Love (Ed.), *Developing effective internal evaluation: New directions for program evaluation* (No. 20, pp. 71–92). San Francisco: Jossey-Bass.

Newman, F. & Howard, K. (1986). Therapeutic effort, treatment outcome, and national health policy. *American Psychologist, 41,* 181–187.

Newman, F., Kopta, S. M., McGovern, M. P., Howard, K. I. & McNeilly, C. L. (in press). Evaluating trainees relative to their supervisors during the psychology internship. *Journal of Consulting and Clinical Psychology.*

Nietzel, M. T., Russell, R. L., Hemmings, K. A. & Gretter, M. L. (1987). Clinical significance of psychotherapy for unipolar depression: A meta-analytic approach to social comparison. *Journal of Consulting and Clinical Psychology, 55,* 156–161.

Norcross, J. C. (1985). For discriminating clinicians only. *Contemporary Psychology, 30,* 757–758.

Norcross, J. C. (Ed.) (1986a). *Casebook of eclectic psychotherapy.* New York: Brunner/Mazel.

Norcross, J. C. (Ed.) (1986b). *Handbook of eclectic psychotherapy.* New York: Brunner/Mazel.

Norcross, J. C. (1986c). Eclectic psychotherapy: An introduction and overview. In J. C. Norcross (Ed.), *Handbook of eclectic psychotherapy* (pp. 3–24). New York: Brunner/Mazel.

Norcross, J. C. (Section Editor) (1986d). Training integrative/eclectic psychotherapists. *International Journal of Eclectic Psychotherapy, 5,* 71–94.

Norcross, J. C. (1988). Supervision of integrative psychotherapy. *Journal of Integrative and Eclectic Psychotherapy, 7,* 157–166.

Norcross, J. C. & Prochaska, J. O. (1982). A national survey of clinical psychologists: Views on training, career choice, and APA. *The Clinical Psychologist, 35* (4), 1–6.

Norcross, J. C. & Prochaska, J. O. (1988). A study of eclectic (and integrative) views revisited. *Professional Psychology: Research and Practice, 19,* 170–174.

Norcross, J. C. & Stevenson, J. F. (1984). How shall we judge ourselves? Training evaluation in clinical psychology programs. *Professional Psychology: Research and Practice, 15,* 497–508.

Norcross, J. C. & Thomas, B. L. (1988). What's stopping us now? Obstacles to psychotherapy integration. *Journal of Integrative and Eclectic Psychotherapy, 7,* 74–80.

Norcross, J. C. & Wogan, M. (1983). American psychotherapists of diverse persuasions: Characteristics, theories, practices and clients. *Professional Psychology: Research and Practice, 14,* 529–539.

Nuechterlein, K. & Dawson, M. (1984). A heuristic vulnerability/stress model of schizophrenic episodes. *Schizophrenia Bulletin, 10,* 300–312.

Oberndorf, C.P. (1938). Psychoanalysis of married couples. *Psychoanalytic Review, 25,* 453–475.

O'Farrell, T. J. & Birchler, G. R. (1987). Marital relationships of alcoholic, conflicted, and nonconflicted couples. *Journal of Marital and Family Therapy, 13,* 259–274.

Olson, D. H. & Killorin, E. (1985). *Clinical rating scale for the circumplex model.* St. Paul: Family Social Science, University of Minnesota.

Orlinsky, D. E. & Howard, K. I. (1978). The relation of process to outcome in psychotherapy. In S. L. Garfield & A. E. Bergin (Eds.), *Handbook of psychotherapy and behavior change: An empirical analysis,* 2nd ed New York: John Wiley.

Orlinsky, D. E. & Howard, K. I. (1986). Process and outcome in psychotherapy. In S. L. Garfield & A. E. Bergin (Eds.), *Handbook of psychotherapy and behavior change,* 3rd ed. (pp. 311–384). New York: John Wiley and Sons.

Orlinsky, D. E. & Howard, K. I. (1987). A generic model of psychotherapy. *Journal of Integrative and Eclectic Psychotherapy, 6,* 6–28.

Parloff, M. B. (1986). Frank's "common elements" in psychotherapy: Nonspecific factors and placebos. *American Journal of Orthopsychiatry, 56,* 521–530.

Parloff, M. B., Waskow, I. E. & Wolfe, B. E. (1978). Research on therapist variables in relation to process and outcome. In S. L. Garfield & A. E. Bergin (Eds.), *Handbook of psychotherapy and behavior change,* 2nd ed. (pp. 233–282). New York: John Wiley and Sons.

Parry, G. & Shapiro, D. A. (1986). Social support and life events in working class women: Stress buffering or independent effects? *Archives of General Psychiatry, 43,* 315–323.

Pasamanick, B., Scarpitti, F. R. & Dinitz, S. (1967). *Schizophrenics in the community: An experimental study in the prevention of hospitalization.* New York: Appleton-Century-Crofts.

Patterson, G. R. (1982). *Coercive family process.* Eugene, OR: Castalia Publishing Co.

Patterson, G. R. & Forgatch, M. S. (1985). Therapist behavior as a determinant for client noncompliance: A paradox for the behavior modifier. *Journal of Consulting and Clinical Psychology, 53,* 846–851.

Patterson, M. L. (1982). A sequential functional model of nonverbal exchange. *Psychological Review, 89,* 231–249.

Paul, G. L. (1969). Behavior modification research: Design and tactics. In C. M. Franks (Ed.), *Behavior therapy: Appraisal and status* (pp. 29–62). New York: McGraw-Hill.

Paul, G. L. (1978). The implementation of effective treatment programs for chronic mental patients: Obstacles and recommendations. In J. A. Talbott (Ed.), *The chronic mental patient.* Washington, DC: American Psychiatric Association.

Paul, G. L. & Lentz, R. J. (1977). *Psychosocial treatment of chronic mental patients.* Cambridge, MA: Harvard University Press.

Pearlin, L. I. & Johnson, J. (1977). Marital status, life strains, and depression. *American Sociological Review, 42,* 704–715.

Pennebaker, J. W., Kiecolt-Glaser, J. K. & Glaser, R. (1988). Disclosure of traumas and immune function: Health implications for psychotherapy. *Journal of Consulting and Clinical Psychology, 56,* 239–245.

Percell, L. P., Berwick, P. T. & Beigel, A. (1974). The effects of assertive training on self-concept and anxiety. *Archives of General Psychiatry, 31,* 502–504.

Perls, F. S. (1969). *Gestalt therapy verbatim.* Moab, Utah: Real People Press.

Perry, S., Frances, A., & Clarkin, J. F. (1985). *A DSM-III casebook of differential therapeutics: A clinical guide to treatment selection.* New York: Brunner/Mazel.

Perry, W. (1970). *Forms of intellectual and ethical development in the college years: A scheme.* New York: Holt, Rinehart & Winston.

Pfohl, B. & Andreasen, N. (1986). Schizophrenia: Diagnosis and classification. In A. Frances & R. Hales (Eds.), *Psychiatry update: Annual review,* Vol. 5 (pp. 7–24). Washington: American Psychiatric Press.

Phillips, G. L. & Kantner, C. N. (1984). Mutuality in psychotherapy supervision. *Psychotherapy, 21,* 178–183.

Pilkonis, P., Imber, S., Lewis, P. et al. (1984). A comparative outcome study of individual, group, and conjoint psychotherapy. *Archives of General Psychiatry, 41,* 431–437.

Piper, W. E., Debbane, E. G., Bienvenu, J. P. & Garant, J. (1984). A comparative study of four forms of psychotherapy. *Journal of Consulting and Clinical Psychology, 52,* 268–279.

Polster, E. & Polster, M. (1973). *Gestalt therapy integrated.* New York: Brunner/Mazel.

Pomerleau, O. F. (1979). Behavioral medicine: The contribution of the experimental analysis of behavior to medical care. *American Psychologist, 34,* 654–663.

Pomerleau, O. F. & Pomerleau, C. S. (1984). *Break the smoking habit: A behavioral program for giving up cigarettes.* W. Hartford, CT: Behavioral Medicine Press.

Pope, B. (1979). *The mental health interview: Research and application.* New York: Pergamon.

Pratt, J. H. (1907). The class method of treating consumption in the homes of the poor. *Journal of the American Medical Association, 49,* 755–759.

Probst, L. R. (1980). The comparative efficacy of religious and nonreligious imagery for the treatment of mild depression in religious individuals. *Cognitive Therapy and Research, 4,* 167–178.

Probst, L. R., Ostrom, R. & Watkins, P. (1984, June). *The efficacy of religious cognitive-behavioral therapy for the treatment of clinical depression in religious individuals.* Paper presented at the Society for Psychotherapy Research, Lake Louise, Alberta, Canada.

Prochaska, J. O. (1984). *Systems of psychotherapy: A transtheoretical analysis,* 2nd ed. Homewood, IL: Dorsey Press.

Prochaska, J. O. & DiClemente, C. C. (1982). Transtheoretical therapy: Toward a more integrative model of change. *Psychotherapy: Theory, Research, and Practice, 19,* 276–288.

Prochaska, J. O. & DiClemente, C. C. (1986). The transtheoretical approach. In J. C. Norcross (Ed.), *Handbook of eclectic psychotherapy* (pp. 163–200). New York: Brunner/Mazel.

Proschaska, J. O., Velicer, W. F., DiClemente, C. C. & Fava, J. (1988). Measuring processes of change: Applications to the cessation of smoking. *Journal of Consulting and Clinical Psychology, 56,* 520–528.

Prusoff, B. A., Weissman, M. M., Klerman, G. L. et al. (1980). Research diagnostic criteria subtypes of depression: Their role as predictors of differential response to psychotherapy and drug treatment. *Archives of General Psychiatry, 37,* 796.

Rachelson, J. & Clance, P. (1980). Attitudes of psychotherapists toward the 1970 APA standards for psychotherapy training. *Professional Psychology, 11,* 261–267.

Rachman, S., Hodgson, R. & Marks, I. M. (1971). Treatment of chronic obsessive-compulsive neurosis. *Behavior Research and Therapy, 9,* 237–247.

Rachman, S. J. & Wilson, G. T. (1980). *The effects of psychological therapy.* New York: Pergamon Press.

Rapee, R. (1987). The psychological treatment of panic attacks: Theoretical conceptualization and review of evidence. *Clinical Psychology Review, 7,* 427–438.

Regier, D. A., Myers, J. K., Kramer, M., Robin, L. N., Blazer, D. G., Haugh, R. L., Eaton, W. W. & Locke, B. Z. (1984). The NIMH epidemiologic catchment area program. *Archives of General Psychiatry, 41,* 934–941.

Rehm, L. P. (1984). Self-management therapy for depression. *Advances in Behavioral Research and Therapy, 6,* 83.

Reichenbach, H. (1964). *The rise of scientific philosophy.* Berkeley: University of California Press.

Remer, P., Roffey, B. H. & Buckholtz, A. (1983). Differential effects of positive versus negative self-involving counselor responses. *Journal of Counseling Psychology, 30,* 121–125.

Rhoades, L. J. (1981). *Treating and assessing the chronically mentally ill: The pioneering research of Gordon L. Paul* (DHHS Publication No. ADM 81–1100). Rockville MD: Science Reports Branch, Division of Scientific and Public Information, National Institute of Mental Health.

Rice, L. N. & Greenberg, L. S. (1984). *Patterns of change.* New York: The Guilford Press.

Riehl, A. (1986). Influence of partnership on the outcome of psychotherapy. *Psychotherapie Psychosomatica, 45,* 37–45.

Riggio, R. E. & Friedman, H. S. (1983). Individual differences and cues to deception. *Journal of Personality and Social Psychology, 45,* 899–915.

Rivlin, L. G., Wolfe, M. & Beyda, M. (1973). Age-related differences in the use of space. In W. F. E. Preiser (Ed.), *Environmental design research.* Stroudsburg, PA: Dowden, Hutchinson & Ross.

Robbins, E. S. & Haase, R. F. (1985). Power of nonverbal cues in counseling interactions: Availability, vividness, or salience? *Journal of Counseling Psychology, 32,* 502–513.

Robertson, L. S. (1976). The great seat belt campaign flop. *Journal of Communication, 26,* 41–45.

Robertson, M. (1984). Teaching psychotherapy in an academic setting. *Psychotherapy: Theory, Research, and Practice, 21,* 209–212.

Robertson, M. (1986). Training eclectic psychotherapists. In J. C. Norcross (Ed.), *Handbook of eclectic psychotherapy* (pp. 416–435). New York: Brunner/Mazel.

Robins, L. N., Helzer, J. E., Croughan, J. & Ratcliff, K. S. (1981). National Institute of Mental Health Diagnostic Interview Schedule: Its history, characteristics, and validity. *Archives of General Psychiatry, 38,* 381–389.

Robinson, E. A. & Jacobson, N. S. (1987). Social learning theory and family psychopathology: A Kantian model in behaviorism? In T. Jacob (Ed.), *Family interaction and psychopathology: Theories, methods, and findings* (pp. 117–162). New York: Plenum.

Roessler, R. (1973). Personality, psychophysiology, and performance. *Psychophysiology, 10,* 315–327.

Rogers, C. R. (1951) *Client-centered therapy.* Boston: Houghton Mifflin.

Rogers, C. R. (1957). The necessary and sufficient conditions of therapeutic personality change. *Journal of Consulting Psychology, 21,* 95–103.

Rosen, B., Katzoff, A., Carrillo, C. & Klein, D. (1976). Clinical effectiveness of "short" versus "long" stay psychiatric hospitalization. I. Inpatient results. *Archives of General Psychiatry, 33,* 1316–1322.

Rosenberg, S. E., Silberschatz, G., Curtis, J. T., Sampson, H. & Weiss, J. (1986). A method for establishing reliability of statements from psychodynamic case formulations. *American Journal of Psychiatry, 143,* 1454–1456.

Rosenblatt, A. & Mayer, J. (1975). Objectionable supervisory styles: Students' views. *Social Work, 18,* 184–189.

Rosenthal, N. R. (1977). A prescriptive approach for counselor training. *Journal of Counseling Psychology, 24,* 231–237.

Rosenthal, R., Blanck, P. D. & Vannicelli, M. (1984). Speaking to and about patients: Predicting therapists' tone of voice. *Journal of Consulting and Clinical Psychology, 52,* 679–686.

Rotter, J. B. (1966). Generalized expectancies for internal versus external control of reinforcement. *Psychological Monographs: General and Applied, 80* (1, Whole No. 609).

Rounsaville, B. J., Chevron, E. S., Prusoff, B. A., Elkin, I., Imber, S., Sotsky, S. & Watkins, J. (1987). The relation between specific and general dimensions of the psychotherapy process in interpersonal psychotherapy of depression. *Journal of Consulting and Clinical Psychology, 55,* 379–384.

Rounsaville, B. J., Chevron, E. S., Weissman, M. M., Prusoff, B. A. & Frank, E. (1986). Training therapists to perform interpersonal psychotherapy in clinical trials. *Comprehensive Psychiatry, 27,* 364–371.

Rounsaville, B. J., O'Malley, S., Foley, S. & Weissman, M. M. (1988). The role of manual guided training in the conduct and efficiency of interpersonal psychotherapy for depression. *Journal of Consulting and Clinical Psychology, 56,* 681–688.

Rush, A. J. (1988, June). *Overview of literature on recurrence of depression and bulimea.*

A paper presented at the annual meeting of the Society for Psychotherapy Research, Santa Fe, NM.

Rush, A. J., Beck, A. T., Kovacs, M. & Hollon, S. (1977). Comparative efficacy of cognitive therapy and pharmacotherapy in the treatment of depressed outpatients. *Cognitive Therapy and Research, 1,* 17–37.

Sachs, J. S. (1983). Negative factors in brief psychotherapy: An empirical assessment. *Journal of Consulting and Clinical Psychology, 51,* 557–564.

Sanchez-Craig, M. & Lei, H. (1986). Disadvantages to imposing the goal of abstinence on problem drinkers: An empirical study. *British Journal of Addiction, 81,* 505–512.

Sandler, J., Holder, A. & Dave, C. (1973). *The patient and the analyst.* New York: International Universities Press.

Sank, L. I. & Shaffer, C. S. (1984). *A therapist's manual for cognitive behavior therapy in groups.* New York: Plenum.

Saper, B. (1987). Humor in psychotherapy: Is it good or bad for the client? *Professional Psychology: Research and Practice, 18,* 360–367.

Saunders, S. M., Howard, K. I. & Orlinsky, D. E. (in press). The therapeutic bond scales: Psychometric characteristics and relationship to treatment effectiveness. *Journal of Consulting and Clinical Psychology.*

Schaefer, C., Coyne, J. C. & Lazarus, R. S. (1981). The health-related functions of social support. *Journal of Behavioral Medicine, 4,* 381–406.

Schooler, N. R. & Keith, S. J. (1984). NIMH protocol for treatment strategies in schizophrenia study. Unpublished manuscript: National Institute of Mental Health, Rockville, MD.

Schooler, N. R., Levine, J., Severe, J. B., Brauzer, B., DiMascio, A., Klerman, G. L. & Tuason, V. B. (1980). Prevention of relapse in schizophrenia: An evaluation of fluphenazine decanoate. *Archives of General Psychiatry, 37,* 16–24.

Schradle, S. B. & Dougher, M. J. (1985). Social support as a mediator of stress: Theoretical and empirical issues. *Clinical Psychology Review, 5,* 641–661.

Schramski, T. G., Beutler, L. E., Lauver, P. J. & Arizmendi, T. A. (1984). Factors that contribute to posttherapy persistence of therapeutic change. *Journal of Clinical Psychology, 40,* 78–85.

Schuckit, M. A., Zisook, S. & Mortola, J. (1985). Clinical implications of DSM-III diagnosis of alcohol abuse and alcohol dependence. *American Journal of Psychiatry, 142,* 1403–1408.

Schulberg, H. C. & Baker, F. (1969). Unitization: Decentralizing the mental hospitalopolis. *International Journal of Psychiatry, 7,* 213–223.

Schulberg, H. C. & McClelland, M. (1987). Depression and physical illness: The prevalence, causation, and diagnosis of comorbidity. *Clinical Psychology Review, 7,* 145–167.

Seltzer, L. F. (1986). *Paradoxical strategies in psychotherapy: A comprehensive overview and guidebook.* New York: John Wiley and Sons.

Shakir, S. A., Volkmar, F. R., Bacon, S. & Pfefferbaum, H. (1979). Group psychotherapy as an adjunct to lithium maintenance. *American Journal of Psychiatry, 136,* 455–456.

Shapiro, D. (1965). *Neurotic styles.* New York: Basic Books, Inc.

Shapiro, D. A. & Shapiro, D. (1982). Meta-analysis of comparative therapy outcome studies: A replication and refinement. *Psychological Bulletin, 92,* 581–604.

Shapiro, P. N. & Penrod, S. (1986). Meta-analysis of facial identification studies. *Psychological Bulletin, 100,* 139–156.

Shaw, B.F. (1983, July). *Training therapists for the treatment of depression: Collaborative study.* Paper presented at the meeting of the Society for Psychotherapy Research, Sheffield, England.

Shaw, B. F. & Dobson, K.S. (1988). Competency judgments in the training and evaluation of psychotherapists. *Journal of Consulting and Clinical Psychology, 56,* 666–672.

Shoham-Salomon, V., Avner, R. & Zevlodever, R. (1988, June). *"You are changed if you do and changed if you don't": Cognitive mechanisms underlying the operation of therapeutic paradoxes.* A paper presented at the Society for Psychotherapy Research, Santa Fe, NM.

Shoham-Salomon, V. & Rosenthal, R. (1987). Paradoxical interventions: A meta-analysis. *Journal of Consulting and Clinical Psychology, 55,* 22–27.

Siegman, A. W. & Feldstein, S. (Eds.) (1985). *Multichannel integrations of nonverbal behavior.* Hillsdale, NJ: Lawrence Erlbaum Associates.

Sifneos, P. (1972). *Short-term psychotherapy and emotional crisis.* Cambridge, MA: Harvard University Press.

Silberschatz, G., Fretter, P. B. & Curtis, J. T. (1986). How do interpretations influence the process of psychotherapy? *Journal of Consulting and Clinical Psychology, 54,* 646–652.

Simons, A. D., Garfield, S. L. & Murphy, G. E. (1984). The process of change in cognitive therapy and pharmacotherapy for depression. *Archives of General Psychiatry, 41,* 45.

Sinfield, A. (1981). *What unemployment means.* Oxford: Martin Robertson Press.

Skinner, B. F. (1953). *Science and human behavior.* New York: Macmillan.

Skinner, B. F. (1971). *Beyond freedom and dignity.* New York: Knopf.

Skinner, H. A. (1986). Construct validation approach to psychiatric classification. In T. Millon & G. L. Klerman (Eds.), *Contemporary directions in psychopathology: Toward the DSM-IV* (pp. 307–330). New York, Guilford Press (See page 325 for two studies on how clinicians think.)

Slater, J. & Depue, R. A. (1981). The contribution of environmental events and social support to serious suicide attempts in primary depressive disorder. *Journal of Abnormal Psychology, 90,* 275–285.

Sloane, R. B., Staples, F. R., Cristol, A. H., Yorkston, N. J. & Whipple, K. (1975). *Psychotherapy versus behavior therapy.* Cambridge MA: Harvard University Press.

Smith, E. W. (1972). Postural and gestural communication of A and B "therapist types" during dyad interviews. *Journal of Consulting and Clinical Psychology, 39,* 29–36.

Smith, M. L. & Glass, G. V. (1977). Meta-analysis of psychotherapy outcome studies. *American Psychologist, 32,* 752–760.

Smith, M. L., Glass, G. V. & Miller, T. I. (1980). *The benefits of psychotherapy.* Baltimore: Johns Hopkins University Press.

Smoller, J.W. (1986). The etiology and treatment of childhood. In G.C. Ellenbogen

(Ed.), *Oral sadism and the vegetarian personality* (pp. 5–12). New York: Brunner/ Mazel.

Snyder, C. R. & Forsyth, D. R. (Eds.) (in press). *Handbook of social and clinical psychology: The health perspective.* New York: Pergamon.

Snyder, L. H. & Ostrander, E. R. (1972, June). *Spatial and physical considerations in the nursing home environment: An interim report of findings.* Paper presented at the Cornell University Conference on Nursing Homes, Ithaca, New York.

Sorenson, R. L., Gorsuch, L. & Mintz, J. (1985). Moving targets: Patients' changing complaints during psychotherapy. *Journal of Consulting and Clinical Psychology, 53,* 49–54.

Spencer, J. & Mattson, M. (1979, December). Criteria for admission to a psychiatric hospital. *QRB/Quality Review Bulletin.*

Spielberger, C. D., Gorsuch, R. L. & Lushene, R. E. (1970). *The State-Trait Anxiety Inventory (STAI) test manual for form X.* Palo Alto: Consulting Psychologists Press.

Spitzer, R. L., Endicott, J. & Robins, E. (1978). Research diagnostic criteria: Rationale and reliability. *Archives of General Psychiatry, 35,* 773–382.

Stafford, E. M., Jackson, P. R. & Banks, M. H. (1980). Employment, work involvement and mental health in less qualified young people. *Journal of Occupational Psychology, 53,* 291–304.

Stampfl, T. G. & Levis, D. J. (1967). Essentials of implosive therapy: A learning theory-based psychodynamic behavioral therapy. *Journal of Abnormal Psychology, 72,* 496–503.

Staples, F. R. & Sloane, R. B. (1976). Truax factors, speech characteristics, and therapeutic outcome. *Journal of Nervous and Mental Disease, 163,* 135–140.

Stein, D. M. & Lambert, M. J. (1984). On the relationship between therapist experience and psychotherapy outcome. *Clinical Psychology Review, 4,* 127–142.

Stein, L. I. & Test, M. A. (1980). Alternative to mental hospital treatment: I. Conceptual model, treatment program, and clinical evaluation. *Archives of General Psychiatry, 37,* 392–397.

Stein, S. P., Karasu, T. B., Charles, E. S. & Buckley, P. J. (1975). Supervision of the initial interview. *Archives of General Psychiatry, 32,* 265–268.

Steinbrueck, S. M., Maxwell, S. E. & Howard, G. S. (1983). A meta-analysis of psychotherapy and drug therapy in the treatment of unipolar depression with adults. *Journal of Consulting and Clinical Psychology, 51,* 856–863.

Stern, S. (1984). Professional training and professional competence: A critique of current thinking. *Professional Psychology: Research and Practice, 15,* 230–243.

Stevenson, J. F. & Norcross, J. C. (1987). Current status of training evaluation in clinical psychology. In B. Edelstein & E. Berler (Eds.), *Evaluation and accountability in clinical training* (pp. 77–115). New York: Plenum.

Stiles, W. B. (1978). Verbal response modes and dimensions of interpersonal roles: A method of discourse analysis. *Journal of Personality and Social Psychology, 36,* 693–703.

Stiles, W. B. (1979). Verbal response modes and psychotherapeutic technique. *Psychiatry, 42,* 49–62.

Stoltenberg, C. (1981). Approaching supervision from a developmental perspective: The counselor complexity model. *Journal of Counseling Psychology, 28,* 59–65.

Stricker, G. (1988). Supervision of integrative psychotherapy: Discussion. *Journal of Integrative and Eclectic Psychotherapy, 7,* 176–180.

Strong, S. R. (1978). Social psychological approach to psychotherapy research. In S. L. Garfield & A. E. Bergin (Eds.), *Handbook of psychotherapy and behavior change,* 2nd ed. (pp. 101–135). New York: John Wiley and Sons.

Strong, S. R. (1987). Social-psychological approach to counseling and psychotherapy: "A false hope"? *Journal of Social and Clinical Psychology, 5,* 183–194.

Strupp, H. H. (1975). Training the complete clinician. *The Clinical Psychologist, 28*(4), 1–2.

Strupp, H. H. (1980a). Success and failure in time-limited psychotherapy: A systematic comparison of two cases (Comparison 1). *Archives of General Psychiatry, 37,* 595–603.

Strupp, H. H. (1980b). Success and failure in time-limited psychotherapy: A systematic comparison of two cases (Comparison 2). *Archives of General Psychiatry, 37,* 708–716.

Strupp, H. H. (1981). Toward the refinement of time-limited dynamic psychotherapy. In S. H. Budman (Ed.), *Forms of brief therapy* (pp. 219–242). New York: Guilford.

Strupp, H. H. (1986). The nonspecific hypothesis of therapeutic effectiveness: A current assessment. *American Journal of Orthopsychiatry, 56,* 513–520.

Strupp, H. H. & Binder, J. L. (1984). *Psychotherapy in a new key.* New York: Basic Books, Inc.

Strupp, H. H. & Bloxom, A. L. (1973). Preparing lower class patients for group psychotherapy: Development and evaluation of a role-induction film. *Journal of Consulting and Clinical Psychology, 41,* 373–384.

Strupp, H. H., Butler, S. F. & Rosser, C. (1988). Training in psychodynamic therapy. *Journal of Consulting and Clinical Psychology, 56,* 689–695.

Strupp, H. H. & Hadley, S. W. (1977). A tripartite model of mental health and therapeutic outcomes. *American Psychologist, 32,* 187–196.

Strupp, H. H., Hadley, S. W. & Gomes-Schwartz, R. (1977). *Psychotherapy for better or worse: An analysis of the problem of negative effects.* New York: Jason Aronson.

Stuart, R. B. (1975). Behavioral remedies for marital ills. A guide to the use of operant interpersonal techniques. In A. S. Gurman & D. G. Rice (Eds.), *Couples in conflict.* New York: Aronson.

Stuart, R. B. (1982). *Adherence, compliance and generalization in behavioral medicine.* New York: Brunner/Mazel.

Sullivan, H. S. (1954). *The psychiatric interview.* New York: Norton.

Sundland, D. M. (1977, June). *Theoretical orientation: A multi-professional American sample.* Paper presented at the eighth annual meeting of the Society for Psychotherapy Research, Madison, WI.

Swinburne, P. (1981). The psychological impact of unemployment on managers and professional staff. *Journal of Occupational Psychology, 54,* 47–64.

Taube, C. A., Kessler, L. & Feuerberg, M. (1984). Utilization and expenditures for ambulatory mental health care during 1980. *National Medical Care Utilization and Expenditure Survey,* Data Report 5. U.S. Department of Health and Human Services.

Taylor, M. A., Greenspan, B. & Abrams, R. (1979). Lateralized neuropsychological dysfunction in affective disorder and schizophrenia. *American Journal of Psychiatry, 136,* 1031–1034.

Tennen, H., Rohrbaugh, M., Press, S. & White, L. (1981). Reactance theory and therapeutic paradox: A compliance-defiance model. *Psychotherapy: Theory, Research and Practice, 18,* 14–22.

Terrell, R. & Terrell, S. (1984). Race of counselor, client sex, cultural mistrust level, and premature termination from counseling among black clients. *Journal of Counseling Psychology, 31,* 371–375.

Thompson, L. W. & Gallagher, D. (1984). Efficacy of psychotherapy in the treatment of late-life depression. *Advances in Behavioral Research and Therapy, 6,* 127.

Thompson, L., Gallagher, D. & Breckenridge, J. (1987). Comparative effectiveness of psychotherapies for depressed elders. *Journal of Consulting and Clinical Psychology, 55,* 385–390.

Thorpe, S. A. (1987). An approach to treatment planning. *Psychotherapy, 24,* 729–735.

Thyer, B. A. & Himle, J. (1985). Temporal relationships between panic attack onset and phobic avoidance in agoraphobia. *Behavior Research and Therapy, 23,* 607–608.

Tibbits-Kleber, A. L. & Howell, R. J. (1987). Doctoral training in clinical psychology: A students' perspective. *Professional Psychology: Research and Practice, 18,* 634–639.

Tjelveit, A. C. (1986). The ethics of value conversion in psychotherapy: Appropriate and inappropriate therapist influence on client values. *Clinical Psychology Review, 6,* 515–537.

Tracey, T. J. (1986). Interactional correlates of premature termination. *Journal of Consulting and Clinical Psychology, 54,* 784–788.

Tracey, T. J. (1987). Stage differences in the dependencies of topic initiation and topic following behavior. *Journal of Counseling Psychology, 34,* 123–131.

Tracey, T. J. & Dundon, M. (1988). Role anticipations and preferences over the course of counseling. *Journal of Counseling Psychology, 35,* 3–14.

Tracey, T. J., Hays, K. A., Malone, J. & Herman, B. (1988). Changes in counselor response as a function of experience. *Journal of Counseling Psychology, 35,* 119–126.

Tracey, T. J. & Ray, P. B. (1984). The stages of successful time-limited counseling: An interactional examination. *Journal of Counseling Psychology, 31,* 13–27.

Truax, C. B. & Carkhuff, R. R. (1967). *Toward effective counseling and psychotherapy: Training and practice.* Chicago: Aldine.

Truax, C. B., Fine, H., Moravec, J. & Millis, W. (1968). Effects of therapist persuasive potency in individual psychotherapy. *Journal of Clinical Psychology, 24,* 359–362.

Truax, C. B. & Wargo, D. G. (1969). Effects of vicarious therapy pre-training and alternate sessions on outcome in group psychotherapy with outpatients. *Journal of Consulting and Clinical Psychology, 33,* 440–447.

Tsuang, M. T. & Dempsey, M. (1979). Long-term outcome of major psychoses. II. Schizoaffective disorder compared with schizophrenia, affective disorders, and a surgical control group. *Archives of General Psychiatry, 36,* 1302–1304.

Turkat, D. M. (1979). Psychotherapy preparatory communications: Influences upon patient role expectations. *Dissertation Abstracts International, 39,* 4059B.

Turner, S. & Armstrong, S. (1981). Cross-racial psychotherapy: What the therapists say. *Psychotherapy: Theory, Research, and Practice, 18,* 375–378.

Tyler, J. D. & Weaver, S. H. (1981). Evaluating the clinical supervisee: A survey of practices in graduate training programs. *Professional Psychology, 12,* 434–437.

Tyson, C. L. (1979). Physical contact in psychotherapy. *Dissertation Abstracts International, 39,* 4601B.

Ullmann, L. P. (1967). *Institution and outcome: A comparative study of mental hospitals.* New York: Pergamon.

Vaillant, G. E. (1971). Theoretical hierarchy of adaptive ego mechanisms. *Archives of General Psychiatry, 24,* 107–118.

Valentine, M. E. & Ehrlichman, H. (1979). Interpersonal gaze and helping behavior. *Journal of Social Psychology, 107,* 193–198.

Vallis, T. M., Shaw, B. F. & Dobson, K. S. (1986). The cognitive therapy scale: Psychometric properties. *Journal of Consulting and Clinical Psychology, 54,* 381–385.

VandenBos, G. R. & DeLeon, P. H. (1988). The use of psychotherapy to improve physical health. *Psychotherapy, 25,* 335–343.

Vitz, P. C. (1988). *Sigmund Freud's Christian unconscious.* New York: Guilford.

von Essen, C. (1987, June). *The Berlin study of psychotherapy: About the validity of a diagnostic category system.* Paper presented at the annual meeting of the Society for Psychotherapy Research, Ulm, West Germany.

Wachtel, P. L. (1977). *Psychoanalysis & behavior therapy.* New York: Basic Books, Inc.

Warr, P. B. (1978). A study of psychological well-being. *British Journal of Psychology, 69,* 111–121.

Warr, P. B. (1982). Psychological aspects of employment and unemployment. *Psychological Medicine, 12,* 7–11.

Warr, P. B. & Parry, G. (1982). Paid employment and women's psychological well-being. *Psychological Bulletin, 91,* 498–516.

Warren, R. C. & Rice, L. N. (1972). Structuring and stabilizing of psychotherapy for low-prognosis clients. *Journal of Consulting and Clinical Psychology, 39,* 173–181.

Waskow, I. E. & Parloff, M. B. (Eds.) (1975). *Psychotherapy change measures* (Publication No. 74–120). Rockville, MD: National Institute of Mental Health.

Watkins, C. E., Jr., Lopez, F. G., Campbell, V. L. & Himmell, C. D. (1987). What do counseling psychologists think about their graduate training? *Professional Psychology: Research and Practice, 18,* 550–552.

Watzlawick, P. (1978). *The language of change: Elements of therapeutic interaction.* New York: Basic Books.

Weary, G. (1987). Natural bridges: The interface of social and clinical psychology. *Journal of Social and Clinical Psychology, 5,* 160–167.

Weary, G. & Mirels, H. L. (Eds.) (1982). *Integrations of clinical and social psychology.* New York: Oxford University Press.

Weiss, R. L., Hops, H. & Patterson, G. R. (1973). A framework for conceptualizing marital conflict, technology for altering it, some data for evaluating it. In L. A. Hamerlynck, L. C. Handy & E. J. Mash (Eds.), *Behavior change: Methodology, concepts, and practice.* Champaign, IL: Research Press.

Weiss, R. L. & Margolin, G. (1977). Assessment of marital conflict and accord. In A. R. Ciminero, K. S. Calhoun & H. E. Adams (Eds.), *Handbook of behavioral assessment* (pp. 555–602). New York: John Wiley.

Weissman, M. M., Klerman, G. L., Prusoff, B. A. et al. (1981). Depressed outpatients: Results one year after treatment with drugs and/or interpersonal psychotherapy. *Archives of General Psychiatry, 38,* 51.

Weissman, M. M., Prusoff, B. A. & Klerman, G. L. (1978). Personality and the prediction of long-term outcome of depression. *American Journal of Psychiatry, 135,* 797.

Welsh, G. S. (1952). An anxiety index and an internalization ratio for the MMPI. *Journal of Consulting Psychology, 16,* 65–72.

Wetzel, J. W. (1978). The work environment and depression: Implications for intervention. In J. W. Hawks (Ed.), *Toward human dignity: Social work in practice.* New York: NASW Professional Symposium Service.

Wetzel, J. W. & Redmond, F. C. (1980). A person-environment study of depression. *Social Service Review, 54,* 363–375.

Widiger, T. A., Trull, T. J., Hurt, S. W., Clarkin, J. F. & Frances, A. (1987). A multidimensional scaling of the DSM-III personality disorders. *Archives of General Psychiatry, 44,* 557–563.

Wilder, J. F., Levin, G. & Zwerling, I. (1966). A two-year follow-up evaluation of acute psychotic patients treated in a day hospital. *American Journal of Psychiatry, 122,* 1095–1101.

Wiley, M. O. & Ray, P. B. (1986). Counseling supervision by developmental level. *Journal of Counseling Psychology, 33,* 439–445.

Williams, S. L., Kinney, P. J. & Falbo, J. (in press). Generalization of therapeutic changes in agoraphobia: The role of perceived self-efficacy. *Journal of Consulting and Clinical Psychology.*

Wilkins, W. (1979). Expectancies in therapy research: Discriminating among heterogeneous nonspecifics. *Journal of Consulting and Clinical Psychology, 47,* 837–845.

Wilkins, W. (1984). Psychotherapy: The powerful placebo. *Journal of Consulting and Clinical Psychology, 52,* 570–573.

Wills, R., Faitler, S. & Snyder, D. (1987). Distinctiveness of behavioral versus insight-oriented marital therapy: An empirical analysis. *Journal of Consulting and Clinical Psychology, 55,* 685–690.

Wilson, D. O. (1985). The effects of systematic client preparation, severity, and treatment setting on dropout rate in short-term psychotherapy. *Journal of Social and Clinical Psychology, 3,* 62–70.

Wilson, G. T. (1981). Behavior therapy as a short-term therapeutic approach. In S. H. Budman (Ed.), *Forms of brief therapy* (pp. 131–166). New York: Guilford.

Wolberg, L. R. (Ed.) (1965). *Short-term psychotherapy.* New York: Grune and Stratton.

Wolfe, B. E. & Goldfried, M. R. (1988). Research on psychotherapy integration: Recommendations and conclusions from an NIMH workshop. *Journal of Consulting and Clinical Psychology, 56,* 448–451.

Woody, R. H. & Roberston, M. (1988). *Becoming a clinical psychologist.* Madison, CN: International Universities Press, Inc.

Worthington, E. L. (1984). An empirical investigation of supervision of counselors as they gain experience. *Journal of Counseling Psychology, 31,* 63–75.

Worthington, E. L. (1987). Changes in supervision as counselors and supervisors gain experience: A review. *Professional Psychology: Research and Practice, 18,* 189–208.

Wynne, L. C. (1983). A phase-oriented approach to treatment with schizophrenics and their families. In W. R. McFarlane (Ed.), *Family therapy in schizophrenia* (pp. 251–266). New York: Guilford Press.

Yalom, I. D. (1975). *The theory and practice of group psychotherapy,* 2nd ed. New York: Basic Books, Inc.

Yalom, I. D. (1985). *The theory and practice of group psychotherapy,* 3rd ed. New York: Basic Books, Inc.

Yalom, I. D., Houts, P. S., Newell, G. & Rand, K. H. (1967). Preparation of patients for group therapy. *Archives of General Psychiatry, 17,* 416–427.

Yogev, S. (1982). An eclectic model of supervision: A developmental sequence for the beginning psychotherapy student. *Professional Psychology, 13,* 236–243.

Yost, E., Beutler, L. E., Corbishley, M. A. & Allender, J. R. (1986). *Group cognitive therapy: A treatment approach for depressed older adults.* New York: Pergamon Press.

Zook, A., II & Sipps, G. J. (1987). Machiavellianism and dominance: Are therapists in training manipulative? *Psychotherapy, 24,* 15–19.

Zwick, R. & Attkisson, C. C. (1985). Effectiveness of a client pretherapy orientation videotape. *Journal of Counseling Psychology, 32,* 514–524.

Name Index

Abelson, R. P., 33–34
Abramowitz, S. I., 176, 177
Abrams, D. D., 52
Abrams, R., 39
Abramson, L. Y., 217
Ackerman, N. W., 116
Adland, M. L., 137
Adler, A., 7
Aldwin, C., 88
Alexander, J. F., 169, 189
Alexander, L., 175, 296
Allen, G. J., 303–304, 305
Allen, J., 151
Allender, J. R., 10, 88, 154, 251
Anchor, K. N., 174, 202
Anderson, M. P., 9
Anderson, W., 277
Andrasik, F., 10
Andreasen, N., 44
Andrews, G., 88, 136, 224
Aneshensel, C. S., 88
Applebaum, A., 234
Arizmendi, T. G., 61, 62, 69, 76, 84, 86, 91, 174, 176, 181, 182, 186, 187, 196, 198, 275
Arkowitz, H., 8, 88, 214, 222, 272, 281
Armstrong, S., 176
Arnold, R. C., 295, 305
Arthur, J., 93
Ashinger, P. A. G., 87
Atkinson, B. M., 10, 86
Atkinson, D. R., 176
Attkisson, C. C., 188
Auerbach, A., 173, 176, 225
Auerbach, S. M., 169
Authier, J., 295
Autry, J. H., 10, 40
Avner, R., 277
Azrin, N. H., 190

Bachrach, H., 176
Bachrach, L. L., 107
Bacon, S., 137
Baekeland, F., 145
Baer, J. S., 51, 262

Baer, P. E., 265
Baker, F., 111
Baker, T. B., 52
Bamford, C. R., 190, 217, 218, 234
Bandura, A., 8, 73, 251
Banks, M. H., 95
Barbaree, H. E., 54
Barlow, D. H., 46–48, 35–36, 126, 214, 215, 228, 244, 274, 280
Barnett, P. A., 88, 90, 94
Barrett, J., 201, 204
Bartko, J. J., 39
Barton, C., 189
Battle, C. C., 188
Bauman, N. C., 198
Beasley, C., 151
Beck, A. T., 8, 10, 49, 148, 189, 214, 216, 225, 228, 242–243, 244, 251, 281, 306
Bedell, R., 104
Bednar, R. L., 118
Behrman, J. A., 146
Beidel, D. C., 9, 68
Beitman, B. D., 18–19, 26, 213, 254, 263
Bell, J., 115
Bell, P. A., 200, 201
Bellack, A. S., 49, 135, 136, 148, 217
Bemis, K. M., 10, 306
Benjamin, L. S., 38, 54
Bennun, I., 129
Bergin, A. E., 11, 80, 158, 159, 182, 196
Berkowitz, R., 135
Berman, J. S., 242, 251
Berry, D. S., 174, 175
Berzins, J. I., 179
Bescript, M. A., xv
Beutler, L. E., xv, 5, 9, 10, 11, 14, 17, 18, 22, 31, 61, 62, 69, 71, 72, 76, 84, 86, 88, 91, 118, 135, 136, 142, 154, 174, 176, 177, 179, 181, 182, 183, 186, 187, 190, 195, 196, 198, 199, 202, 214, 217–219, 222, 229, 230, 232, 234, 240, 241, 243, 251, 255, 258, 260, 262, 265, 268, 273, 274, 275, 281–282, 290, 291, 296, 297, 299, 301, 303, 304, 306
Bienvenu, J. P., 154

Biglan, A., 93
Billings, A. G., 42, 85, 90
Binder, J. L., 7, 10, 19, 177, 180, 214, 220–221, 225, 229, 232, 248, 259, 282–283
Biondo, J., 183
Birchler, G. A., 52
Birley, J. L. T., 134
Bishop, D., 39
Bishop, S., 135, 136
Blackburn, I. M., 135, 136
Blanchard, E. B., 10
Blanck, P. D., 174, 202
Bland, R. C., 44
Blanton, S., 302–303
Blase, J. J., 175, 176
Blatt, S. J., 78
Blau, T. H., 254, 275–276
Blazer, D. G., 86
Blier, M. J., 176
Bloxom, A. I., 188, 189
Blumenfield, M., 302
Bond, J. A., 71, 248
Bootzin, R. R., 227
Bordin, E. S., 173
Borduin, C. M., 116, 118
Borkovec, T., 10, 73, 274
Boster, F. J., 68
Bowlby, J., 115
Boyd, J. L., 135
Boyer, J. T., 246, 296, 297, 299, 304
Brasted, W. S., 291
Brauzer, B., 134
Breckenridge, J., 10
Brehm, J. W., 17, 183, 200
Brehm, S. S., 17, 174, 183, 200, 275
Breuer, J., 9, 115
Brickman, P., 51
Brockington, I. F., 44
Broderick, C. B., 116
Brodsky, A. M., 204
Brody, C. M., 176
Bromer, E. J., 85, 94
Brown, G. W., 88, 92, 134
Brownlee-Duffeck, M., 273
Brunink, S., 213
Buchanan, D. R., 198
Buckholtz, A., 202
Buckley, P. J., 305
Budman, S. H., 71, 118, 126, 142, 145, 146, 154
Buglass, D., 121
Buller, D. B., 197
Burgoon, J. K., 68, 197
Burgoon, M., 68, 247
Burlingame, G. M., 18, 118, 146
Butcher, J. N., 24, 144, 156, 190
Butler, S. F., 291, 296, 306

Byrne, D., 77

Caffey, E., 109
Calhoun, K. S., 10
Calvert, S. J., 18, 69, 243
Campbell, V. L., 291
Cannon, D. S., 52
Caplan, G., 87
Carkhuff, R. R., 175, 189, 295
Carpenter, W. T., 39, 43, 45
Carr, A., 234
Carrillo, C., 150
Carson, R. C., 178, 179
Carstairs, G. M., 92
Casey, N. A., 111
Catalano, R., 95
Chambers, A., 10, 274
Chambless, D. L., 47
Charcot, J. M., 9
Charles, E. S., 305
Charone, J. K., 181
Cherniss, C., 305
Chevron, E. S., 10, 49, 148, 170, 171, 214, 219–220, 229, 231, 242, 262, 282, 296, 306
Childress, R., 188, 201
Christensen, H., 136, 224
Christie, J. E., 135, 136
Clance, P., 291
Clarke, D. M., 10
Clarke, J., 121
Clarke, K. M., 296
Clarkin, J. F., xv, 11, 16, 18, 23, 24, 37, 39, 54, 70, 89, 102, 107, 116, 119, 125, 129, 138, 155, 158, 179, 241, 292, 298, 300, 302
Coates, B., 199
Coates, D., 51
Cobb, J., 121–122
Cobb, S., 87
Cohen, C. I., 85
Cohen, J., 111
Cohen, M., 175, 176, 296
Cohn, E., 51
Collins, J. F., 111
Comstock, B. A., 108
Conklin, L., xv
Conn, D., 68
Connell, M. M., 85, 94
Connors, G. J., 51
Cook, P. E., 76
Cooper, A., 249, 270, 276, 296
Cooper, H. M., 116, 118
Corbishley, A., 10, 181
Corbishley, M. A., 10, 88, 154, 190, 217, 218, 234, 251
Corrigan, J. D., 58, 62, 174, 175, 186
Corsini, R. J., 213
Costello, C. G., 88

Covi, L., 136, 198
Coyne, J. C., 88, 222, 234, 273
Coyne, L., 151
Crago, M., 18, 22, 61, 62, 69, 76, 86, 142, 174, 176, 181, 182, 186, 187, 196, 198, 199, 202, 243, 275
Cramer, P., 78
Cristol, A. H., 9, 190, 213, 243
Crits-Christoph, P., 175, 176, 249, 270, 276, 296
Cronkite, R. C., 90
Crowne, D., 68
Cumming, J. D., 11, 171, 242, 250
Curtis, H., 176
Curtis, J. T., 232, 249, 270, 276, 296

Daldrup, R. J., 10, 154, 195, 214, 217–219, 230, 241, 246, 247, 248, 273, 281–282, 296, 297, 299, 304, 306
Dangler, R. F., 10
Dasberg, H., 306
Dave, C., 160
Davenport, Y. B., 137
Davidson, S., 88
Davis, C. S., 199
Davis, J. D., 202
Davis, J. M., 136
Davis, K. L., 296
Davison, G. C., 251
Dawson, M., 42
Debbane, E. G., 154
Deci, E. L., 183
DeJulio, S. S., 31
DeLeon, R. H., 142
Dell, D. M., 58, 62, 174, 175, 186, 201
Delworth, U., 299, 301, 302
Demby, A., 126
Dempsey, M., 39, 44
Dennis, H., 109
Depue, R. A., 88
Derogatis, L. R., 136
DeRubeis, R. J., 10, 292, 306
de Turck, M. A., 197
Dickey, B. A., 111
Dickman, H. R., 111
Dicks, H. V., 116
DiClemente, C. C., 18, 65–66, 241, 255, 257, 258, 259, 260, 262
DiMascio, A., 134, 136, 224
Dinitz, S., 108
Dixon, D. N., 63, 174
Dobson, K. S., 148, 291, 292, 296, 306
Doehrman, M., 306
Dohrenwend, B. P., 87
Dohrenwend, B. S., 87
Dollard, J., 8
Donovan, D. M., 51, 262

Dooley, D., 95
Dougher, M. J., 87
Dowd, E. T., 73, 275, 276, 277
Druleu, K. A., 53
DuBrin, J. R., 145
Dubro, A. F., 227
Duff, E., 95
Dunbar, P. W., 265
Dundon, M., 60, 63

Eaton, W. W., 86
Eberlein-Vries, R., 135
Ebert, M. H., 137
Ebrahimi, S., 10, 274
Edelstein, B. A., 291
Edinger, J. A., 174
Edwards, D. J. A., 8, 9
Edwards, G., 51
Ehrlichman, H., 198
Eisenberg, N., 76, 77, 78
Ekman, P., 197, 198, 247
Ekstein, R., 306
Elkin, I., 10, 170, 171, 190, 219, 242, 296
Elkins, D., 181, 182
Ellenbogen, G. C., 33
Elliott, R., 269
Ellsworth, P. C., 197
Ellsworth, R., 105, 111
Emery, G., 8, 10, 148, 189, 214, 216, 225, 228, 244, 251, 281, 306
Emmelkamp, P., 47, 125, 190
Endicott, J., 39, 107, 108, 150, 158
Endicott, N. A., 158
Engle, D., 10, 154, 195, 214, 217–219, 230, 241, 246, 247, 248, 273, 281–282, 296, 297, 299, 304, 306
Equatios, E., 305
Ersner-Herschfeld, R., 152
Evans, M. D., 306
Exline, R. V., 199
Eysenck, H. J., 34, 40–41, 75, 158
Eysenck, S. B. G., 75

Failtler, S., 235
Fairweather, G., 111, 160
Falbo, J., 216
Falloon, I. R. H., 103, 135
Fava, J., 65–66, 259, 262
Feighner, J. P., 39
Feldstein, M., 126
Feldstein, S., 247
Felner, R. D., 62, 68, 86, 87, 196
Feuerberg, M., 24
Fiedler, F. E., 9
Fine, H., 174
Fischer, C. S., 88
Fisher, D. C., 298

Fisher, J. D., 200, 201
Fishman, H. C., 215, 221–222, 229, 231, 283
Flaherty, J. A., 85, 91
Flanery, R. C., 190
Fleming, J., 305
Fletcher, B. C., 95
Flynn, H., 105–106
Foley, S., 225, 292
Folkman, S., 75, 76
Follette, V., 148
Follette, W. C., 118, 119, 120, 179
Foon, A. E., 183
Ford, R. Q., 78
Foreman, S. A., 68, 185
Forer, B. R., 198
Forgatch, M. S., 120
Forsyth, D. R., 60, 169, 275
Forsyth, N. L., 60, 275
Forte, R. A., 197
Fowler, L., xv
Frances, A., 11, 16, 18, 23, 24, 37, 39, 54, 70, 102, 107, 129, 138, 155, 158, 179, 241, 292, 298, 300, 302
Frank, E., 306
Frank, J. D., 10–11, 15, 171, 188, 213
Frankel, A. S., 201, 204
Frankhauser, M., 113
Franklin, J., 217
Freebury, M. B., 71
Freeman, A., 10, 281
Fremont, S. K., 277
Fretter, P. B., 249, 270, 276, 296
Fretz, B. R., 174
Freud, S., 7, 9, 83–84, 94, 115, 142, 160, 302–303
Friedlander, M. L., 269
Friedman, A. F., 34, 40–41
Friedman, H. S., 197
Friedman, L. S., 93
Fuchs, C. Z., 10
Fuhriman, A., 18

Gadow, K. D., 116, 135, 136
Gallagher, D., 10, 243
Garant, J., 154
Garfield, S. L., 6, 10, 11, 15, 22, 31, 32, 39, 57, 58, 61, 62, 86, 145, 148, 196, 213, 291
Gaston, L., 68, 243, 281
Gebhard, M. E., 160
Geer, C. A., 176
Geller, M. H., 178, 179
Genack, A., 176
Gendlin, E. T., 247, 248
George, W. H., 262
Gilderman, A. M., 135
Gillis, J. S., 39, 183, 188, 201
Gilmore, M., 39

Gino, A., 52
Gittelman, R., 134, 135
Glaser, R., 74
Glass, G. V., 119, 159, 213
Glen, A. I. M., 135, 136
Gleser, G. C., 75, 76, 78, 79, 246
Glick, I. D., 89, 105, 108, 125, 150
Goldberg, D. P., 269
Goldfried, M. R., 5, 8, 251, 299, 300
Goldman, M., 197, 198
Goldman, R. L., 296
Goldstein, A. P., 11, 15, 16, 17, 61, 68, 145, 174, 196, 295
Goldstein, D., 273
Goldstein, M. J., 91–92
Gomes-Schwartz, R., 160
Gonzales, M., 176
Goodstein, L. D., 203
Goodwin, F. K., 137
Gordon, J. R., 262
Gorsuch, L., 229
Gotlib, I. H., 88, 90, 94
Gottlieb, B. H., 87
Goulding, M., 189, 248
Goulding, R., 189, 248
Grater, H. A., 305
Greenberg, L. S., 10, 128, 129, 154, 195, 214, 217–219, 230, 241, 246, 247, 248, 281–282, 296, 306
Greene, L. R., 201, 205
Greenspan, B., 39
Gretter, M. L., 115, 119
Grigg, A. E., 203
Gross, M., 109
Guest, P. D., 9, 10, 222, 296, 301, 303
Gunderson, J. G., 104, 105
Gurel, L., 111
Gurman, A. S., 71, 118, 145, 146, 154, 174
Guy, W., 109
Guze, S. B., 39

Haas, G. L., 116, 119, 125, 306
Haase, R. F., 174, 197, 198
Hadley, S. W., 10, 40, 160
Hadzi-Pavlovic, D., 136, 224
Hafner, R. J., 121
Hafner, R. R., 121
Hagaman, R., 181
Hakstian, A. R., 49, 135
Hale, J. L., 197
Halgin, R. P., 296, 298, 299
Halleck, S. L., 300
Halloran, P., 232
Hamblin, D. L., 181, 190, 217, 218, 229, 234
Hamilton, E. W., 217
Handley, P., 303
Hannah, M. T., 222, 272

Hannan, M., 126
Hansell, J., 71, 248
Harding, C. M., 44, 45
Hardy, E., 299, 301, 302
Hardy, G. E., 293
Hargreaves, W., 105, 108, 150
Harris, T. O., 88
Hart, G. M., 302
Harvey, J. H., 182
Hassenfield, I., 301
Hatcher, S. L., 220, 229, 234, 253
Haugh, R. L., 86
Hauser, S. T., 176
Hautzinger, M., 93
Hay, W., 52
Hays, K. A., 295, 301
Hazelrigg, M. D., 116, 118
Hector, M. A., 296
Heesacker, M., 174
Heide, F. J., 73, 174
Heine, R. W., 178
Heinrichs, D. W., 43, 45
Heitler, J. B., 188
Hellman, I. D., 177
Helms, J. E., 269, 270
Hemmings, K. A., 115, 119
Henderson, A. S., 121
Henisz, J., 105–106
Henry, W. E., 300
Heppner, P. P., 63, 174, 302
Hepworth, S. J., 95
Herbert, D. L., 33–34
Herbert, J. D., 33–34
Herman, B., 295, 301
Hermansson, G. L., 198
Hersen, M., 49, 135, 136, 148
Herz, M., 108, 150
Hess, A. K., 300, 302, 304
Hester, R. K., 106
Heverly, M., 104
Hewson, D., 88
Hickey, R. H., 111
Higbee, K. L., 68
Hill, C. E., 269, 270
Hill, J. A., 182
Himle, J., 47
Himmelhoch, J. M., 49, 135, 136, 148
Himmel, C. D., 291
Hobson, R. F., 269
Hobson, R. R., 269
Hodgson, R., 51
Hoehn-Saric, R., 188
Hoette, S., 273
Hoffman, N., 93
Hogan, R. A., 302
Hogarty, C., 109
Hogarty, G., 109

Holder, A., 160
Holland, J. L., 160
Holliday, P. B., 188
Holliday, S., 88
Hollon, S. D., 49
Hollon, S. E., 306
Holroyd, J. C., 204
Holroyd, K., 273
Holt, R. R., 95
Hooley, J. M., 93–94, 262
Hops, H., 190
Hops, S., 93
Horgan, C. M., 24
Horney, K., 7
Horn-George, J. B., 174, 202
Horowitz, L. M., 38, 54, 232
Horowitz, M., 11, 159, 171, 220, 229, 232, 242, 250
Horwitz, A., 85, 160
Houston, B. K., 183
Houts, P. S., 187, 188
Howard, G. S., 119, 136
Howard, K. I., 11, 22, 24, 38, 43, 102, 143, 174, 182, 186, 187, 198, 233, 262, 284
Howell, R. J., 291
Hubble, M. A., 198
Huebner, D. A., 220, 229, 234, 253
Hughes, J., 197, 198
Hunt, D. E., 303
Hurt, S. W., 39, 70, 179
Hurt, W. S., 54
Hutter, M., 88
Hyer, L., 111

Ihlevich, D., 75, 76, 78, 79, 246
Imber, S., 119, 170, 171, 188, 219, 242, 296
Ittelson, W. H., 200
Ivey, A. E., 295

Jackson, P. R., 95
Jacob, J. L.., 87
Jacob, T., 52, 94
Jacobs, M. K., 188
Jacobson, G. F., 144
Jacobson, N. S., 10, 118, 119, 120, 148, 179, 221, 262
Jarrett, R. B., 148–149
Jessor, R., 183
Jobe, A. M., 181, 182
Johnson, J., 91
Johnson, M., 176
Johnson, S. M., 128, 129, 218, 248
Johnston, D. W., 122
Jones, E. E., 11, 171, 175, 176, 242, 250
Jones, R., 190
Juhnke, R., 198
Jung, C. G., 7

Kagan, N., 305
Kahn, J., 88
Kahn, M., 227
Kalafat, J., 290
Kalehzan, M., 232
Kaltreider, N., 220, 229, 232
Kanter, C. N., 305
Karasek, R. A., 95
Karasu, T. B., 305
Karuza, J., 51
Kasl, S. V., 95
Katzoff, A., 150
Kaul, T., 118
Kazdin, A. E., 15
Keith, S. J., 135
Kendell, R. E., 44
Kerig, P. K., 175, 176
Kernberg, O. F., 149, 234, 306
Kerr, B. A., 201
Kessler, D. R., 89
Kessler, L., 24
Kessler, R. C., 87, 88–89
Kiecolt-Glaser, J. K., 74
Kiesler, C., 106, 108
Kiesler, D. J., 12, 300
Killilea, M., 87
Kilo, C., 273
Kimble, C. E., 197
King, J. W., 296
Kinney, P. J., 216
Kirkish, P., 190, 217, 218, 234
Kirlahan, D. R., 51
Kirschenbaum, D. S., 190
Kirshner, L. A., 176
Kivlahan, D. R., 262
Klar, H., 107
Klein, D. F., 134, 135
Klein, D. N., 39
Kleinke, C. L., 197, 198, 199
Klerman, G. L., 10, 49, 134, 135, 136, 137–
    138, 148, 150, 214, 219–220, 224, 229,
    231, 262, 282
Klett, J., 109
Kniskern, D. P., 118
Koenigsberg, H., 234, 306
Kohut, H., 173, 179
Kolb, D. L., 199, 240
Kopel, S., 152
Kopta, S., 104, 143
Korman, M., 291
Koss, M. P., 24, 144, 156, 190
Kovacs, M., 49, 136, 148
Kramer, M., 86
Krause, M., 143
Krause, N., 182, 183
Kreiger, P., 204
Kreitman, N., 121

Kriebel, G., 39
Krupnick, J. L., 175, 176, 220, 229, 232
Kuipers, L., 135
Kurtz, R., 10, 32, 291

Lachman, M. E., 183
LaCrosse, M. B., 174
Lamb, H. R., 109
Lambert, M. J., 11, 31, 158, 159, 196, 295, 305
Lane, T. W., 306
Langer, E. J., 33–34
Larson, D. G., 213
Larson, D. W., 217
Larson, V. A., 169, 172, 181, 284
Last, C. G., 48
LaTorre, R. A., 187
Lauver, P. J., 84, 91
Lawton, M. P., 111
Lazarus, A. A., 5, 6, 11, 17
Lazarus, R. S., 75, 76, 88
Leeman, C. P., 104, 105
Lefcourt, H. M., 182, 183
Leff, J., 44, 92–93, 135
Lentz, R. J., 45, 109–110, 251
Leonard, K. E., 52
Levenson, A. I., 190, 217, 218, 234
Levenson, A. J., 108
Levin, G., 107
Levine, J., 134
Levis, D. J., 8
Lewin, K., 117
Lewinsohn, P. M., 217
Lewis, J. M., 114
Lewis, K. N., 58, 62, 174, 175, 182, 186
Lewis, P., 119
Lieberman, M. A., 9, 91, 160
Linden, M., 93
Linehan, M. M., 124, 149, 160, 234
Linn, L. S., 111
Linn, M., 109
Lipkin, M. D., 39
Lipman, R. S., 136, 198
Llewellyn, C. E., Jr., 179
Locke, B. Z., 86
Loevinger, J., 78
Loganbill, C., 299, 301, 302
London, P., 240
Longabaugh, R., 39
Loomis, R. J., 200, 201
Lopez, F. G., 291
Lopez, S., 86
Lord, C. J., 108
Lorion, R. P., 62, 68, 86, 87, 196
Lotterman, A., 306
Luborsky, L., 7, 9, 10, 19, 53, 71, 173, 175,
    176, 177, 180, 220, 225, 229, 248, 249,
    270, 276, 291, 296

358

Luborsky, L., 9
Lundwall, M. A., 145
Lytle, R., 10, 274

MacDonald, A. P., Jr., 183
Madanes, C., 189
Maguire, G. P., 269
Maharini of Jaipus, 305
Mahoney, M. J., 118, 135, 136, 262, 304
Mahrer, A. R., 248, 269
Malan, D. H., 19, 142, 149, 153, 220, 229
Malone, J., 295, 301
Mann, B., 202
Marachi, J., 129
Margison, F. R., 269
Margolin, G., 10, 221
Margolis, M., 175, 296
Marks, I., 10, 121–122
Marlatt, G. A., 51, 262
Marmar, C. R., 68, 185, 220, 229, 232, 243, 281
Maroney, R. J., 111
Marsden, D., 95
Marshall, W. L., 54
Martelli, M. F., 169
Martin, P. J., 63
Maslow, A., 289
Mason, J., 47
Massman, P. J., 242, 252
Masters, K. S., 118
Matarazzo, R. G., 291, 292, 295, 305
Mathews, A. M., 10, 274
Mattes, J., 150
Mattick, R., 136, 224
Mattson, M., 105–106
Maurer, R. E., 174, 198
Mavissakalian, M., 136
Maxwell, S. E., 119, 136
Mayer, J., 305
Mayerson, N. H., 187, 188, 189, 192
McArthur, L. Z., 174, 175
McClelland, M., 37, 38, 49
McConnaughy, E. A., 177
McCrady, B. S., 52, 227
McCroskey, J. C., 68
McCullough, L., 39
McDonald, R., 121–122
McFarland, K., 198
McGill, C. W., 135
McGlashan, T., 45, 105
McLachan, J. C., 243
McLean, P. D., 49, 135
McLellan, A. T., 53, 173, 225
McLemore, C., 38, 54
McNabb, C., 301
McNamara, T. P., 33
Meara, N. M., 296

Megargee, E. I., 75–76
Meichenbaum, D. J., 68, 188, 244, 251
Mendelsohn, G. A., 76, 178, 179
Menn, A. Z., 108
Mercuri, L. G., 169
Meredith, K., 190, 217, 218, 234, 246, 273, 296, 297, 299, 304
Mesnikoff, A., 108
Messer, S. B., 8, 214
Miles, M. B., 9, 160
Millan, D., 150
Miller, G. R., 68
Miller, I. W., III, 183
Miller, N. E., 8
Miller, P. A., 76, 77, 78
Miller, R. C., 242, 251
Miller, T. I., 119, 159, 213
Miller, W. R., 52, 106
Millis, W., 174
Millon, T., 76, 179–180
Mintz, E. E., 197
Mintz, J., 176, 229
Minuchin, S., 215, 221–222, 229, 231, 283
Mirels, H. L., 174, 275
Mischel, W., 199
Mitchell, K. M., 86
Mitchell, R., 18, 69, 76, 243
Mittleman, B., 116
Mock, J. E., 198
Monck, E. M., 92
Mongeau, P., 68
Monroe, S. M., 85, 94
Montgomery, L. M., 227
Moore, J. E., 63
Moos, H. B., 135
Moos, R., 42, 85, 90, 104, 105, 111
Moran, T. J., 39
Moravec, J., 174
Morey, L., 33, 43, 51
Morgan, R., 176
Morley, W., 144
Morrison, T. L., 177
Mortola, J., 51
Mosher, L. R., 108
Moskowitz, S., 305
Moss, S., 269
Mowrer, O. H., 8
Munby, M., 122
Munoz, R., 39
Murphy, G. E., 148
Murphy, K. C., 202
Murray, J., 176
Muzekari, L. H., 204
Myers, J. D., 87
Myers, J. K., 86

Namenek, T. M., 86

Nash, E. H., 188
Naster, B. J., 190
Nathan, P. E., 52
Neigher, W. D., 290
Neimeyer, G. J., 176
Nelson, G., 302, 305
Nelson, H. F., 52
Nelson, R. O., 33–34, 274
Nesselroade, J. R., 111
Neu, C., 224
Newell, G., 187, 188
Newhart, B., 158
Newman, F., 102, 104
Newton, I., 7
Nietzel, M. T., 115, 119
Noble, F. C., 198
Noel, N. E., 52
Norcross, J. C., 5, 6, 11, 32, 115, 116, 118, 135, 136, 262, 288, 289, 290, 296, 297, 298, 304, 305, 306
Norman, W. H., 183
Nuechterlein, K., 42
Nuñez, J. A., 86

Oberndorf, C. P., 116
O'Brien, C. P., 53, 173, 176, 225
O'Brien, G. T., 48
O'Dowd, T., 269
O'Farrell, T. J., 52
Oliker, S. J., 88
O'Malley, S., 225, 292
Orlinsky, D. E., 11, 22, 24, 143, 174, 182, 186, 187, 233, 284
Orn, H., 44
Oro'-Beutler, M. E., 246, 273, 296, 297, 299, 304
Orwin, R. G., 227
Osborn, M., 269
Osteen, V., 93
Ostrom, R., 182

Pace, T. F., 73, 275, 276, 277
Packard, T., 88
Padawer, W., 300
Pagel, M., 118, 119, 120, 179
Parker, J. H., 44
Parloff, M. B., 10, 11, 15, 187, 213
Parry, G., 85, 87, 88, 95
Parsons, B. V., 189
Pasamanick, B., 108
Patterson, D., 291, 292, 295, 305
Patterson, G. R., 103, 120, 126, 190
Patterson, M. L., 174, 198, 199
Pattison, J. H., 136
Paul, G. L., 31, 45, 109–110, 251
Paul, S. C., 18
Pavlov, I. P., 8

Paykel, E. S., 136, 224
Payne, R. L., 95
Pearlin, L. I., 91
Pennebaker, J. W., 74
Penrod, S., 175
Pepper, M. P., 87
Perls, F. S., 248
Perry, S., 11, 16, 18, 23, 24, 37, 102, 138, 241, 292, 298, 300
Perry, W., 299
Peterson, L., 273
Pfefferbaum, H., 137
Pfohl, B., 44
Phillips, G. L., 305
Pierce, A., 175
Pilkonis, P., 119
Pinsof, W. M., 118
Piper, W. E., 154
Pollack, S., 181
Polster, E., 218, 248
Polster, M., 218, 248
Polster, R. A., 10
Pomerleau, C. S., 189
Pomerleau, O. F., 189
Pope, B., 202
Potter, R., 190, 217, 218, 234
Pratt, J. H., 117
Presley, A. S., 121
Press, S., 183
Price, R. H., 87, 88–89
Probst, L. R., 182
Prochaska, J. O., 5, 18, 26, 32, 65–66, 118, 135, 136, 241, 255, 257, 258, 259, 260, 261, 262, 279, 291
Proshansky, H. M., 200
Prusoff, B. A., 136, 148, 170, 171, 219, 224, 242, 296, 306

Quitkin, F., 134, 135

Rabinowitz, V. C., 51
Rachelson, J., 291
Rachman, S. J., 213
Rand, K. H., 187, 188
Rapee, R., 273
Ray, P. B., 202, 203, 302
Razani, J., 135
Reahl, J. E., 160
Redmond, F. C., 90
Redondo, J. P., 126
Regier, D. A., 86
Rehm, L. P., 10, 148
Remer, P., 202
Rice, L. N., 189, 246, 247
Richman, J. A., 85, 91
Rickels, K., 198
Riehl, A., 91

Rifkin, A., 134, 135
Riggio, R. E., 197
Ring, J., 68, 126, 281
Rivlin, L. G., 200
Robbins, E. S., 174, 197
Robertson, L. S., 68
Robertson, M., 118, 135, 136, 262, 290, 291, 296, 298, 304
Robins, L. N., 86
Robins, E., 39
Robinson, S. E., 198
Rockland, L., 306
Roehlke, H. J., 302
Roessler, R., 76
Roffey, B. H., 202
Rogers, C. R., 7, 174
Rohrbaugh, M., 183
Rosen, B., 150
Rosen, M., 104
Rosenberg, S. E., 232
Rosenblatt, A., 305
Rosenthal, N. R., 303
Rosenthal, R., 161, 174, 202, 277
Ross, M. W., 121
Rosser, C., 291, 296
Rotter, J. B., 182
Rounsaville, B. J., 10, 49, 148, 170, 171, 214, 219–220, 225, 229, 231, 242, 262, 282, 292, 296, 306
Ruffner, M., 68, 247
Rupert, P., 305
Rush, A. J., 8, 10, 49, 148–149, 189, 214, 216, 225, 228, 244, 251, 262, 281, 306
Russell, R. L., 115, 119

Sachs, J. S., 160
Safran, J., 247
Salusky, S., 148
Sampson, H., 232
Sanders, R., 160
Sandler, J., 160
Sank, L. I., 10, 154
Saper, B., 276
Sarkissian, M. G., 296, 306
Sarris, J., 301
Saunders, S. M., 186
Scarpitti, F. R., 108
Schaefer, C., 88
Schiavo, R. S., 189
Schmaling, K. B., 148
Schmidt, L. D., 58, 62, 174, 175, 186
Schneider, S., 39, 144
Schooler, N. R., 134, 135
Schoonover, R. A., 111
Schrader, S. S., 116
Schradle, S. B., 87
Schramski, T. G., 84, 91

Schretlen, D., 190, 217, 218, 234
Schroeder, H., 213
Schuckit, M. A., 51
Schulberg, H. C., 37, 38, 49, 111
Schwartz, J., 105, 111
Scoggin, F., 181, 190, 217, 218, 234
Seltzer, L. F., 161, 276
Seltzer, M., 234, 306
Sermas, C. E., 108
Severe, J. B., 134
Shadish, W. R., Jr., 227
Shaffer, C. S., 10, 154
Shakir, S. A., 137
Shanfield, S., 181, 199
Shapiro, D., 159, 251
Shapiro, D. A., 11, 85, 87, 88, 158, 159, 251, 293
Shapiro, P. N., 175
Shaw, B. F., 8, 10, 148, 189, 214, 216, 225, 228, 244, 251, 281, 291, 292, 296, 306
Sheffield, J., 77
Sherman, L., 93
Shevrin, H., 71, 248
Shoham-Salomon, V., 161, 277
Siegman, A. W., 247
Silberschatz, G., 232, 249, 270, 276, 296
Simon, K. E., 281
Simon, R., 160
Simonds, S. F., 273
Simons, A. D., 148
Sims, J. H., 300
Sinfield, A., 95
Singer, B., 9
Sipps, G. J., 284
Skinner, A. E., G., 202
Skinner, B. F., 8
Skinner, H., 43, 51
Slater, J., 88
Slavson, S. R., 118
Sloane, R. B., 9, 190, 202, 213, 243
Smith, E. W., 199
Smith, J. E., 136
Smith, M. L., 119, 159, 213
Smith, T., 17, 174
Smoller, J. W., 33
Snyder, C. R., 169
Snyder, D., 235
Sokolovsky, J., 85
Sollod, R. M., 118, 135, 136, 262
Solomon, J., 176
Sommer, G., 144
Sorenson, R. L., 229
Sotsky, S., 170, 171, 219, 242, 296
Spencer, J., 105–106
Spiegel, S. B., 269, 270
Spitzer, R. L., 39, 107, 108, 150
Spohn, H., 151

Spray, S. L., 300
Springer, T., 118, 126
Stafford, E. M., 95
Stamfl, T. G., 8
Staples, F. R., 9, 190, 202, 213, 243
Stein, L. I., 108
Stein, N., 11, 15, 16
Stein, S. P., 305
Steinbrueck, S. M., 119, 136
Steiner, S. C., 85, 94
Steinmetz, J. L., 217
Stern, R., 121–122
Stern, S., 290
Sterne, A. L., 63
Stevenson, J. F., 291
Stiles, W. B., 269
Stockwell, T., 51
Stoltenberg, C., 302
Stone, A. R., 188
Stone, G. B., 160
Stone, J. D., 88
Stout, R., 39, 52
Strachan, A. M., 91–92
Strauss, J. S., 39, 44, 45
Strickler, M., 144
Strong, S. R., 17, 171, 174
Strupp, H. H., 7, 10, 19, 68, 160, 177, 180,
    188, 189, 213, 214, 220–221, 225, 229,
    232, 248, 259, 282–283, 290, 291, 296,
    306
Stuart, R. B., 68, 190
Sturgeon, D., 135
Suedfeld, , 298
Sullender, W., 108
Sullivan, E. V., 303
Sundland, D. M., 25, 213, 266–268
Swinburne, P., 95
Szollos, S. J., 303–304, 305

Tarbox, A. R., 51
Taube, C. A., 24
Taylor, M. A., 39
Teasdale, J. D., 262
Tennant, C., 88
Tennen, H., 183
Tepper, D. T., Jr., 197, 198
Terrell, R., 176
Terrell, S., 176
Test, M. A., 108
Thomas, B. L., 290, 298
Thompson, L., 10, 243
Thornby, J. L., 108
Thorpe, S. A., 71, 240
Thyer, B. A., 47
Tibbits-Kleber, A. L., 291
Tichenor, V., 269, 270
Tjelveit, A. C., 181

Todd, T., 176
Tolman, E., 8
Tracey, T. J., 60, 63, 145, 183, 202, 203, 275,
    295, 301
Tracy, D. C., 296
Trick, O. L., 188
Truax, C. B., 174, 188–189, 295
Trull, T. J., 54, 70, 179
Tsuang, M. T., 39, 44
Tuason, V. B., 134
Turk, D. C., 68, 188
Turkat, D. M., 188
Turner, S. M., 9, 68, 176
Twemlow, S. W., 111
Tyler, J. D., 300
Tyndall, J. H., 174, 198
Tyson, C. L., 204

Ullmann, L. P., 111
Ureno, G., 232
Usdin, G., 114

Vaillant, G. E., 78, 88
Valentine, M. E., 198
Vallis, T. M., 306
VandenBos, G. R., 142
Vannicelli, M., 174, 202
Vaughn, C., 92–93
Velicer, W. F., 65–66, 259, 262
Videka-Sherman, L., 91
Vitkus, J., 38, 54
Volkmar, F. R., 137
von Essen, C., 176, 177

Wachtel, P. L., 8
Waddell, M. T., 35, 126, 214, 215, 228, 244,
    274, 280
Wakefield, J. A., 34, 40–41
Wallerstein, R., 220, 229, 232, 306
Wargo, D. G., 189
Warr, P. B., 95
Warren, R. C., 189
Waskow, I. E., 187
Watkins, C. E., Jr., 291
Watkins, J., 170, 171, 219, 242, 296
Watkins, P., 182
Watson, J., 83–84
Weary, G., 171, 174, 182, 275
Weaver, S. H., 300
Webster, A. C., 198
Weingarten, E., 160
Weishaar, M., 8
Weiss, J., 232
Weiss, R. L., 190
Weissman, M. M., 10, 49, 136, 148, 214, 219–
    220, 224, 225, 229, 231, 262, 282, 292,
    306

Welsh, G. S., 76
Wetzel, J. W., 90
Wetzler, S., 227
Whalley, L. J., 135, 136
Whipple, K., 9, 190, 213, 243
White, L., 183
Widiger, T. A., 39, 54, 70, 179
Wilder, J. F., 107
Wiley, M. O., 302
Wilkins, W., 15
Williams, B. E., 303–304, 305
Williams, S. L., 216
Wills, R., 235
Wilmer, D. M., 144
Wilner, N., 220, 229, 232
Wilson, D. O., 187, 189, 191
Wilson, G. T., 142–143, 149, 152, 213
Wing, J. K., 92, 134
Winokur, G., 39
Winokur, M., 306
Withersty, D., 188
Wogan, M., 32
Wolberg, L. R., 145

Wolfe, B. E., 5, 187
Woodruff, R. A., 39
Woody, G. E., 53, 173, 225
Woody, R. H., 298
Worthington, E. L., 301, 302
Wortman, C. B., 87, 88–89
Wycoff, J. P., 296
Wynne, L. C., 124–125

Yalom, I. D., 9, 118, 129, 160, 187, 188
Yogev, S., 302
Yorkston, N. J., 9, 190, 213, 243
Yoshikawa, J. C., 197
Yost, E., 10, 88, 154, 251

Zakin, D. F., 220, 229, 234, 253
Zastowny, T. R., 145
Zevlodever, R., 277
Zisook, S., 51
Zook, A., II, 284
Zwerling, I., 107
Zwick, R., 188
Zwilling, M., 224

Subject Index

Abstraction, level of, in problems versus syndromes, 35–36
Action(s)
    phase of, 18, 65
    statements versus, 304
Acute day hospital treatment, 107
Acute patient, restrictive settings for, 105–107
Acute psychiatric hospitalization, 105–106
Adolescent, individuating, 133
Affiliative alcoholics, 51
Agoraphobia
    behavioral treatment of, 214, 215–216
    and four steps, 280
    diagnosis and treatment planning for, 46–48
    as symptom illustration of format selection, 120–122
Alcohol abuse, diagnosis and treatment planning for, 50–53
Ambition, as attribute of self, 173
Ambivalent personalities, 180
Antianxiety agents, 137–138
Antidepressant medications, 135–137
Antimanic medications, 137
Antipsychotic medications, 134–135
Anxiety Disordered Interview Schedule (ADIS), 228
Anxiety disorders, diagnosis and treatment plan-

    ning for, 45–48, 49
Arousal, therapeutic, maintenance of, 272–274
Assessment
    of conflict-based foci, 229–234
    needs, as training obstacle, 300–301
    of symptom-based foci, 227–229
Assignment, prescriptive, DSM and, 35
Attentional focus, intratherapy and extratherapy, 268
Attributions, and compatibility, 182–184
Avoidance, what and how of, 272
Axis I, 22, 36, 53, 148, 193
    inadequate reflection of variations in problem complexity by, 36–37
Axis II, 22, 36, 53–54, 70, 179, 193
Axis III, 36
Axis IV, 36, 37

Beck Depression Inventory, 228
Behavioral treatment of agoraphobia, 214, 215–216
    and four steps, 280
Behavior Therapy, 8, 240
Bipolar Disorders, 49, 137
Borderline Personality Disorder, 53, 79, 160, 204

Camberwell Family Interview (CFI), 92
Change(s)
in expectation, 62–63
focal targets of, selection of, 25–26, 211–237
of gaze, selective, 197
instigation of, 254, 255, 256, 259–261
states of, 18–19
Chronic care partial hospitals, 109
Chronic patient, restrictive settings for, 107–108
Client Centered Therapy, 7
Clinical experience, level of, supervision and, 302
Clinical supervision, 300–304
Clinician reluctance to recommend no treatment, 155–158
Cognitive Change Therapies, 8
Cognitive style, supervision and, 303
Cognitive Therapy, 10, 240
of depression, 214, 216–217
and four steps, 281
Coherent framework, supervision and, 303–304
Common Factors, 15, 21
Competence, exposure rather than, in training, 291
Complex problems, procedural menus for treatment of, 245–253
Complex symptom patterns, 226
Compliance, motivation and, 67–69
Compliance-based paradoxical interventions, 276
Conducting therapeutic work, 26–27, 265–284
Conflict, marital, and social support, 94
Conflict-based foci, assessment of, 229–234
Conflict-focused therapies, brief, indications for, 146, 147
Construct-related validity, lack of, in DSM-III, 38–39
Contemplation, phase of, 18, 65
Contemporary eclectic theories, 10–12
Content, as training obstacle, 297–298
Context(s)
interpersonal, of patient's environment, DSM and, 37–38
life-stage, format and, 124
treatment, 23–24, 99–163
and maintaining therapeutic alliance, 204–205
and role induction methods, 194–196
Contracting, therapeutic, 189–191
Conventional training, critique of, 290–293
Coping, nature of, 74–76
Coping ability, 58, 63–66, 80
Coping style(s)
classification of, 76–80
cyclic, 76, 79–80, 81, 258, 260
and level of experience, 250–252
externalizing, 76, 258, 260
and level of experience, 252–253
internalizing, 258, 260

and level of experience, 246–248
matching of, to level of experience, 245
patient personality and, 74–80
repressive, 258, 260
and level of experience, 248–250
Core conflictual focus, 19
Course of disorder, format and, 124–125
Crisis intervention, indications for, 144–145
Criterion-related validity, lack of, in DSM-III, 38–39
Cyclic coping style(s), 76, 79–80, 81, 258, 260
and level of experience, 250–252
Cyclothymia, 49
Cyclothymic Personality, 79
Day hospital treatment, acute, 107
Decision tree for Differential Diagnosis of Mood Disturbances, 137
Decisional alternatives, 223
Defense Mechanism Inventory, 76
Defiance-based paradoxical interventions, 276
Deficit, DSM and areas of, 37
Denial, 76
Dependency Syndrome, 51
Dependent personalities, 179–180
Depression(s), see also Major Depression
Cognitive Therapy of, 214, 216–217
and marital/family environment, 93–94
nonpsychotic, 49–50
time-limited therapies for, 146–149
Depressive Disorders, 49
Detached personalities, 179–180
Development of emotional disturbance, 94–95
Diagnosis(es)
as patient variable, 21–22, 30, 31–55
and duration and frequency, 153–154
role for, in treatment planning, 40–55
Diagnostic concepts, critique of, 32–36
Diagnostic Related Groupings (DRGs), 155
Differential referral, 293–294
Differential Therapeutics, 15, 16–17, 18, 21, 23
Differential treatment considerations, and duration and frequency, 152–155
training in, 289–307
Dimensional assessment, 139
Dimensional model of personality disorders, 54
Directive interventions/treatments, 268
selection of, 275–278
Directiveness, techniques by, 271
Direct observations, 269
Disorder, course of, format and, 124–125
Diversion, 76, 78
Dose-effect relationships, in outpatient psychotherapy, 143–144
DSM-I, 34
DSM-II, 34, 179
DSM-III, 31–40, 43–44, 49, 53–55, 136, 228, 229

DSM-III-R, 34, 35-36, 37, 43-44, 46, 48, 49, 50-51, 55, 65, 74-75, 137, 138-139, 160, 227, 229
DSM-IV, 33, 34, 37
Duration, 24, 45, 141-152; *see also* No treatment
 frequency and, interrelationships of, 152-155
 history of therapy, 142-143
 of least restrictive treatments, indications for, 144-150
 of restrictive treatments, 150-152
Dysfunctional Attitude Scale, 228
Dysthymia, 49
Dysthymic disorder, 79

Early-stage problem drinkers, 51
Eclecticism, in psychotherapy research, 9-10
Eclectic psychotherapy, history of, 6-10
Eclectic theories, 6-9
 contemporary, 10-12
Efficacy, treatment, DSM and, 35
Efficiency, treatment, format and, 125-126
Electroconvulsive therapy (ECT), 113, 133
Engagement, phase of, 254, 255, 256, 257
Enhancing and maintaining therapeutic alliance, 186-206
Environment(s)
 and circumstances, 22-23, 30, 83-97
 of patient, interpersonal context of, DSM and, 37-38
 work/school, 94-96
Environmental factors, in length of stay, 151
Environmental resources, 86-96
Environmental stressors, 84-86
Evocative interventions/treatments, 268
 selection of, 275-278
Exclusion of problems, by diagnostic systems, 38
Expectation(s), 58-63, 80
 changes in, 62-63
 social role, 61-62
 treatment, 59-61
Experience(s)
 clinical, supervision and level of, 302
 inadequate, training and, 290-291
 psychotherapy, types of, 239-253
 variations in, 240-242
Experiential psychotherapy, 217-219, 240
Exposure
 arousal by, 273
 rather than competence, in training, 291
Expressed emotion (EE), 92-93, 96, 134
Expressive Psychoanalytic Psychotherapy, 19
Externalizing coping style(s), 76, 78, 81, 258, 260
 and level of experience, 252-253
Extrapunitive focus, 75, 76, 78
Extratherapy attentional focus, 268
Extratherapy processes, intratherapy versus,

278-279
Extraversion, 75
Eysenck Personality Inventory, 76

Faculty, as training obstacle, 298
Family environment
 depression and, 93-94
 schizophrenia and, 91-93
 and support, 89-91
Family format, 115-117
 indications for, 127-129
Family Therapy
 and four steps, 283
 structural, 215, 221-222
Feeling of self efficacy, 73
Feighner criteria, 39
Final goal of treatment, mediating goals versus, 41-42
First-rank symptoms (FRS), 39
Flexible System, 39
Focal chains in treatment, 226
Focal targets of change, selection of, 25-26, 211-237
Focal treatment goals
 formulation of, 224-234
 and objectives, fitting of, to patient, 223
Focus (i)
 conflict-based, assessment of, 229-234
 core conflictual, 19
 intratherapy and extratherapy attentional, 268
 symptom-based, assessment of, 227-229
 therapeutic, selection of, 225-227
Focused Expressive Psychotherapy (FEP), 214, 217-219
 and four steps, 281-282
Format(s), 23-24, 113-140
 and diagnosis, 45
 and duration and frequency, 154-155
 family, 115-117
 indications for, 127-129
 marital, individual versus, for symptomatic spouse, 131-132
 psychosocial, 114-133
 factors in selection of, 118-126
 historical perspective on, 114-118
 reactive indications for, 126-131
 typical issues in, 131-133
 relative indications for, 126-131
Four steps, treatment manuals and, 279-283
Framework, coherent, supervision and, 303-304
Frequency, 24

Generalized Anxiety Disorder (GAD), diagnosis and treatment planning for,
Gestalt Therapy, 10, 117, 189, 271, 306
Global Assessment of Functioning (GAF), 65, 97

Goals
  focal   formulation of, 224–234
  and objectives, fitting of, to patient, 223
Group format, 117–118
  indications for, 129–131
  versus individual, for YAVIS patient, 132–133
Habits, versus transient responses, 71
Habitual symptoms, 226
Heterogeneous group, indications for, 130
High reactance, 200, 274
HMOs, 102, 155
Homogeneous group, indications for, 130–131
Hospital(s)
  day, acute treatment at, 107
  partial, chronic care, 109
  psychiatric, 104–105
Hospitalization
  acute psychiatric, 105–106
  alternatives to, 108–109
  length of, 150–152
  long-term, 108

Ideal training models, 293–297
Idealized transference relationship, 173
Ideals, as attribute of self, 173
Inadequate experience, training and, 290–291
Independent/narcissistic personalities, 179–180
Indirect observations, 266–268
Individual format, 114–115
  group versus, for YAVIS patient, 132–133
  indications for, 126–127
  versus marital, for symptomatic spouse, 131–132
Individuating adolescent, 133
Instructional methods, 188, 192
Insufficient evaluation, in training, 291–292
Integrative model, 20–27
Integrative psychotherapy, 295–297
Integrative training, obstacles in, 297–300
Intense interventions, 275
Interactive dimensions, 270–271
Internalizing coping style(s), 76–77, 78, 81, 258, 260
  and level of experience, 246–248
Interpersonal context of patient's environment, DSM and, 37–38
Interpersonal Psychotherapy (IPT), 10, 170, 214, 219–220, 231, 240, 306
  and four steps, 282
Interpersonal reactance, 70, 72–74
Interpersonal response patterns, and compatibility, 177–184
Interpersonal strivings, 178–180
Intervention(s),
  crisis, indications for, 144–145
  depth/level of, see Level of experience/intervention

directive, 268
evocative, 268
  therapist styles versus, 196 In-Therapy Environmental Management, 187, 196–205
Intratherapy attentional focus, 268
Intratherapy versus extratherapy processes, 278–279
Intropunitive focus, 75, 76
Introversion, 75
Intrusive interventions, moderately, 275

Learning methods, observational and participatory, 188–189
Length of hospitalization, 150–152
Length of stay (LOS), 108
Level of clinical experience, supervision and, 302
Level of experience/intervention, 26
  matching of coping style to, 245
  selection of, 238–264
  techniques by, 271
  by therapeutic phase/task, 259
Life-stage context, format and, 124
Life strains, 85
Long-term hospitalization, 108
Long-term therapies, indications for, 149–150

Maintenance
  phase of, 18, 65
  and relapse prevention, 262–263
  of therapeutic alliance, 186–206
  of therapeutic arousal, 272–274 74
Major Depression, xvii, 49, 139, 156
Management, medical, treatment mode of, 133–139
Manualized therapies
  comparison of, 214–222
  and four steps, 279–283
Marital conflict, and social support, 94
Marital environment, depression and, 93–94
Marital format, individual versus, for symptomatic spouse, 131–132
Matching
  of coping style, to level of experience, 245
  of focal goals and objectives, to patient, 223
  of mediating goals to treatment phase, 255–262
  of therapy, to patient, model for, 222–224
Mediating goals, 19, 26, 226
  definition of, 254–255
  final goal versus, 41–42
  matching of, to treatment phase, 255–262
  and phases of psychotherapy, 253–263
  selection of, 238–264
  treatment format and mode and, 122–124
Medication(s)
  history and classes of, 134–138
  referring patients for, 138–139

Melancholia, 136
Menus, procedural/treatment, 241
    for treating complex problems, 245–253
    for treating symptoms, 243–245
Methods, psychotherapy, differences among, 212–222
Millon Clinical Multiaxial Inventory, 76
Minnesota Multiphasic Personality Inventory, 76
Mode(s), 23–24
    and format, 113–140
    psychosocial, 114–133
    historical perspective on, 114–118
    of medical management, 133–139
Model(s)
    of differential treatment selection, 14–27
    contributing viewpoints on, 14–19
    as integrative model, 20–27
    roots of, 15–19
    of disorder, diagnostic label and, 41
    for matching therapy to patient, 222–224
    training, ideal, 293–297
Moderately intrusive interventions, 275
Monoamine oxidase inhibitors (MAOs), 135, 138
Mood disorders, diagnosis and treatment planning for, 48–50
Motivation and compliance, 67–69
Multimodal Psychotherapy, 11
Multitheory, superficial, in training, 292
Mutual gaze, 197

Nature of treatment, importance of, 109
Needs assessment, as training obstacle, 300–301
Negative effect of treatment, 159–161
Nondiagnostic patient variables, and duration and frequency, 152–153
Nonpsychotic depressions, 49–50
Nonverbal styles, 197–200, 203
Nosology, politics of, 33–35
No treatment, decision for, 155–161

Objectives, of treatment, fitting of, to patient, 223
Observational learning methods, 188–189, 192
Observations
    direct, 269
    indirect, 266–268
Office treatment, 103
Outpatient psychotherapy, dose-effect relationships in, 143–144
Overcontrolling focus, 75–76

Panic Disorder, 46, 137
Paranoid Personality, 79
Partial hospitals, chronic care, 109
Participatory learning methods, 188–189, 192

Passive Aggressive Personality, 79
Patient(s)
    acute, restrictive settings for, 105–107
    chronic, restrictive settings for, 107–108
    interpersonal context of environment of, DSM and, 37–38
    matching of therapy to, model for, 222–224
    referring of, for medication, 138–139
Patient factors, in length of stay, 151
Patient personal characteristics, 22, 30, 57–81
Patient personality, 66–80
Patient predisposing/predetermining variables, 21–23, 29–97
    nondiagnostic, and duration and frequency, 152–153
Patient preference, and format, 126–127
Pattern search, 254, 255, 256, 257–259
Personal beliefs, compatibility and, 180–182
Personality
    aspects of, 58
    patient, 66–80
Personality disorders, diagnosis and treatment planning, for, 53–54
Personality patterns, 80
Personality styles, response-specific, 67, 69–74
Persuasion, and therapeutic alliance, 171–174
Phase(s)
    problem-solving, 18, 259, 272
    therapeutic
    altering treatment menus to fit, 223
    format and, 124–125
    level of experience by, 256
    mediating goals and, 253–263
Politics of nosology, 33–35
Postpartum Depression, 156
Post Traumatic Stress Disorder (PTSD), xvii, 3, 32, 57, 154, 227, 233, 244, 249
Precontemplation, phase of, 18, 65
Predetermining/predisposing patient variables
    and maintenance of therapeutic alliance 203–204
    prescriptive application of, 193–194
Prescription, of role induction methods, 192–196
Prescriptive decisions, 203–205
Prescriptive Psychotherapy, 15, 16
Prescriptive supervision, 301–303
Prevention of emotional disturbance, work/school and, 94–95
Probative interventions, 275
Problem complexity, 70, 71–72
    inadequate reflection of variations in, 36–37
    treatment mode and format and, 119–122
Problems severity, 64–65, 272
Problems
    complex, procedural menus for treatment of, 245–253

exclusion of, by diagnostic systems, 38
versus syndromes, 35
Problem-solving phase, 18, 259, 272
Problem-solving process, 65–66
Procedural menus, 241
for treating symptoms, 243–245
Procedures, dimensions of specific, 266–279
Professional manual, DSM-III as, 34
Psychoactive Substance Use Disorders, 50
Psychoanalytic Psychotherapy, 10, 240
Psychodynamic psychotherapy, 220–221
Psychosocial modes, 114–133
historical perspective on, 114–118
Psychosocial treatments, DSM diagnostic systems
as not equivalent to indicators of, 39–40
Psychotherapy
experiential, 217–219, 240
integrative, 20–27, 295–297
outpatient, dose-effect relationships in, 143–144
theories of, see Theory(ies) Psychotherapy, 14, 31
Psychotherapy experiences, types of , 239–253
variations in, 240–242
Psychotherapy methods, differences among, 212–222
Psychotherapy research, eclecticism in, 9–10
Psychotic Symptoms, 156

Rationalization, 76
Reactance, interpersonal, 70, 72–74
high, 200, 274
level of, 272
Recurrent obstacles, in integrative training, 297–300
Referral
differential, 293–294
of patients, for medication, 138–139
Rehabilitation programs, 109
Relapse prevention, maintenance and, 262–263
Relationship variables, 24–25, 165–206
and duration and frequency, 153
Relative indications
for format, 126–131
for no treatment, 158–161
Repressive coping style(s), 76, 78–79, 81, 258, 260
and level of experience, 248–250
Research, psychotherapy, eclecticism in, 9–10
Research Diagnostic Criteria (RDC), 39, 136
Resources, environmental, 86–96
Response-specific personality styles, 67, 69–74
Restrictive settings
for acute patient, 105–107
for chronic patient, 107–108
least, 102–103
Restrictive treatments
duration of, 150–152

least, indications for duration of, 144–150
Role Induction methods, 187–196
prescription of, 192–196

Schemas, 217
Schizoaffective Disorder, 139
Schizoid alcoholics, 52
Schizophrenia, 139
diagnosis and treatment planning for, 43–45
and family environment, 91–93
School environment, 94–96
Selection
of depth/level of intervention, 242–253
and mediating goals of psychotherapy, 238–264
of directive and evocative treatments, 275–278
of focal targets of change, 25–26, 211–237
of format, factors in, 118–126
of therapeutic focus, 225–227
Selective changing of gaze, 197
Sensitization, 76
Setting, treatment, 23, 45, 101–112
and duration and frequency, 154–155
psychiatric hospital as, 104–105
versus treatment programs, 109–111 Severity,
problem, 64–65, 272
Simple symptoms, 226
Single theory, in training, 292
Site of difficulty, treatment at, 102–103
Situational cues/stimuli, 197, 200–202, 203
Social role expectations, 61–62
Social support systems, 87–94
marital conflict and, 94
Socioeconomic status (SES), 22, 86–87, 96–97, 184, 192
Somatic treatments, DSM diagnostic systems as
not equivalent to indicators of, 39–40
Soteria, 108
Spouse, symptomatic, 131–132
State(s)
of change, 18–19
of patient's efforts, coping ability and, 58
Strategies, tailoring of, 25–27, 207–285·
Strength, DSM and areas of, 37
Stressful events, definition of, 85
Stressors, environmental, 84–86
Structural Family Therapy, 215, 221–222
Students, as training obstacle, 298–99
Styles
nonverbal, 197–200, 203
therapist, versus interventions, 196
verbal behavioral, 197, 202–203
Superficial multitheory, in training, 292
Supervision
clinical, 300–304
prescriptive, 301–303

Support
  family environment and, 89–91
Symptom illustration, agoraphobia as, 120–122
Symptom patterns, complex, 226
Symptom-based foci, assessment of, 227–229
Symptom-focused therapies, brief, indications
  for, 146, 147
Symptoms
  habitual or simple, 226
  treatment of, procedural menus for, 243–245
Systematic Eclectic Psychotherapy, 15, 17–18,
  21, 71

Tailoring strategies and techniques, 25–27, 207–
  285
Targets of change, focal, selection of, 25–26,
  211–237
Task, level of experience by, 256
Technical Eclecticism, 11, 15
Technique(s), see also Strategies
  by depth of intervention and directiveness, 271
  dimensions of, 223
  tailoring of, 25–27, 207–285
T-groups, 117
Theory(ies)
  eclectic, 6–9
  contemporary, 10–12
  single, in training, 292
Therapeutic alliance,
  enhancement of, 25
  and maintenance of, 186–206
  persuasion and, 171–174
Therapeutic arousal, maintenance of, 272–274
Therapeutic contracting, 189–191, 192
Therapeutic focus, selection of, 225–227
Therapeutic move, no treatment as, 161
Therapeutic styles, 196–203
Therapeutic work, conducting of, 26–27, 265–
  284
Therapist approval and reassurance, 269
Therapist-patient personal compatibility, 25,
  169–185; see also Therapeutic alliance
  dimensions of, 174–184
Therapy(ies),
  long-term, indications for, 149–150
  manualized
    comparison of, 214–222
    and four steps, 279–283
    matching of, to patient, model for, 222–224
Therapy approach, supervision and, 302
Therapy structure, 269
Time-Limited Dynamic Psychotherapy (TLDP),
  19, 214, 220–221, 232, 306
  and four steps, 282–283
  indications for, 145–149
Training
  conventional, critique of, 290–293

  in differential treatment selection, 289–307
  integrative, recurrent obstacles in, 297–300
Training directions, 287–307
Training models, ideal, 293–297
Transactional Analysis, 117, 189
Transtheoretical Psychotherapy, 18, 26
Treatment(s)
  of complex problems, procedural menus for,
    245–253
  decision for no, 155–161
  directive, 268
  duration of, 150–152
  selection of, 275–278
  evocative, 268
  focal chains in, 226
  likelihood of no effect of, 159
  nature of, importance of, 109
  negative effect of, 159–161
  non-necessity of, 158–159
  somatic and psychosocial, 39–40
  of symptoms, procedural menus for, 243–245
Treatment efficiency, format and, 125–126
Treatment expectations, 59–61
Treatment frequency, 24
Treatment planning
  representative diagnoses and, 42–55
  role for diagnosis in, 40–55
Treatment programs, treatment settings versus,
  109–111
Treatment states, adapting procedures to, 223
Tricyclic antidepressants (TCAs), 135, 138
Types of psychotherapy experiences, 239–253
  variations in, 240–242

Undercontrolling focus, 75
Unintrusive interventions, 275
Unipolar Depressive Disorders, 137

Validity, construct- and criterion-related, lack of,
  in DSM-III, 38–39
Verbal behavioral styles, 197, 202–203

Ward Atmosphere Scale (WAS), 104
Ways of Coping Questionnaire, 76
Weakness, DSM and areas of, 37
Work, therapeutic, conducting of, 26–27, 265–
  284
Work environment, 94–96

YAVIS patient, 132–133
Young Loneliness Inventory, 228